The First Transplant Surgeon
The Flawed Genius of Nobel Prize Winner, Alexis Carrel

The First Transplant Surgeon

The Flawed Genius of Nobel Prize Winner, Alexis Carrel

David Hamilton

St Andrews University, Scotland

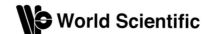 **World Scientific**

NEW JERSEY · LONDON · SINGAPORE · BEIJING · SHANGHAI · HONG KONG · TAIPEI · CHENNAI · TOKYO

Published by

World Scientific Publishing Co. Pte. Ltd.
5 Toh Tuck Link, Singapore 596224
USA office: 27 Warren Street, Suite 401-402, Hackensack, NJ 07601
UK office: 57 Shelton Street, Covent Garden, London WC2H 9HE

Library of Congress Cataloging-in-Publication Data
Hamilton, David, 1939– , author.
  The first transplant surgeon : the flawed genius of Nobel prize winner, Alexis Carrel /
David Hamilton.
    p. ; cm.
  Includes bibliographical references and index.
  ISBN 978-9814699365 (hardcover : alk. paper) -- ISBN 9814699365 (hardcover : alk. paper) --
  ISBN 978-9814699372 (pbk. : alk. paper) -- ISBN 9814699373 (pbk. : alk. paper)
  I. Title.
  [DNLM: 1. Carrel, Alexis, 1873–1944. 2. Surgeons--France--Biography.
3. Organ Transplantation--history--France. WZ 100]
  R507.C34
  617.4'1092--dc23
  [B]
                                                        2015023649

British Library Cataloguing-in-Publication Data
A catalogue record for this book is available from the British Library.

Copyright © 2017 by World Scientific Publishing Co. Pte. Ltd.

Printed in Singapore by Mainland Press Pte Ltd.

The Author

David Hamilton was a transplant surgeon in the Western Infirmary, Glasgow, and in retirement is an Honorary Senior Lecturer at the Bute Medical School at St Andrews University. He trained in immunology with Nobel Prize winner Sir Peter Medawar in London and was also the first director of the Wellcome Unit for History of Medicine at Glasgow University. Added to his works on Scottish medical history, his books on the history of organ transplantation are *The Monkey Gland Affair* (1986) and *A History of Organ Transplantation* (2012).

Prologue

In April 1914, the world's best-known surgeons gathered in New York for a meeting of their International Surgical Association. The meeting was a prestigious forum for new developments, and to acknowledge the new vitality of American surgery, it was their first meeting outside of Europe. Woodrow Wilson, the President of the United States, had agreed to give the speech of welcome.

The meeting's long programme highlighted three surgical topics. The first was the treatment of stomach ulcers, the second was limb amputation and the third, perhaps surprisingly, was 'Grafts and Transplantation of Organs'. At this session the best-known contributor was America's own Alexis Carrel who, two years earlier, had gained a Nobel Prize for his transplantation studies. This was a lively international surgical venture at the time, but then mysteriously disappeared from the surgical agenda after World War I.

Carrel, a Frenchman, but based at New York's Rockefeller Institute from 1906, had a surprise announcement for the conference: he told the delegates that he knew of a way to thwart rejection and allow organ grafts to survive. Decades ahead of his time, he knew that radiation or drugs would reduce the body's response to the foreign tissue and prolong the life of the grafts. These strategies where not revived until they re-appeared, with success, in the late 1950s.

Carrel made many other contributions. At the time of his Nobel Prize, he had been first to develop routine methods of culturing cells outside the body, and following this, in World War I, he gained further fame for his Carrel–Dakin method of treating wounds. In the 1930s, with

WORLD'S SURGEONS IN SESSION HERE

Dr. Depage, President of International Congress, Protests Against Cruelties of War.

TRANSPLANTATIONS FAIL

Organs Cannot Be Successfully Transferred to Another Animal of Same Species, Says Carrel.

The Fourth Congress of the International Surgical Association, which was organized in Brussels in 1905, and has met triennially in that city since its

The *New York Times* coverage of the New York International Surgical Association meeting in 1914 highlighted Carrel's contribution.

the help of the young aviator Charles Lindbergh, he devised a pump to keep organs alive outside the body.

But there was a darker side to his life and works. There were complaints that he failed to credit the work of others and scientific findings by Carrel that could not be confirmed, notably his claim to have produced a long-lived 'immortal' strain of cells. His other writings, notably his book *Man, the Unknown,* in which he advocated authoritarian and eugenic measures, soon had few supporters. In 1941 he moved to German-occupied France, funded by the collaborationist Vichy government to develop his ideas. After the War, his conservative views were recalled when right-wing groups in France discovered and praised his book. Others who spoke highly of Carrel included Islamist writers and ideologues, who found that the West earlier had a distinguished internal critic.

Carrel was a genius, but a flawed one.

This book is a new account of Carrel's scientific career and his involvement in the bio-politics of the day. Medical historians have shown reverence for his scientific achievements and discreetly avoided study of much else in his career. Scientific biography has traditionally depicted any eminent savant as not only intellectually gifted, but also in possession of personal qualities of greatness in heart, mind and deed. Conventional accounts of Carrel assume that, as a well-known scientist and a Nobel laureate, he had these gifts, and any concerns could be minimised or favourable explanations given. But attitudes have changed. It is no longer necessary to look for multiple attainments in a successful scientist, and it is a liberating notion that scientific creativity can be associated with quite ordinary, or even unfortunate, other qualities. The hagiographic myths often attached to scientists do not serve good history, and a more satisfying historical approach is that scientists can be treated as being part of the normal world. In Carrel's case, we can still honour his remarkable achievements in science, but decline to put a gloss on the many awkward findings. Moreover, seeking a proper historical account is important in understanding the scientific life. Surgeons and scientists have often escaped the attentions of probing biographers; Carrel was both a surgeon and a scientist, and his complex life should be looked at anew.

For this present work, the commendably bulky archival sources and Carrel's many publications have been looked at closely, instead of using the many myths which have accumulated and burden the many secondary sources dealing with his life. On the scientific side, this book, for the first time, gives the full story of his early Nobel Prize-winning organ transplant work, which shows that his mastery of the subject and his insights were even greater than has been supposed. The puzzle of why his entirely practical 'road map' announced in 1914 for the development of organ transplantation was not followed through is looked at closely for the first time, and an explanation offered.

≈

The early influences on his career are of interest. His Jesuit schooling, in spite of his later protestations, had a clear input to his attitudes and assumptions, notably his growing conviction that mankind had moral failings and needed a spiritual renaissance. From this upbringing, he believed in the power of prayer and also that monastic seclusion and contemplation assisted scientific creativity. Another early interest was in the military life. He served in the army during student days and contemplated a military career at that time. He enrolled willingly in both European wars as a surgeon, and he held the view that armed conflict between nations was unavoidable, and that 'might is right'. His political views were authoritarian, and in his laboratory his black-uniformed staff followed detailed protocols. His cellular biology work showed a desire to be in control, and he wished to discipline cells and organs and drive them into novel actions.

In looking at any scientist, their 'style' in their day-to-day work can be studied with profit. Formerly, a personal style was not looked for, since the older view of scientific progress was that a savant like Carrel would be a virtuoso user of the 'scientific method'. Little more needed to be said, particularly of a Nobel Prize winner, who was presumed to use the method remarkably effectively. But belief in the existence of a scientific method, as a creative force, has been downgraded. The first steps in creativity are not derived from using a formula, but instead come from theoretical suggestions — hypotheses — that are then stress-tested by experiment, followed by detached observation and dispassionate analysis of the assembled data. Successful hypotheses originate from time to time in the mind of gifted savants, and not in others; the cerebral mechanism for producing ideas which make sense of the world remains elusive. Since a single 'method' is not in use, it encourages curiosity about the details of the savant's scientific practice.

With this in mind, Carrel's style can be studied with more than the usual profit. He made the necessary bold hypotheses, and on many occasions he was right. But on other occasions when advancing new ideas, he was casual about looking critically at his data and could proceed without obtaining adequate supporting evidence. He did this deliberately, since he believed that intuition was a powerful tool, offering a direct route to hidden truth. This belief was elevated by Carrel to almost dangerous levels, but many of his premature claims were forgotten or were dealt with charitably.

On more mundane matters of style, he liked to have something to *show*. As a young surgeon in France he spoke regularly at the Lyon medical meetings, giving demonstrations of the results of his experimental blood vessel surgery in animals. After emigrating to America, he soon showed similar experiments to admiring visiting surgeons. In World War I, serving in France, he proudly demonstrated his complex and visually-attractive Carrel–Dakin wound treatment method to celebrity visitors. From the 1920s, Carrel's 'immortal' chicken heart cells, one of the best-known biological experiments of all time, were on show in a special part of his laboratory. His pioneering micro-cinematographic films of living cells were borrowed, exhibited and admired, and his most successful bit of scientific theatre was his elegant organ perfusion pump of the mid-1930s. It was a triumph of the glass-blowers' skill, and reached the cover of *Time* magazine in 1938. He was showman — a surgical showman — always with something to show.

In his scientific writings, he had a distinctive approach. Many of his published papers give little numerical data, and it seemed sufficient for him to state that he had achieved his goal. Another style, unusual for the times, was that when a new project showed promise, he made the results widely known, with rapid, brief, multiple publication in generalist medical journals in America and simultaneously in France. He was not content that scientific claims would naturally reach their own level of acceptance and sought to bring them to the notice of others by additional means. This included enlisting the help of the newspapers and journals, the only 'media' of the day, who in America's Progressive Era were seeking new local heroes to rival the European stars of the Pasteur and Koch Institutes. Good news was expected from the staff at the new Rockefeller Institute for Medical Research in New York, and Carrel regularly provided it, using his shrewd understanding of what journalists and the public desired. He rivalled Einstein as the newspapers' favourite scientist, and eventually became known, like Einstein, by his last name only. Journalists obtained folksy stories about him and his surgical skill, which he did not discourage, and his popularising flair can be seen in bringing America's most famous citizen, Charles Lindbergh, into his laboratory. Carrel's book *Man, the Unknown* was the non-fiction best-seller of the 1930s, and thereafter he reached out to the public with a series of articles for the *Readers' Digest*. He confidently managed this public position as an international scientific celebrity until disaster at the end.

❧

Much of his life was spent in America, where he cut himself off from the unhappy events which terminated his surgical training in France. But his attitude and links to his native France are important in understanding his later career. In spite of his regular criticism of his native land, and its medical men, Carrel's grumbles conceal a deep attachment to France, not to the France of the day, but to an older France, and what the nation of France might become. He retained his French citizenship and regularly published in French journals. Nor was he geographically cut off from France, as it might seem, since during the long academic summer break, he returned each year to join his wife, who lived in France, at their island home in Brittany. In summer he visited medical and scientific institutions, and he and his wife had some involvement in France's complex interwar politics. His view of genetics and his support for spiritualism mark him out as a Frenchman. His one worldly ambition, nearly fulfilled, was to be elected to the French Academy as one of their 30 'Immortels', which was, and is, France's highest academic award. His final, puzzling move to France during World War II to work in German-occupied Paris was not impulsive, and instead it was a personal mission to revive France along Carrelian lines.

❧

In attempting a reassessment from the rich sources available, one finding stands out, and it influences and colours any assessment. There is much in Carrel's actions and writings which is contradictory. These puzzles start early. As a trainee surgeon in Lyon he claimed to have witnessed a miraculous cure at the shrine at Lourdes, but when talking to the newspapers he denied attributing it to divine intervention. His most famous innovation, a new method of joining blood vessels, is described differently in different publications, and on other occasions in his surgical and tissue culture work, the crucial experimental data is similarly elusive. In his famous organ perfusion work in the mid-1930s with Lindbergh, it was not clear whether a physiological study or organ replacement or even an artificial heart was envisaged. He regularly deplored the interest of the press in his work, yet gave non-attributable briefings to favourite journalists. His understanding of genetics was that inheritance of acquired characteristics was possible, but he does not come out as a Lamarckian, thus leaving unclear his view of the role of nature-versus-nurture. Much of his book *Man, the Unknown* is notably opaque. In it, he blamed the products of science and technology for the ills of mankind, yet urged that the antidote was to bring in more science. In his writings he extolled Catholic teachings, notably brotherly love, yet he embraced eugenics and some application of euthanasia. He talked and wrote of family love and sexuality, yet lived apart from his wife in a childless marriage. His aphorisms often contradict each other, and his friends chided him for his rambling discourse. He could praise his New York Jewish colleagues, yet blame 'Bolsheviks and Jews' for the European war. He urged a return to the spiritual life, but considered that conventional church-going was useless. Catholic commentators, understandably keen to enrol a great scientist to their cause, can pick and choose from his writings to show he was a visionary believer who gave 'hope for mankind', but other sceptics, finding useful quotations, have concluded that he was fascist and eugenicist. As World War II approached, Carrel professed alternate admiration and dislike for the Nazis, and then created the greatest mystery of his career by settling in Occupied France. Allegations that he was a collaborator with the German invaders are still debated. Recently, Islamist thinkers have been pleased to quote him as sharing their view of Western decadence, yet far-right politicians and thinkers in the West see him as an early defender of the white races against outside threats. Those with a particular agenda when writing on Carrel can claim him as 'one of us', and with neat symmetry, and using selective quotation, others can defend him, proving he was not 'one of them'.

When this rich, conflicting evidence is assembled, and the many contradictions noted, it explains much, notably the diversity of historical verdicts on Carrel and why his legacy is revived and revised so regularly.

A perceptive colleague noticed and warned future biographers of the 'terrible responsibility of those who would accurately and fairly interpret Carrel's thoughts'. The assessment in this book accepts the numerous contradictions and discourages any attempt to resolve them; the ambiguity in the layers of evidence is instead emphasised. Even looking at him, there was a puzzle: Carrel had one blue eye, and the other was brown.

∼

What are we to make of Carrel? Biographers often seek to rescue their subject from obscurity or to raise them to greater levels of respect. The task in this book is a little different. Carrel's remarkable scientific achievements do, at last, require a detailed examination, but an attempt to find the historical Alexis Carrel is also needed. There is no need to over-state his contributions, nor any reason to minimise his faults. He can be seen as a genius, but an elusive, flawed one.

Acknowledgements

My study of the important collection of Carrel's papers at the Rockefeller University Archives was assisted by grant-in-aid which gave an enjoyable period of study at the Archive Center at Sleepy Hollow, New York. There, the skilled archivists, notably Lee Hiltzik, guided me to the many collections of relevance. With a research grant from the Carnegie Trust for the Universities of Scotland, I visited Washington's Georgetown University, where I was made welcome at the Booth Family Center for Special Collections by John Buchtel and Scott Taylor, who assisted my studies of the Alexis Carrel Papers. The Charles Augustus Lindbergh Collection at Yale University Library's Manuscripts and Archives department proved to have new insights into Carrel's research and his life, and Sim Smiley and Amy Schmidt at the US National Archives at College Park searched and found the American security agencies' interest in Carrel in World War II. The Bibliotheque municipale de Lyon found some of the documents relevant to Carrel's early career.

Nearer home, London's Royal Society of Medicine Library has a unique collection of European medical journals, held from earliest times, and being still on open shelving, it allows searching which is often rewarded by serendipitous discovery. The Wellcome Library in London has a unique collection of books and documents relevant to the history of medicine and the nearby British Library has some even rarer items. At the Library of the Royal College of Surgeons in Edinburgh, Marianne Smith offered advice, and traced some rare sources, as did Carol Parry at the Library of the Royal College of Physicians and Surgeons in Glasgow.

At home, St Andrews University Library's Interlibrary Loans department regularly obtained distant works for my study.

Of particular assistance with the French literature on Carrel are the recent accounts by Andrés H. Reggiani, *God's Eugenicist: Alexis Carrel and the Sociobiology of Decline* (2007), and Alain Drouard's two books, *Une inconnue des sciences sociales: La Fondation Alexis Carrel 1941–1945* (1992) and *Alexis Carrel (1873–1944) De la mémoire à l'histoire* (1995). I had help with French translation from Sam Bootle and then Sarah Townsend of the Department of French at St. Andrews University, and David Smith, of Troon, dealt with German sources.

The growth of online information has made intensive historical research possible from the home or office using the power of Google searching and particularly Wikipedia entries. These lead to online sources like the early *New York Times* archive and to the generous journals like the *Journal of Experimental Medicine*, who have opened up their back numbers without charge.

On the controversy over Carrel's 'immortal' cells, Leonard Hayflick and Jan Witkowski gave their insights, and at Lourdes, Alessandro de Franciscis searched and found details of Carrel's visit in 1902. Alain Drouard in Paris and Louis P. Fischer in Lyon helped with questions on Carrel's early life in France and provided useful images, as did Jean-Bernard Kazmierczak in Nice, the National Library of Medicine in Washington, Timothy DeWerff at the Century Association in New York and Erica Mosner, archivist at the Institute for Advanced Study, Princeton.

At an early stage, Iain McIntyre, the Edinburgh surgeon, historian and editor, was a helpful and reassuring reader, and my wife Jean shared my enthusiasm for this project, helping to unravel the enigma of Carrel and, as a keen reader, preventing many errors. Here in St Andrews, Julie Falkner assisted me greatly by producing fine versions from my draft texts.

Lim Sook Cheng at World Scientific Publishing quickly accepted and encouraged publication of the book and guided it to publication.

Contents

CHAPTER ONE

Lyon Days

Carrel was born on 28 June 1873 in Lyon in southern France, the nation's second-largest city. The family lived in a house in the Quai de la Pêcherie on the river in the merchant area of the city.[1] This prosperous area was south of the crowded textile factories in the Croix Rousse district, known as the 'hill that works', and to the west over the river were the churches on 'the hill that prays'. Alexis was christened Marie-Joseph-Auguste Carrel-Billiard. Of the three siblings, he was one-and-a-half years older than his brother Joseph, later a local composer and writer, and three years younger than his sister Marguerite. His father, Alexis Carrel-Billiard, worked as a broker in Lyon's important silk-processing industry, which imported raw materials from their colonies, and the family had been involved in Lyon's silk and textile industry since the 18th century. On his mother's side, the Ricards were merchants, politicians and magistrates. The family were devout Catholics and Alexis' nephew became bishop of Clermont-Ferrand. They had bourgeois attitudes and kept apart from the radicalism and anticlericalism then prominent in Lyon. But Alexis' father died of pneumonia in 1897, and as was customary, young Alexis, aged

---

[1] But his birth-place was in the Lyon suburb of Sainte-Foy-lès-Lyon, where his mother had gone to her mother's house for the delivery. For the many accounts of Carrel's early life, see 'Bibliography' later. The first biography was Robert Soupault's *Alexis Carrel* (Paris: Libraire Plon, 1952), and the most recent is Alain Drouard, *Alexis Carrel (1873–1944): De la mémoire à l'histoire* (Paris: Éditions L'Harmattan, 1995).

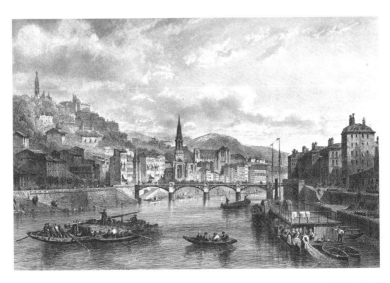

The city of Lyon circa 1850:   Carrel's family lived on the right bank of
this, the La Saöne river.

five, took his father's name.[2] Thereafter, until leaving France, he used the
hyphenated surname Carrel-Billiard, simplifying it only later to Carrel.

Though he was to be a critic later of France and French society, it
seems that this was a happy time. Later in life, when concerned about
national decline, he wrote that:

> Tonight I long for or rather I see the Christmas nights of other years ...
> that charming little life gone forever ... that balanced world, happy above
> all, made up of those people. ... Why have we so degenerated? ... Perhaps
> because our life was too happy ...[3]

The death meant that the family were left in difficulty. They moved
to a smaller house, but the constraints ceased when money was inherited

---

[2] Study of Nobel Prize winners shows a preponderance of first-born children. Also
over-represented are those with early loss of a parent: see R.D. Clark and G.A. Rice
(1982) 'Family constellations and eminence: the birth orders of Nobel Prize winners'
The Journal of Psychology 110: 281–87, and Marvin Eisenstadt, *Parental Loss and
Achievement* (New York: International Universities Press, 1989).
[3] Carrel to his brother Joseph in 1938, Alexis Carrel Papers, box 38 file 41, Georgetown
University Library, Booth Family Center for Special Collections (GULBFC).

in 1900 after Carrel's grandfather's death. As a result, his mother could move to La Bâtie, a comfortable country chateau, in the town of Saint-Martin-en-Haut, 30 miles north of Lyon. Alexis also received a legacy from his grandfather. This gave him a modest income thereafter, one large enough to support him in his first poorly-paid posts in America, and further money came to him after his mother died in 1905. This private income explains much in his life thereafter: at the time, private means were almost essential for a career in medical research.[4] Carrel came into other money later. His Nobel Prize in 1912 gave him a substantial cash payment, and he married a rich widow in 1913. To add to this, he later wrote an internationally best-selling book. In short, he never lacked money, and had the freedom of action that this allows.

School Days

French education was largely secular at the time, but Alexis was sent as a day boy to a Jesuit school, the Collège des Jésuites de Saint-Joseph, a short distance from his home. Now called the Lycée Saint-Marc, it was, and is, one of the many respected schools run by the Society of Jesus, the religious order allied to the Roman Catholic Church. Known then as the 'schoolmasters of Europe', the Jesuits' pedagogy sought, as well as teaching an ethical code, to encourage 'individualism, leadership and reflection'. The teaching was suffused with moral instruction and also encouraged 'eloquentia perfecta' — excellence in writing and speaking. But the teaching of mathematics and the sciences was not a priority.[5] The Jesuits' recall an aphorism of Ignatius Loyola, their founder, who said: 'Give me the child till he is seven, and I will show you the man.' This schooling gave an obvious input to Carrel's later thoughts and writings. Although he later had an ambivalent attitude to organised religion, and criticised the Jesuits, he retained much of their outlook. A more practical youthful influence came in summer when the family spent time at his grand-parents' home

---

[4] The eminent American surgeons Harvey Cushing and William Halsted, both known for their research contributions at this time, came from well-off families.

[5] For a revisionist account, see Mordechai Feingold, *Jesuit Science and the Republic of Letters* (Cambridge: MIT Press, 2003).

in Sainte-Foy, and they were joined there by Uncle Joseph Ricard, an army officer. There he set up a simple experimental laboratory and Alexis was interested in both his military life and the experiments.

At school, Alexis had a good academic record, but not an outstanding one, and in 1890, he took his Science baccalaureate examination, having taken it in Letters in 1889. At this point, he thought of joining the army, like his uncle, but, because he was short-sighted, this career was closed to him. This military bent was fulfilled later, not only during a year of military service in his student days, but also through French army appointments in both World War I and II. A liking for the discipline of military life can be detected in other aspects of his career, notably in the administration of his laboratories and even in his research projects. Instead, at age 17, Carrel enrolled on 1 October 1891 in the faculty of medicine in the local University of Lyon. About 120 students started medical training each year, and 60 others were taught in Lyon at a separate school for military surgeons.

Lyon Student

After two years' basic studies in anatomy and physiology, Carrel started clinical training in 1893. This Lyon medical teaching involved a series of competitive examinations over four years followed by further tests for those wishing to enter a hospital career. When he took the examination for entry to the first two years of 'externat' training, he did well. Next year in 1894, he failed in an attempt to reach the next grade as an 'internat'. Not discouraged, Carrel took one year out for military service from November 1894 to autumn 1895, where he served as a 'médecin-auxiliaire' in the 'chasseurs alpins', a mountain regiment trained to protect the border with Italy. After this year out, and a reservist until 1900, he waited until 1896, when he was successful in his second attempt at the exams for an intern surgical post. This involved rotating between the seven surgical units of the Lyon hospitals, many of them in the magnificent ancient Hôtel-Dieu, a hospital of 1,065 beds.

In some accounts of Carrel's life, it is suggested that medical teaching, surgery and research in Lyon at the time was not particularly distinguished,

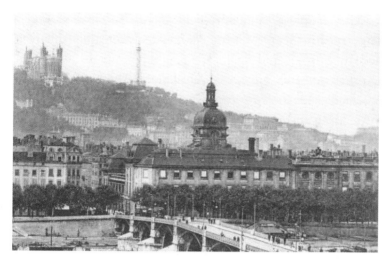

Carrel trained at the venerable Hôtel-Dieu hospital on Le Rhöne river in Lyon.

but this is not the case. In the 1870s reform of the universities, France, including Lyon, had caught up with Germany's prominence in medicine, notably in accepting the importance of adding laboratory studies to clinical work.[6] Thereafter in Europe, France and Germany vied with each other for the world leadership in medicine and surgery. France had the legacy of Claude Bernard's introduction of scientific methods to the study of living tissue, showing that life mechanisms were not impenetrable but could be understood in physical and chemical terms. Added to this, the world was in awe of Pasteur's achievements in Paris in establishing the microbial origins of infectious disease, and that there were methods for prevention. Europe's university-based medical schools and institutes had earlier been copied throughout the world and in America, much earlier, Philadelphia made a start using the Edinburgh medical school as their model. America now studied the continental European medical school research ethos. The rest of the medical world had to be fluent in German and French and this was an extra reason for the American visits. William

---

[6] See Thomas Neville Bonner, *Becoming a Physician: Medical Education in Britain, France, Germany and the United States 1750–1945* (Oxford: Oxford University Press, 1995) and Alain Bouchet *La Médecine à Lyon* (Lyon: Editions Hervas, 1987).

Halsted, the Hopkins surgeon, spent formative time in France and Germany, as did George Crile.[7] Harvey Cushing, like many others, travelled to Europe and spent time in Lyon in 1900, visiting the distinguished research-minded surgical staff. Abraham Flexner toured Europe's medical schools to investigate and report on best practices for future American medical teaching. He enthused about how France had gone further in ensuring that medical education was linked with clinical medical practice and praised the public hospitals of Lyon. He thought anatomical teaching at Lyon was superior to that in Paris and picked out the medico-legal and hygiene departments for praise.[8]

This rite of passage for young Americans would start to fade about 1905, and World War I finally destroyed the European dominance.

Lyon Medicine

As the second city in France, Lyon medicine shared in the competitive and innovative European milieu, particularly in surgery, and Carrel soon had a part in it. In Lyon at this time, the hospitals' notable surgeons were Antonin Poncet (1849–1913), Louis Léopold Ollier (1830–1900),[9] and Mathieu Jaboulay (1860–1913).[10] They made the city famous, rivalling Paris in medical practice and research. Jaboulay published on techniques of blood vessel and testis surgery, and pioneered abdominal surgery, being remembered for his stomach by-pass operations and, as described later, he carried out the first attempts at human kidney transplantation. Poncet had the Lyon chair of operative medicine and wrote extensively on urology and the surgery of tuberculosis, and Ollier was famed for his bone grafting methods. All these talented men in Lyon vigorously followed and expanded their countryman Claude Bernard's advocacy of experimental

---

[7] From 1912 onwards, Halsted kept up a close friendship with the Lyon surgeon René Leriche, even translating Leriche's papers for publication in American journals.

[8] Abraham Flexner, *Medical Education in Europe* (Washington: Carnegie Foundation, 1912): 56. René Leriche's views on the strengths and weaknesses of Lyon surgery are found in Angelo M. May and Alice G. May, *The Two Lions of Lyons* (Kabel Publishing, 1994): 196.

[9] For Ollier, see René Leriche (1952) 'A tribute to Dr Halsted' *Surgery* 32: 538–41.

[10] F. Collet (1960) 'Testut et Jaboulay' *Cahiers Lyonnais d'histoire de la médecine* 5: 3–10.

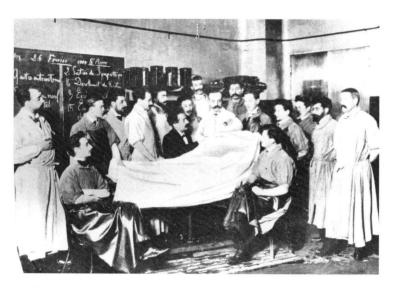

Professor Jaboulay in theatre with a group of assistants in February 1903. Carrel, no longer in favour, may be second from the right.

investigation. Ollier's studies of bone growth were innovative, and as chief surgeon at the Hôtel Dieu, he was ahead of his time in giving up general surgery to specialise in orthopaedics. Among the Lyon physicians was Léon Bouveret (of his eponymous disease and syndrome)[11] and Raphaël Lépine (1840–1919), who contributed to the understanding of diabetes. Lépine was a reforming dean of the Medical School after World War I, attracting Rockefeller Foundation funds to Lyon in the 1920s. These Lyon teachers authored a remarkable number of standard texts, notably those of Testut and Morat. Leo Testut (1849–1925), a surgeon and professor of anatomy, wrote his four-volume, beautifully illustrated *Traité d'anatomie humaine* (1899), which was the best-selling text of the time and was translated and used widely even until the 1950s. The physiologist Jean-Pierre Morat (1846–1920), who studied under Claude Bernard, produced his remarkable six-volume *Traité de physiologie* in 1904, which was much translated elsewhere.[12]

---

[11] Bouveret's Syndrome results from a gallstone entering and blocking the duodenum.

[12] For the surgeon Pollosson's works, see *Titres et travaux scientifiques du Docteur Pollosson* (Lyon, 1929).

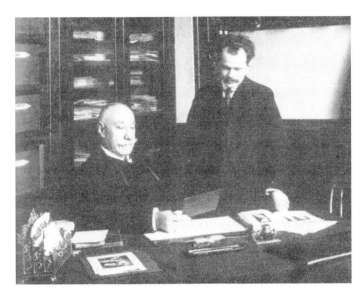

Lyon's famous surgeon Antonin Poncet with the young René Leriche in 1912. (*Cahiers Lyonnais d'histoire de la médecine* April 1959.)

It is clear that the Lyon medical school during Carrel's student days was innovative and thriving. Because Carrel's career did not prosper in Lyon, he later often spoke dismissively of Lyon medicine. His biographers have often accepted his view that the medical school was at a low ebb: all the evidence is that this was not the case.

Surgical Training

After three years on the extern grade, Carrel was an intern from 1896, and these trainee surgeons, who lived in the hospital, did much of the routine and emergency surgical work. Carrel's surgical work would be mainly dealing with trauma, fractures, skin ulcers, hernias and abscesses. He moved every six months between the units run by the distinguished Lyon surgeons, and Carrel, a natural surgeon, may thus have gained considerable skills in general surgery via this impressive training scheme.[13]

---

[13]This impressive rotation through the surgical units is listed in Soupault, *Carrel* (note 1): 17. There was a 'chef du clinique', possibly the senior intern, who would take much responsibility and instruct the juniors.

Such rotations did not exist in Britain or America, where prolonged apprenticeship to individual senior surgeons was the tradition.

The established Lyon senior surgeons, who had their private practice, were available for any difficulties. The interns gave the simple anaesthetics of the day and assisted the senior surgeons in the major surgery in the hospital, and in the many operations carried out in patients' homes. Abdominal operations were in the development stage, and although Lyon's Jaboulay was a pioneer, these were only occasionally attempted. Operations on the chest or blood vessels in human patients were almost unknown.

But there were attempts at experimental blood vessel surgery in the Lyon laboratories by Jaboulay. At this time, from Germany, came the news of the first attempts at animal organ transplants. Carrel was soon to join these efforts, as did Jaboulay.

Personal Life

Carrel had a heavy black beard at this time, but removed it later in America.[14] He was of short stature, dressed well, did not smoke and disapproved of drinking. Hobbies were not important to him, but he fenced at a club and rode horses. He was not known to have any girlfriends, and confided in his diary that he dreaded the 'ennui' of a conventional marriage. Though he had some male friends, no hint of closer relations can be found then or later. His assertive nature, which was to feature later, was in evidence as a student, gaining him a nickname of 'coton poudre', or 'guncotton' shortened to 'cotton'. Others noticed an 'appartenance de bourgeoisie aisé, une politesse stricte, réserve distante, un peu d'égoïsme'. At this time, Carrel joined in with a weekly discussion group called the 'Conférence Joseph de Maistre', named after the early monarchist philosopher who was a critic of democracy and opposed the French Revolution. The group of about 10 had medical and non-medical student members. It was organised by Adolphe Berthet, later a composer,

---

[14] An early photograph of the bearded Carrel appears in *Cahiers Lyonnais d'histoire de la médecine*, April 1959, p. 77.

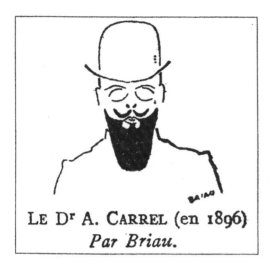

LE Dᴿ A. CARREL (en 1896)
Par Briau.

A portrait of Carrel from
Le Crocodile of January 1925.
(*Courtesy of Alain Drouard.*)

and Carrel was to re-create and enjoy this format again later in America. He kept up a correspondence with some of the members for years afterwards, sharing deeply conservative views.[15] Carrel's contributions to their debates would be robust. The topics of the day in Lyon included politics and religion, and although France's Roman Catholic Church had traditional strength, Lyon was notably anti-clerical and the city's medical and university circles were particularly hostile to Catholicism. Within the Church in Lyon, there was a modernisers group called the 'School of Lyon' and one of the members, also in Carrel's discussion group, was Marcel Rifaux, a medical student. In 1905 he wrote his *L'Agonie du Catholicism*, complaining of the Catholic Church's 'anthropomorphism, autocracy, ridiculous legends, sanctuaries with shameless commercialism, fraudulent relics, and abuse of titles.'[16] It caused offense in conventional circles, and since Carrel's introspective diaries show he was having

---

[15] For Carrel's friends, see Drouard (note 1): 4.
[16] Marcel Rifaux (1872–1938) continued to write, and was later director of a psycho-therapeutic clinic at Chalor-sur-Saüne, near Lyon.

religious doubts, the controversy would suit him.[17] Another debate was whether science was hostile to religious belief, since Claude Bernard's reductionism seemed to eliminate the need for any mysterious God-given life force in living tissues. Adding to this, the group would be well aware of the French philosopher Ernest Renan's *L'Avenir de la science* (Paris 1890), which suggested that science had replaced religion in solving the problems of the world.[18] Carrel recalled later that at this time he also developed a lasting interest in telepathy and clairvoyance and hoped to demonstrate its existence using scientific methods.[19] Immigration was a local issue in the city, and in 1896, Lyon students demonstrated against the presence of large numbers of foreign students coming in from the French empire, and affecting their chance of promotion.[20] The Dreyfus case, in which Alfred Dreyfus, a low-ranking Jewish military officer, was wrongly convicted of treason in 1894, would be a dominant issue at the young men's meeting, dividing them, like the rest of France, between those unable to accept that there could be injustice in high places, and those calling for reform.

On one occasion, Carrel and his friends, disguised in shabby clothing and armed with clubs, attempted to disrupt a local meeting. This may have been an event organised by the Ligue des droits de l'homme, an early human rights group which emerged after the Dreyfus *cause célèbre*.[21]

---

[17] Carrel's diary details his early religious doubts; see Alexis Carrel, *Jour après jour: journal 1893–1944* (Paris: Plon, 1956), which is examined closely in Drouard (note 1): 53–8, and in Joseph T. Durkin, *Hope for Our Time: Alexis Carrel on Man and Society* (New York: Harper and Row, 1965).

[18] For Ernest Renan's influence on young French students at this time, see the French-born American scientist René J. Dubos, *The Dreams of Reason: Science and Utopias* (New York: Columbia University Press, 1961): 8–9.

[19] Carrel's interest in telepathy during his student days is noted in Carrel's book *Man, the Unknown* (New York: Harper & Brothers, 1935): 124.

[20] Xenophobia among French medical students is mentioned in Donna Evleth (1995) 'Vichy France and the continuity of medical nationalism' *Social History of Medicine* 8: 95–116.

[21] For Carrel's hostility to the Ligue, see Andrés H. Reggiani, *God's Eugenicist: Alexis Carrel and the Sociobiology of Decline* (New York: Berghahn Books, 2007): 12.

Also in 1894, when Carrel was a young extern, there was a major incident in Lyon's history. The French President Sadi Carnot, rising in popularity but under political pressure, visited the city, and the ceremonials included the award of the Légion d'honneur to the local surgeon Louis Ollier. But later that day, Carnot was stabbed in the abdomen by an Italian anarchist, and Carnot was taken to the Prefecture (the Town Hall), where resuscitation was attempted by Ollier and his colleague Poncet, though no abdominal exploration was carried out. Post-mortem examination showed that the cause of death was bleeding from damage to the portal vein near the liver, then, as ever, a difficult surgical challenge. The events were much discussed in Lyon. Carrel is said to have developed an interest in blood vessel surgery at this time, but it would be eight years before Carrel took up such work, and he had other interests in the interim.

Publications

As an intern from 1896 onwards, Carrel was quick to start publishing. In Lyon's medical community, it was clear to aspiring surgeons that they should 'publish or perish', which meant writing papers and giving presentations to the local medical societies. Carrel showed the energy he displayed later, and his ambition appears in his introspective diaries. He wrote:

> Science can conduct me to an important position in the world....
> I want for myself intellectual satisfaction and a flattering of my self-love.
> Can I in this kind of life and in these times achieve happiness? I do not
> believe so, because I crave too much, because a thing once possessed
> loses for me all value.[22]

Most of Carrel's reports were in the respected journal *Lyon Médical*, which dated from 1850. His first publication in this journal was in 1896 on 'bilocular' stomach, and then in 1897 he described a local chickenpox epidemic. There were three more papers that year, including

---

[22] Carrel *Diary*, box 39 file 70, GULBFC (note 3).

a study of Cheyne-Stokes respiration, the ominous sign in serious illness, and in the following year he published five papers, including one on a leg aneurysm, and one on thumb tendonitis, in a Paris journal. In 1899 there was a remarkable total of nine more, including an eight-page article, again published in Paris, on breast tuberculosis, and with five added in 1900.[23] In 1902 came his famous paper on blood vessel surgical methods, as described later, and there were also three more publications in that year.

The European clinical research tradition was 'generalist' at the time, encouraging involvement in a number of unrelated projects, and Carrel's publications show this conventional breadth. Only later did he discard this assumption and, taking a different view, focus instead on the sharply defined area of blood vessel surgery and the closely related study of organ transplantation.

The Meetings

Carrel's publications were mostly the result of his presentations to the four local medical societies which were part of Lyon's impressive medical milieu. The two largest were the Société des Sciences médicales de Lyon (founded 1789) and the Société nationale de Médecine de Lyon. They met on alternate weeks. Membership was restricted to the senior staff, but younger staff gave contributions when introduced by senior members. Two or three papers were given at each meeting, and the meetings offered a platform for the surgical interns to show their talents, hoping for promotion to the one or two local established surgical posts which came up each year. The meetings, as elsewhere in France, had a tradition of robust discussion, and any defects in a presentation were ruthlessly exposed. These 'beauty contests' among the young men could also reflect credit on the senior surgeons, who used their junior staff's presentations to show off the work of their units. Following the meetings, the speakers' texts appeared quickly

---

[23]There are many incomplete bibliographies of Carrel's numerous publications, but the best are Sutter's original attempt in Soupault, *Carrel* (note 1) and the more recent listing in Reggiani, *God's Eugenicist* (note 21).

in *précis* form in the *Lyon Médical*. This journal (founded 1869) appeared monthly and at this time had an impressive size, reaching over 1,000 pages per year.

Carrel contributed on many occasions to these meetings and was a confident performer. He was in a race for promotion among the young, talented trainee Lyon surgeons, and all were being watched closely by the senior surgeons. Carrel could hardly have done more to achieve his ambition. He gave many presentations, he had surgical talent, he knew the right people, his research work was well known, and it reflected credit on his seniors.

Research Opportunities

With his four intern years finished, Carrel was qualified as a 'Docteur de la faculté de Lyon', and while waiting for the more senior surgical positions, notably of 'chirurgien des hôpitaux', to come up, Carrel had obtained a post, one with added surgical work. In February 1899 he joined the talented Leo Testut's anatomy department as 'l'adjuvat' and was soon rewarded by promotion to 'prosecteur', and his skill at dissection was noticed. Ambitious young men were also encouraged to write a 'thèse', a work of usually about 100 pages. By 1901, Carrel managed to produce a 303-page thesis based on Poncet's considerable clinical experience of thyroid cancer surgery. It was well-received and was published first in Lyon and then in Paris.[24] He soon obtained experimental surgical facilities in a new medical research laboratory belonging to Auguste Lumière, who, with his brother Louis, had, in Lyon, made the first motion pictures. Later, in 1901, his friend Marcel Soulier, son of Lyon's Prof. Marcel Soulier, gave Carrel facilities in his father's laboratory for surgical experiments using dogs. Until this stage, Carrel had worked mostly on clinical topics; now with these facilities he moved into the experimental blood vessel surgery which would make him famous.

---

[24] Carrel's thesis was published in full as Alexis Carrel-Billard, *Le goitre cancéreux* (Lyon: Paul Legendre, 1900 and Paris: Baillière, 1901).

Promotion Opportunities

The Lyon hospitals were run by the city, and when a surgical vacancy appeared, the method of appointment — the 'concours' — followed civil service procedures. A day was set, essays on surgical subjects given to the candidates, and this was followed by a public examination by a 'jury' of seven or eight local surgeons, plus two physicians. On the day, the candidates had to speak at short notice for 20 minutes on topics given to them. During the week-end prior to the *concours*, the candidates were expected to call on the members of the panel at their homes. Carrel's first attempt at promotion to the hospital surgeon post was in 1901. There were 12 candidates, and included Léon Bérard (1870–1956). Bérard was four years older and had also been a prosector and 'chef de clinique chirurgical'. Bérard had failed to gain promotion in two

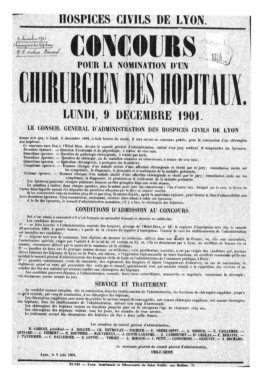

Public announcement of the 1901 *'concours'* process to select a surgeon for the Lyon hospitals. (*Courtesy of the Archives municipales de Lyon.*)

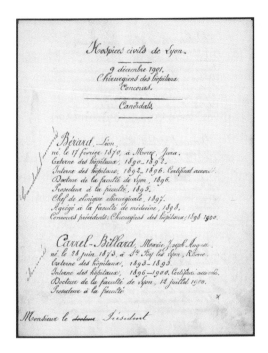

Carrel's entry for the 1901 surgical *concours* competition. (*Courtesy of the Archives municipales de Lyon*.)

previous *concours* in 1898 and 1900, but now Bérard got the post.[25] To fail at a first or second attempt was common: with patience, Carrel could be rewarded.[26]

During this time of waiting, he coached younger men in the 'conférences d'internat' for their first hurdle — the *concours* examination for intern posts. One of the students he taught was René Leriche (1879–1955), six years his junior, and later Europe's leading vascular surgeon.[27] Leriche always admired Carrel's surgical skill, 'equal to

---

[25] From 1923, Léon Bérard headed a pioneering cancer treatment centre in Lyon.

[26] Drouard, *Alexis Carrel* (note 1) p. 65 gives an interesting list of notable Lyon surgeons who were unsuccessful in their early 'concours' attempts, but had success later. It is often stated wrongly that it had a pass/fail format and Carrel 'failed'.

[27] René Leriche later had rapid promotion in Lyon, and became professor of experimental surgery in 1920. He moved to Strasbourg, then in 1928 to the chair of experimental medicine at the Collège de France in Paris, operating at the American Hospital. See

Jaboulay', he said, and the paths of the two men were later to cross and intersect. But they were never particularly close.

The Paper

Using his opportunity for operating on dogs in Soulier's lab, in 1902 Carrel published a paper in *Lyon Médical* describing a method of joining blood vessels. This short publication was to give him lasting fame, and is seen as the origin of modern blood vessel and organ transplantation surgery. This historic paper has been quoted many times, but deserves a closer look.

There had been little interest in the surgery of blood vessels until this time. This disinterest is largely explained by a lack of a clinical need. Between times of war, injuries to the large blood vessels in the chest and abdomen were uncommon in civilian life. Any deep wounds to the chest and abdomen were not routinely explored surgically, and an 'expectant' strategy was used instead. However, if a limb's major blood vessel was badly damaged, the main artery above the leak could be tied off. This can be a surprisingly successful treatment, and was standard practice in military surgery even into World War II. After such 'proximal ligation', particularly in a young person, the small vessels of the 'collateral' circulation above the blockage can open up and restore the supply to the limb below the tied-off artery.

'Hardening' and narrowing of the arteries by atheroma was not yet a common clinical problem, particularly as life expectancy at the time was lower. It was also wrongly taught at the time that, when present, arterial disease diffusely affected the blood vessels, rather than showing a patchy distribution, and hence was not suitable for surgical treatment. Radiology of the blood vessels was yet to come.

But the surgeons had one more familiar vascular challenge. This was the aneurysmal weakening and ballooning of the large arteries in the chest or abdomen or limbs, common at the time, through damage to the wall

---

Fredric Jarrett (1979) 'René Leriche (1879–1955): father of vascular surgery' *Surgery* 86: 736–41, René Leriche, *Souvenirs de ma vie morte* (Paris: Seuil, 1956) and May and May, *Two Lions* (note 8).

by syphilis. When threatening to rupture, or starving the distal tissues of blood, the ancient method of simply tying off the affected artery above the swelling was in regular use.[28] In New Orleans, Rudolph Matas had a unique exposure to the challenge of these aneurysms, and he and William Halsted at Johns Hopkins were trying to refine a better method for dealing with aneurysms. But because the simple ligation techniques were available, attempting removal and repair of damaged or diseased lengths of artery was not favoured.

Methods

For those experimenting on how to join blood vessels together, there was a debate on the best method to use. The first attempts at stitching them together usually led to leakage of blood, or clotting within the vessels. But in Lyon in 1896, six years prior to Carrel's famous paper, Prof. Jaboulay and his assistant Eugène Briau reported re-joining a divided donkey carotid artery by direct stitching, and their method was not unlike the modern technique, putting their rather crude needle and thread through all coats of the vessel.[29] The suture used is not mentioned, but their illustration in *Lyon Médical* suggests 'horizontal mattress' sutures of coarse thread or perhaps catgut. These stitches were passed through the vessels and back again nearby with the knot tied on one side only. Carrel later called these 'Jaboulay stitches', and they are still widely used in surgery when needed. The donkey carotid was large enough for this strategy to be a success, but Jaboulay reported no further experiments. Perhaps regular success was not achieved.[30] Only J.B. Murphy in Chicago in 1897 had made attempts at joining human arteries and had repaired a gun-shot

---

[28] See D.A. Cooley (1999) 'The history of surgery of the thoracic aorta' *Cardiology Clinics* 17: 609–13.

[29] M. Jaboulay and E. Briau (1896) 'Recherches expérimentales sur la suture et la greffe artérielles' *Lyon Médical* 81: 97–9.

[30] The many pre-Carrel reports on attempts to join blood vessels, notably by Dörfler, are reviewed in Harris B. Shumacker Jr. and H.Y. Muhms (1969) 'Arterial suture techniques and grafts: past, present and future' *Surgery* 66: 419–33 and by Steven G. Friedman *A History of Vascular Surgery* (Malden: Blackwell Futura, 2005).

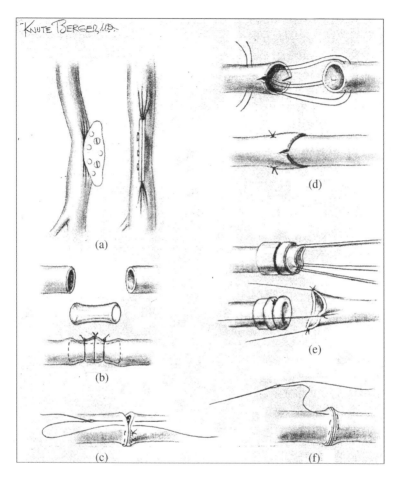

Early twentieth century methods of joining blood vessels: method C was used in Lyon by Jaboulay. (*Illustration by Knute E. Berger, M.D.*)

wound in a human femoral artery. He also reported extensive experimental work with blood vessel surgery in dogs and large animals.[31]

There was an alternative to the stitching method. It was developed by the German surgeon Erwin Payr, who pulled the two vessels over a short

---

[31] J.B. Murphy (1897) 'Resection of arteries and veins injured in continuity — end-to-end suture — experimental and clinical research' *Medical Record (New York)* 51: 73–88. This long paper has a useful historical review. Murphy inserted the proximal vessel inside the distal, and his silk sutures penetrated the entire wall.

BULLETIN DU LYON MÉDICAL

RECHERCHES EXPÉRIMENTALES SUR LA SUTURE
ET LA GREFFE ARTÉRIELLES.

La réunion immédiate des plaies artérielles au moyen de la suture a été réalisée expérimentalement par Jassinowsky (*Arch. f. klin. chirurg.*, 1891), et plus récemment par Heidenhain *(Cent. f. chirurg.*, 1895).

Les expériences suivantes, pratiquées chez des chiens, démontrent que grâce à un procédé spécial de suture, il est possible de rétablir le courant sanguin dans une artère complètement sectionnée ; nous avons fait la suture simple, bout à bout, ou bien nous avons interposé au moyen de deux sutures un fragment artériel détaché ; le rétablissement de la circulation sanguine s'est opéré sans hémorrhagie au niveau de la jonction.

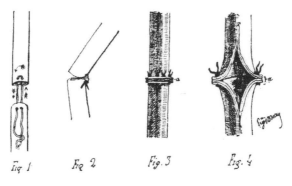

$\overline{lig}\,1$ $\overline{lig}\,2$ $lig.3$ $lig.4$

Jaboulay's paper on his method of joining blood vessels. (*From Reference 29.*)

length of hollow tubing and tied them onto it; the tube served as an inner conduit for the blood. And there was another reason for an interest in Europe in blood vessel surgery and methods of joining blood vessels. Organ transplantation was on the surgeon's agenda: the news from Germany was that it was possible. In 1902, Payr's stent method was used for the first ever experimental animal kidney transplant, reported by Ullmann from Vienna in 1902.[32]

---

[32] E. Ullmann (1902) 'Experimentelle Nierentransplantation' *Wiener Klinische Wochenschrift* 15: 281–82.

Carrel's Method

Carrel's 1902 paper reported that, having tried the Payr method, he had returned, like Jaboulay locally, to direct stitching to join blood vessels together.[33] Carrel's improvement in the stitching method included use of smaller needles ('No. 13 Kirby'),[34] and he used finer linen or cotton thread obtained from the local lace-making industry.[35] He did not put the stitches through the entire wall of the larger vessels to be joined, but described that he skimmed their surfaces. In this way, the thread suture did not penetrate into the blood stream inside the new junction of the vessels, diminishing

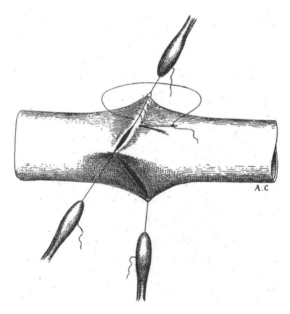

Carrel's 'triangulation' technique is helpful when joining small vessels. (*From Reference 33.*)

---

[33] Dr Carrel [sic] (1902) 'La technique opératoire des anastomoses vasculaires et la transplantation des viscères' *Lyon Mèdical* 99: 859–62. There is a translation of this paper in Toni Hau, *Renal Transplantation* (Austin: Silvergirl, 1987): 4–5.

[34] These needles were made by Kirby, Beard & Co. Ltd of Birmingham, England, makers later of the Kirbygrip.

[35] Carrel had surgical talent, and when he became a public figure later, popular accounts emerged which told of how he developed his methods from lace-making lessons from a Mme Leroudier, a lacemaker in Lyon.

the chances of internal clotting. To assist the accurate insertion of these stitches in smaller vessels, he used his 'triangulation' technique. He placed three equidistant, loose preliminary untied stitches which held the vessels together. With the assistant picking up two of these three 'stay' sutures at a time, and gently pulling them apart, the vessels were stretched and the two vessel edges were presented to the operator, allowing for accurate, close stitching. It is still occasionally useful. In his paper, Carrel included three illustrations of this triangulation technique, drawn by himself, and these have became iconic images in the history of surgery.

In his paper, Carrel thanked Prof. Soulier for allowing him to use the 'new laboratory', and he was grateful for the valuable collaboration of 'Messrs. Morel and Marcel Soulier'. But the only experimental use of the technique mentioned is of one attempt with a dog kidney graft, placed in the neck. It seems this was not a success: a little urine appeared after a while, but the venous anastomosis failed.[36]

He finished the paper with hints of work in progress.

> The experiments we are now undertaking concerning the transplantation of the thyroid, kidney and pancreas are not sufficiently advanced to enable us to draw any conclusions.

Carrel's text shows a confident stance. It is written in the first person, and he says the method is 'simple'. It also reads as if little had gone before, and there are no references. It was merely reporting a technical improvement for those attempting such surgery in small vessels.

Events of 1902

In early 1902, the prospects for Carrel's career looked good. Soulier, who had supported Carrel's dog experiments, was President of the local Société Nationale de Médecine and accordingly chaired their meetings that year.

---

[36] The operation would take some time, and immediate urine production could not be expected. Carrel later described this kidney graft attempt briefly, plus an unsuccessful thyroid gland graft, in Alexis Carrel (1905) 'The transplantation of organs. A preliminary communication' *JAMA* 45: 1645–6; see also William C. Beck (1986) 'Alexis Carrel and Carl Beck — a historical footnote' *Perspectives in Biology and Medicine* 30: 148–51, who heard that only two dogs were involved, plus practice on cadavers.

Not only that, it was the turn of the innovative surgeon Prof. Jaboulay to be president of Lyon's other society — the Société des Sciences médicales de Lyon — and as the year progressed, Carrel spoke a number of times at these meetings.

Lourdes Visit

But by the time of that productive summer, there was a problem hanging over Carrel, making his future uncertain, and it had arisen earlier that year. In May 1902, some months before describing the new method, Carrel was unexpectedly asked to accompany some Lyon pilgrims going by special train to Lourdes, the shrine with a reputation for miraculous healing, 250 miles south-west of the city. It was usual to include a medical attendant in the group because of the poor health of the pilgrims.[37]

Lourdes' reputation came from reports of cures at the shrine, dating from 1858. To deal with criticism from sceptics, the claims were increasingly reviewed by local doctors, rather than priests, and by 1884, more careful medical audits were brought in by the Bureau des Contestations Médicales, which documented immediately any 'medically inexplicable' clinical improvements. The Bureau, which still exists, studies each case, and over the years has documented 7,000 such events. They go no further than making a report. The Bureau leaves it to the bishop of the patient's diocese to look at the religious aspect, and it is left open to him to declare 'a miraculous event'.[38]

But Carrel's interest in going to Lourdes was not new. His diaries show that he had been interested in the events at the shrine for at least a year and had read widely on the subject and discussed it with priests. In 1901 he entered this plan for a new project:

> I shall pass these months in studying and digging deep into the question that chiefly interests me — the question of miracles. I shall study this

---

[37] Carrel's experiences were used for his posthumously published 1949 novel *Le voyage de Lourdes* (Paris: Plon, 1949): his manuscript was said to date from 1902.
[38] The Catholic Church has so far supported 69 claims for miraculous cures at Lourdes. See Ruth Harris, *Lourdes: Body and Spirit in the Secular Age* (London: Allen Lane, 1999). Cases of tuberculosis are prominent in the list of cures, including seven affecting the abdomen.

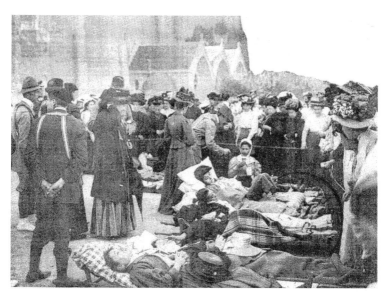

Pilgrims at Lourdes waiting to enter the 'piscine' bath and encounter its healing waters.

question as much as possible, and shall write a volume entirely sincere, which according to my beliefs, will be a glorification of the Virgin of Lourdes.

He went on:

I shall publish the book under my name, no matter what the cost, whatever be its conclusions, and whatever may be the damage I shall sustain from the publication.[39]

This shows that he had a serious interest in the matter of the claims at Lourdes, and it is clear that he was hardly a sceptic. He assumed that it was likely that he would come out in support, and he was even prepared to publish his conclusions and fund the publication himself. He was prepared to provoke controversy, knowing that it might damage his career. This is exactly what happened.[40]

---

[39] Durkin, *Hope* (note 17): 59.

[40] Carrel's biographers often state that his journey to Lourdes was a new venture and not premeditated. They also often wrongly date this Lourdes visit to 1903, taking the error from Soupault's *Carrel* (note 1).

The Cure

In the Lyon train to Lourdes was Marie Bailly, an ill young lady who had a swollen, tender abdomen with palpable masses. There was tuberculosis in the family, and she had lung infections earlier. The clinical diagnosis seemed certain to be abdominal tuberculosis, although no tests were then available to make a firm diagnosis. Normally the ritual at Lourdes was for the pilgrims to enter the water of the pool of the shrine, but Marie Bailly was judged to be too ill for this, and accordingly water was merely sprinkled on her body. By the afternoon, she was clinically improved and her abdominal swelling had reduced. Soon she was able to walk to the Grotto and improved daily thereafter, then returning well to Lyon. She made a full recovery, and later entered a convent, where she lived to the age of 50.[41]

While at Lourdes, Carrel reported what he had seen to the Medical Bureau. As was his intention in the previous year, he was prepared to take a

Carrel made a registry entry on arrival at the Lourdes shrine in May 1902. (*Courtesy of the Bureau des Contestations Médicales de Lourdes.*)

---

[41] Advanced cases of tuberculosis could recover, but did so slowly. One possible secular explanation of Marie Bailly's rapid recovery is that an intra-abdominal abscess drained internally.

LE NOUVELL

UNE GUÉRISON À LOURDES

Nous avons brièvement rapporté hier la conversation que nous avons eue avec M. le docteur Carrel qui assista aux différentes phases du voyage et de la guérison de Mᴵˡᵉ Bailly à Lourdes. Les termes de cette conversation étaient très clairs, très fidèles et ne prêtaient à aucune ambiguïté. Nous recevons cependant de M. le docteur Carrel la lettre suivante :

Monsieur le rédacteur en chef,

Dans votre numéro du 9 juin 1902, vous publiez, au sujet du pèlerinage de Lourdes, une interview d'un de vos rédacteurs.

Malheureusement ma conversation a été rapportée de telle sorte que le sens en est dénaturé. Je vous prie donc de bien vouloir publier la rectification suivante :

Dans l'histoire de Mᴵˡᵉ X..., un seul point est indiscutable. Cette jeune fille, très gravement malade le 28 mai, à une heure de l'après-midi, était guérie le soir à sept heures, et la guérison persiste encore aujourd'hui.

En dehors de ce fait certain, tout le reste est vague. La nature réelle de la maladie est entièrement indéterminée. Par conséquent il est impossible actuellement de tirer de cette observation les conclusions qu'il vous plaît d'en faire ressortir.

Pardon, M. le docteur Carrel ne rectifie rien du tout, la meilleure preuve c'est qu'il répète dans sa lettre ce que nous avons publié et que voici :

The Lyon *Nouvelliste* newspaper report quoting Carrel's experience at Lourdes.

public stance, and on his return to Lyon 10 days later, two Lyon newspapers had the story of the 'miracle'. He allowed himself to be quoted about the case, and the interview appeared in *Le Nouvelliste* on 9 June.[42] Carrel said that the events could not be explained by any normal mechanism. The newspaper understood that he considered that supernatural forces were at

---

[42] The various articles on this Lourdes controversy start in *Le Nouvelliste de Lyon*, 3 June 1902, and continued until 10 June.

work, but after the article appeared, he wrote back to the editor of the newspaper claiming that he had been misquoted. Carrel insisted that his view was merely that the apparent cure had no normal explanation and that he would speculate no further. The paper published his complaint, but stood by its original story.

Lyon took religious matters seriously at the time, and Carrel's stance pleased no one. Lyon's conservative Catholics might have hoped that Carrel had supported divine intervention but the local Catholic modernisers were not supportive of such claims from the shrines. It is of interest that, in spite of the dramatic events, the bishop of Lyon did not take Bailly's case any further towards recognition of a miraculous cure. The largely sceptical local medical profession not only criticised Carrel's view that something inexplicable had happened, but also deplored the personal publicity involved. An important critic of Carrel was the Lyon professor of medicine Victor Augagneur, then also the socialist mayor of the city, and a national political figure later.[43] Augagneur joined the controversy, denying the existence of miracles. Carrel seemed to have no regrets at the newspaper involvement, and had kept the story alive by responding to the claimed inaccuracies. It was the beginning of a lifelong, close relationship with the press.

After this visit, and for the rest of his life, Carrel never wavered in his belief that such rapid healing was possible. He believed it lay latent, but available, in the human body, and it could be activated by intense prayer. He also thought that ordinary methods would eventually be found to liberate this rapid mechanism, and he often claimed to be close to success. He returned many times to Lourdes and registered with the Bureau as an advisor. Carrel grumbled about the Medical Bureau's lack of rigorous analysis, notably having 'a rosary but no medical tools'. He criticised the lack of photographic evidence, and suggested that the Bureau took a

---

[43] See Jack D. Ellis, *The Physician-legislators of France* (Cambridge: Cambridge University Press, 1990). Victor Augagneur was later a member of the French National Assembly, then Governor-General of Madagascar, and finally a French government minister during WWI.

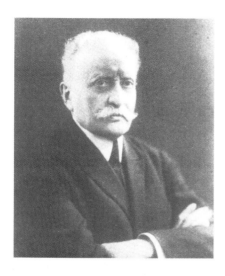

Victor Augagneur, the physician and major of Lyon, was one of Carrel's critics (*fr.wikipedia*).

generally credulous stance.[44] But, after these later visits he told friends and colleagues of further rapid cures.[45] His view was that:

> Miraculous cures seldom occur. Despite their small number, they prove the existence of organic and mental processes that we do not know ... they are stubborn irreducible facts, which must be taken into account.

Summer 1902

This public stance on the case of Marie Bailly was hardly a prudent move for a young man seeking promotion. His famous paper appeared in *Lyon Médical* on 8 June 1902, just at the time of the Lourdes controversy. In the busy few months which followed, his hospital work and research continued apparently unaffected, and he and Morel gave another paper to the Société de Médecine on 16 June, which apparently pleased their supervisor Soulier, chairman of the meeting at that time.[46] Next month, with Soulier again in

---

[44] Carrel's severe criticism of the Bureau appeared in 1909 in the journal *Croix de Paris*; the reaction to the article is described in Durkin, *Hope* (note 17): 112–16.

[45] See for instance Eleanor R. Belmont, *The Fabric of Memory* (New York: Farrar, Straus and Cudahy, 1980): 7.

[46] The *Lyon Médical* 16 June 1902 paper with Morel was entitled 'Opération de Pawlow'.

the chair, on 7 and 21 July 1902, Carrel and Morel gave a presentation and demonstration describing how they had joined end-to-end a dog's carotid artery in the neck to the adjacent jugular vein.[47] This was done with the hope that, by reversing the flow of arterial blood and re-routing it back up the vein, the blood supply to the brain would increase. This experiment was a reasonable suggestion at the time, offering a possible treatment for strokes or mental decline by increasing the brain blood flow.[48] The animal was also exhibited to the medical society. The abnormal neck pulsation could be felt and the turbulent flow of blood in the vein, the 'souffle intermittent', easily heard when listening with a stethoscope, must have impressed the members. It was made clear by Carrel to the meeting that the idea for this operation came from Prof. Jaboulay, and Jaboulay spoke at length in the discussion which followed; in a publication by Jaboulay later that year, the older, famous surgeon was clearly proud of Carrel's technical success. Achieving the operation was a novelty.[49] This experiment influenced much of Carrel's thinking later. He continued to follow Jaboulay's approach in repeatedly trying, and failing, to improve organ activity by altering the pressure, volume or content of the arterial input.

Promotion Denied

But in spite of his considerable research contributions, and his surgical skill, Carrel had lost support, and he was advised that the Lourdes publicity counted against him. Carrel could not have expected otherwise, and indeed had anticipated it, and there is no suggestion that he showed contrition or had private regrets. To add to this, Carrel's confidence and assertiveness may have made him unpopular with the senior staff. He may also have indicated that, as was clear later, he was

---

[47] Carrel, A., Morel (1902). Présentation d'un chien porteur d'une anastomose artério-veineuse *Lyon Médical* 99: 152–3.

[48] For the history of such attempts at increasing blood flow to the brain, see M.G. Hayden, M. Lee, R. Guzman and G.K. Steinberg (2009) 'The evolution of cerebral revascularization surgery' *Neurosurgical Focus* 26: E17.

[49] See Mathieu Jaboulay's 'Clinique Chirurgicale: Chirurgie des artères' *La Semaine Médicale* No. 50, 10 Dec 1902: 405–6.

not particularly interested in routine clinical surgery and instead preferred considerable involvement in research. Another *concours* for a vacant Lyon hospital permanent surgical post was coming up, and there were 10 candidates: M. Durand, who came third in 1901, not Carrel, was appointed.

Aftermath

Carrel published nothing after the soon-to-be-famous July 1902 paper, and he was now absent from the Lyon medical meetings at which he had such a high profile. Carrel's position in the anatomy department came to an end in August 1902. He now supported a new venture, helping fund two other doctors in setting up 'La clinique des accidents du travail', a free clinic to treat accidents at work. It aimed to give specialised prompt attention to such injuries, with rehabilitation following. The clinic got the support of local industry and the insurance companies and it prospered initially, lasting until 1909.[50] In 1903 he gave medical training to some missionaries going to Northern Canada, and was invited to join them, but declined. The 1903 *concours* was coming up but there was no point in entering, particularly as the 'brilliant' Eugène Vignard was now the favourite, and did gain the promotion, at his third attempt.[51] More younger talent was coming up, and not long after, René Leriche was successful in 1906, going on to gain international surgical fame with his blood vessel surgery and add to Lyon's reputation for producing innovative vascular surgeons.[52]

---

[50] The Clinic is described in Drouard, *Alexis Carrel* (note 1): 69–72.

[51] The celebratory announcement of Vignard's promotion, and the interesting structure of the 1903 *concours*, is given in detail in *Lyon Médical* 102, (1904): 548–50. Vignard's later career is unknown, and he had given only two papers at the Lyon medical societies that year.

[52] A. Bouchet (1994) 'Les pionniers Lyonnais de la chirurgie vasculaire: M. Jaboulay, A. Carrel, E. Villard et R. Leriche' *Histoire des Sciences Médicales* 28: 223–38. Eugène Villard (1868–1953) would join Carrel as an invited speaker at the international New York meeting in 1914.

By mid-1903, low in spirits, Carrel moved to Paris. He made half-hearted applications to become a naval surgeon and considered joining the Bulgarian army medical services. Instead he attended lectures at the Sorbonne and College de France. The savants he listened to included Catholic modernisers like Alfred Loisy (1857–1940) and the philosopher of science Léon de Rosney (1837–1914). Also influential in Paris at the time was Henri Berr (1863–1954), who advocated synthesis of disparate disciplines and sought to extend scientific methods into social studies. Carrel would, later in his career, make use of his exposure to these ideas. A biographer noted that in Paris he lived a simple life and took no part in enjoying 'l'alcohol, le tabac, l'amour …'

After staying in Paris over the winter, Carrel decided to emigrate. As he spoke only French, few places in the world were attractive to him. He decided to move to francophone eastern Canada, and sailed from Bordeaux for Montreal by steam ship on 6 May, travelling first class. His mother was dismayed at his decision, and hoped to later join him.

His Motives

In the many accounts of Carrel's life, it is usually said that he emigrated to escape the parochialism of Lyon and Lyon medicine and to seek the greater surgical opportunities in America. Durkin's biography of Carrel explained that

> [Carrel] could not endure what he considered to be the reactionary attitude of French medical men of his time with respect to scientific research.... The United States, on the contrary, he could not praise too highly … new ideas were welcome and financial aid was placed at the disposal of any scientist who could prove his competence.[53]

This was the view encouraged by Carrel later. It requires considerable modification. North America, far from offering scope for an ambitious young research-minded surgeon, had as yet almost nothing to offer. Ambitious Americans instead came to Europe to train, and on return

---

[53] Durkin, *Hope* (note 17): xvii.

complained that there were no comparable facilities or funding at home. The pioneering Johns Hopkins' Hunterian Laboratory for animal experimentation did not open until 1906, and the Rockefeller Institute in New York did not emerge fully until that year also. All the evidence suggests that Lyon at this time had a flourishing medical milieu which favoured research and publication. There was particular strength in experimental surgery, facilities which Carrel had used. His departure came from his failure to gain promotion in Lyon. He was a proud, talented man who took his rebuff badly. Moreover, Carrel's move was not to America but to Canada, and it was a voyage into the unknown.

CHAPTER TWO

New Life in North America

Carrel landed in French-speaking Montreal at the end of May 1904. In the city, he met up with two old French acquaintances, the brothers Adelstan and François de Martigny, who were doctors at the Catholic l'Hôtel-Dieu hospital. One month after he arrived, the second French-language Congrès des Médecins de Langue français de l'Amérique du Nord was held, organised by Adelstan, and Carrel had put in a paper before he left France. Shortly after, two quickly-published publications on his Lyon blood vessel work appeared in French-Canadian medical magazines.[1] The well-connected de Martignys, though good friends then and later, did not arrange a local surgical post. Carrel may have wished to seek better opportunities, but he also looked at other ventures. Some evidence suggests that Carrel made moves to become a cattle rancher in the Ottawa Valley, and Carrel's archives also show another project. In August that year he obtained a letter of introduction from the French authorities in Montreal to the French 'agent consulaire' in Winnipeg in central Canada which said that:

> The cause of colonisation is the object of his [Carrel's] study. He seems to be investigating the causes which have led to the failure of some and the success of the majority of his compatriots in this country. No doubt

---

[1] See Alexis Carrel (1904) 'Les anastomoses vasculaire et leur technique opératoire' *Union Médicale du Canada* 33: 521–7, and 'Les anastomoses vasculaire, leurs techniques opératoires et leurs indications' *Revue Médicale du Canada* 8: 29–32.

his visit will produce some valuable results for the rapid development of our French colonies, especially those of the Quest.[2]

Keeping his options open, de Martigny also assisted Carrel with advice and a written reference for any surgical posts he might apply for. This letter of introduction says that Carrel was skilled in 'surgery of bones, joints and arteries except for [the] abdomen which he does not do.' Not being an abdominal surgeon was less of a handicap than it might seem at the time: this was a new, optional surgical skill.

De Martigny added that

> he has done some really extraordinary things, which had never been done before him, and which have not been done since, such as the suture of arteries and veins and the transplantation of organs. ... You see what splendid results might be expected if his experiments, pushed still further, should permit the attempt to replace a Bright's disease kidney ...

This letter of reference adds that Carrel's difficulties in Lyon were the result of illness. It added that he had a private income, and if Carrel chose to devote himself to research, he had no need of part-time paid clinical work.[3]

Attending the conference was the distinguished Paris surgeon Samuel Pozzi (1846–1918), who was soon to become a close friend and supporter of Carrel. Also attending the conference was Carl Beck (1864–1952) the talented Prague-born surgeon who had been an assistant in Billroth's surgical clinic in Vienna, and who had travelled widely in Europe before settling in Chicago in 1889 as professor of surgical pathology in the Postgraduate Medical College. He brought with him the European tradition of investigative and experimental surgery.[4] Beck knew of Carrel's

---

[2] Letter, 10 August 1904, box 38 folder 64, Alexis Carrel Papers, Georgetown University Library Booth Family Center for Special Collections (GULBFC).
[3] Hugh E. Stephenson Jr and Robert S. Kimpton, *America's First Nobel Prize in Medicine or Physiology: The Story of Guthrie and Carrel* (Boston: Midwestern Vascular Surgery Society, 2001): xiv. Carrel was not known to have health problems then or thereafter.
[4] Beck contributed a remarkable chapter on 'Plastic Surgery' for Albert J. Ochsner's multi-volume, *Surgical Diagnosis and Treatment* (Philadelphia and New York: Lea and

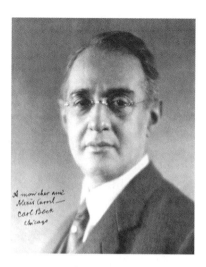

Professor Carl Beck at Chicago gave Carrel his first post in America. (*Courtesy of the Georgetown University Library Booth Family Center for Special Collections.*)

work, since Beck had attempted a dog kidney transplant, without success, in 1903. The two men had corresponded, and now Carrel was in North America, Beck was keen to bring Carrel to work in Chicago. Carrel accepted his offer, and first travelled across Canada, then back into America, to reach Chicago in September 1904.[5]

Chicago Hospitals

On reaching Chicago, he started work in Beck's surgical practice at the Westside and Cook County Hospitals, staying as a guest at Beck's house. They did experimental dog surgery together at the laboratory of Chicago's College of Physicians and Surgeons, and their ambitious project was to

Febiger, 1922). He has eponymous fame for his hypospadias operation of 1898 and for his Beck's Paste (bismuth in paraffin), used to pack bone cavities.
[5] William Baader and Lloyd M. Nyhus (1986) 'The life of Carl Beck and an important interval with Alexis Carrel' *Surgery, Gynecology & Obstetrics* 163: 85–8 and William C. Beck (1986) 'Alexis Carrel and Carl Beck — a historical footnote,' *Perspectives in Biology and Medicine* 30: 148–51.

form a new oesophagus by transposing a loop of bowel into the chest to join up the gullet to the stomach. Beck had in mind the treatment of a problem patient, one who had an oesophageal stricture caused by accidentally swallowing some lye (caustic potash). They reported success in the dogs in 1905.[6] Carrel was involved with conventional surgical work in Beck's clinic, but it seems this was not a success.[7] Carrel's English was still poor, and he lacked enthusiasm for routine surgery. Nor did Carrel admire American medicine and surgery at this time, and he was restive. His diary reveals a sour view of his situation, being repelled by what he saw of American medical practice and teaching posts.

He complained about

> the crowd of imbeciles and villains who corrupt the world of medicine … my friends urge me to stay here. … To be a medical doctor in the United States is the lowest form of business. … To be a professor is interesting only under absolutely exceptional conditions where one can work and accomplish marvellous things: this requires a combination of circumstances that is almost impossible to realise at this time in America.

Nor did he admire the local surgeons:

> I have met C. in the hall of a University. He is an illustrious surgeon, a little man, very morose and vain. When he dies they will make a statue of him. … He demands money everywhere. … The vanity of these people is repulsive.[8]

---

[6] C. Beck and A.C. Carrel (1905) 'Demonstration of specimens illustrating a method of formation of the pre-thoracic esophagus' *Illinois Medical Journal* 7: 463. This procedure is sometimes called the Beck–Jianu operation, rewarding both rival innovators.

[7] An image of Carrel giving an anaesthetic for an operation by Beck is found in Baader and Nyhus (note 5): 86.

[8] From Joseph T. Durkin's translation of Carrel's diaries and letters in his *Hope for Our Time: Alexis Carrel on Man and Society* (New York: Harper and Row, 1965): 61. The disliked surgeon 'C' is unlikely to be Cushing or Crile; Cushing was quite tall and Crile was soon admired by Carrel.

Carrel kept up correspondence with family and friends in Lyon, and he wrote regularly to his brother and mother until her death in April 1905. His brother managed Carrel's financial affairs in Lyon, even buying investments and purchasing land, and he soon started returning to Lyon each summer.

A New Position

One career opportunity arose when Beck and Carrel offered their services in 1905 to the Austrian government to assist with their military surgical needs, but nothing came of it.[9] Carrel had a surgical contact in Managua in Nicaragua and toyed with the idea of moving to Central America, where he could expect to have a wealthy surgical practice. He decided against it because 'the degraded Latins of Central America are as savage as the Indians that they massacred. Countries can only be civilised by Anglo-Saxons'.[10]

Instead, after nine months of clinical work with Beck, Carrel had a chance to return to the experimental work which suited him. He had an introduction in spring 1905 to the Scottish-educated Prof. George N. Stewart (1860–1930) at the nearby University of Chicago's Hull Biological Laboratory.[11] The Laboratory offered facilities for animal experimentation, notably dog surgery, but no salary was available. Carrel dropped clinical work and fell back on his private income for support, never to practise routine human surgery again. Carrel was now 31 years old, and it was three years since his Lyon blood vessel experiments.

---

[9] Beck, *Carrel* (note 5): 151.

[10] Carrel to his brother Joseph, Malinin Collection of the Papers of Alexis Carrel and Charles Lindbergh, FA 208, box 16 folder 1, Rockefeller University Archives, Rockefeller Archives Center (RUA RAC).

[11] Stewart moved to Chicago from Western Reserve University and arranged for fellow Scot J.J.R. MacLeod, future Nobel Prize winner for the discovery of insulin, to succeed him.

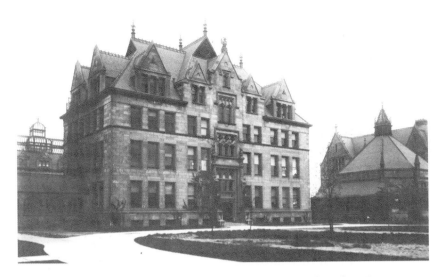

Carrel's blood vessel surgery studies resumed in 1905 at the Physiology Department in Chicago University's Hull Biological Laboratory — now Culver Hall. (*Courtesy of University of Chicago.*)

Enter Guthrie

On his visit with Stewart, Carrel was introduced to a younger Hull departmental member, Charles Claude Guthrie, then aged 25, and who was already using the animal surgery facilities. Guthrie had been working with Stewart on the revival of animals after haemorrhage or shock, and in long, scholarly papers on resuscitation, they showed that the brain could not survive after a period of about 20 minutes lack of oxygen. They were perhaps first to emphasise that the other organs were still viable for a while after the brain was dead, and hence that bodily death was a process, rather than a single event. Guthrie also noticed that there were examples in the literature of the protective effect of cooling organs against damage.[12] All these ideas, doubtless soon shared with Carrel during their daily work together, assisted Carrel's thinking in his later work.

---

[12] F.H. Pike, C.C. Guthrie and G.N. Stewart (1908) 'Studies in resuscitation: 1. The general conditions affecting resuscitation, and the resuscitation of the blood and of the heart' *JEM* 10: 371–418. See also [Editorial] 'Remarkable resuscitations' *The Lancet*, April 9 1904: 1005–6.

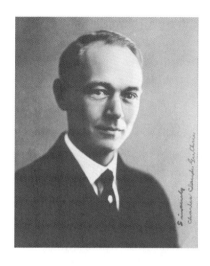

Charles Claude Guthrie joined Carrel in their famous joint work on vascular surgery in Chicago in 1905.

Before Carrel arrived, Guthrie had been looking at methods of stitching bowel together, a technique of relevance to the new growing interest in abdominal surgery. The topic was a Chicago specialty and John B. Murphy, the distinguished surgeon who also worked at Cook County Hospital nearby (and who, as noted earlier, had published on blood vessel surgery) had evolved a novel method of joining the bowel after removal of diseased or damaged segments. In this, he used his own 'Murphy button' method, rather than stitching the bowel together. The two buttons were used to clamp the bowel together, without stitching, not unlike the stapling methods which appeared later in the century. With bowel suturing looking outmoded, when Carrel arrived with his experience in blood vessel stitching, Guthrie was probably pleased to assist the newcomer in the challenge of blood vessel suturing methods. He was also intrigued to be unexpectedly teamed up with a confident smartly-dressed Frenchman, although communication was difficult.

Guthrie later gave an account of their first meeting:

Dr. Karl Beck brought him [Carrel] out to Hull Physiological Laboratory, University of Chicago, in the spring of 1905, and introduced him to Scotsman Dr. George N. Stewart, professor and Head of the

Department. After about half an hour together, Dr. Stewart — Stewart's text *Manual of Physiology* (1895) was the standard student text of the day — brought him across the hall to my laboratory, introduced us, explained that Dr. Carrel would like to do some experimental work on blood vessels; and since I had recently fixed us a cubby-like place to operate and was doing some gastrointestinal experimentation. ... After inspecting the place and discussing work with Dr. Carrel that he would like for us to do together, we agreed to go ahead with it, and so informed Dr. Stewart, who said he was glad, and that from then the matter was in our hands.

Personally, to me Carrel was sophisticated, polished and interesting, engaging, intriguing, pleasing and of likable personality and appearance, with a delightful sense of humour, with a twinkling blue and brown eye as could sometimes be seen through his near-sighted lenses. He dressed neatly and most of the time wore a high buttoned vest and "Ascot."[13]

Guthrie would modify these views later.

Early Experiments

Guthrie had his own projects, notably on resuscitation, which continued, and initially he may have acted simply to assist the surgical techniques already familiar to Carrel. This gave Carrel a skilled assistant, since the blood vessel experimental work suited two people working closely together. In Guthrie, Carrel also had someone who could help with his still-halting spoken English and would help when writing their papers.

The dog experiments started on 12 May 1905, and the first operation was to join the femoral vein to the femoral artery in the leg.[14] This was the Lyon strategy, hoping to improve blood flow in the body by routing

---

[13] See S.P. Harbison (1962) 'Origins of vascular surgery: the Carrel–Guthrie letters' *Surgery* 52: 406–18. Guthrie's papers are held by the State Historical Society of Missouri, Collections C3108 and C3549.

[14] Alexis Carrel and C.C. Guthrie (1906) 'The reversal of the circulation in a limb' *Annals of Surgery* 43: 203–15. Harbison, *Origins* (note 13) and others state wrongly that the first period of the joint Carrel–Guthrie work was only from June to August 1905.

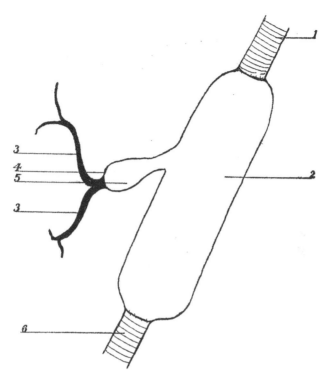

Carrel and Guthrie's first experiments showed that grafts from the adjacent vein (marked '2') could replace the main leg artery in the dog. (*From Reference 14.*)

arterial blood back through the veins. They next swung over a segment of femoral vein and used it to replace a length of the femoral artery. The femoral vein graft distended and pulsated for some hours, which confirmed that the veins could withstand arterial pressure. At this point, recalling his Lyon experiment which showed that the jugular vein could transmit blood flow from the carotid artery, Carrel realised that veins could be successfully used as grafts to replace segments of arteries. Shortly after, Carrel published a brief paper under his own name in the August 1905 edition of *American Medicine* of the use of veins as arterial grafts.[15] In the paper he predicted correctly that this method could be used as a

---

[15] Alexis Carrel (1905) 'Anastomosis and transplantation of blood-vessels' *American Medicine* 10: 284–5. The number of vein graft attempts is not given.

new treatment for aneurysms of arteries, and he said it had not been attempted before.[16] At the end of the paper he thanked Guthrie, who was not a co-author, for help with 'revision of the paper'. Soon after, Carrel sent off another paper under his own name to the *Journal of the American Medical Association* which was published on 25 November 1905.[17] This time, there were clearly results obtained in joint experiments with Guthrie, and Carrel said so in the text. Carrel also submitted the same work in a report to the *Presse médicale*, a French rapid-publication journal.[18]

Many years later, Guthrie said that he became annoyed at that time, and that Carrel treated him only as an assistant, not a collaborator. He recalled that he confronted Carrel:

> As soon as I discovered that he was publishing our results under his own name, I told him that this was at variance with our agreement and therefore I would discontinue working with him. He was profuse in trying to explain how it was unintentional, deepest regret, etc., and that he would immediately take steps to correct it, which he did.[19]

It is, however, odd that Guthrie did not protest, until later, that his name was missing as a co-author in these 1905 papers. Guthrie had no need to 'discover' the Carrel-only papers. Guthrie had clearly assisted with writing the text for both articles and Carrel had thanked him for his surgical help. It seems that later, when Carrel became famous, Guthrie was keen to establish retrospectively that he had immediate involvement

---

[16] Carrel failed to mention vein graft attempts by Glück (1898) and Exner (1903), and he corrected this omission later in *JAMA* 51 (1908): 1663. Easily the best historical account at this time of early vascular surgery was given by Watts (note 57).

[17] Alexis Carrel (1905) 'The transplantation of organs. A preliminary communication,' *JAMA* 45: 1645–6.

[18] Alexis Carrel (1905) 'La transplantation des veines et ses applications chirurgicales' *Presse médicale* 13: 843–4. The *JAMA* (note 17) paper was published on 25 November and the French version on 30 December. The two papers must have been sent off almost simultaneously.

[19] Harbison, *Letters* (note 13): 408. The date of their disagreement is not given by Guthrie when recalling the events later.

with Carrel. These events continued to rankle with Guthrie, and later he was to air his concerns prominently.

New Studies

In August 1905, Guthrie visited Washington University in St. Louis, where he was favoured for the up-coming chair of physiology in the School of Medicine, which was hoped would soon be the 'Johns Hopkins of the West'. When Guthrie returned to Chicago in January 1906, he and Carrel again worked closely together and published together until March, when Guthrie finally left for St. Louis.[20] While Guthrie was away, Carrel's letters describe his work with various unsatisfactory assistants, but although he may have obtained new personal results, to include Guthrie, they continued to publish together. Guthrie, for his part, did some vascular experiments while visiting St. Louis, but now seemed touchy and concerned that he was being excluded from the project. He warned Carrel not to put the Chicago assistants' names on any papers.

In their surgical work they added many extra details, and also made one major change to Carrel's technique. In Carrel's Lyon work and his paper of 1902, he did not put his stitches through the entire wall of the blood vessels to be joined. Guthrie had done so with regular success in joining bowel. Perhaps because of this, they decided to change their blood vessel anastomosis technique and put the stitches through the entire wall of the vessels, as had Jaboulay, Dörfler and even Murphy in Chicago before them, with limited success. In one of Guthrie's letters to Carrel, he describes Carrel's previous 'skimming' technique in his 1902 paper as 'the old method'.[21] There was marked initial leakage from the suture line which

---

[20] These events were reconstructed with the help of four publications — Harbison, *Origins* (note 13); L.G. Walker Jr (1974) 'The Carrel-Guthrie letters revisited' *Surgery* 76: 359–62; L.G. Walker Jr (1988) 'The letters and friendship of Carrel and Cushing' *Surgery Gynecology & Obstetrics* 167: 253–8; and I.M. Rutkow (1980) 'The letters of William Halsted and Alexis Carrel' *Surgery, Gynecology & Obstetrics* 151: 676–88. Walker did not accept the revisionist proposal from Harbison and others that Guthrie was the neglected pioneer in the joint work with Carrel.
[21] See Harbison, *Origins* (note 13): 414.

would usually cease after two to three minutes of gentle pressure on the area. With regular practice of their surgical technique, their results improved.

To add to this quest for regular success, Guthrie looked around in St. Louis and found even finer stitching material, namely silk 'ravelings' — the extra fine threads taken from the silk cloth used to make sieves for flour. Better straight needles were sourced from England — their improved, finer 'No. 16 Kirby'. Better smooth-jawed clamps were used to control flow — the 'small Crile or serrefine' — or they used linen slings to hold and gently control the vessels. Asepsis was unusually strict, but they did not use surgical gloves, although Halsted at Baltimore had started to do so as early as 1894. They constantly irrigated the area with saline solutions, and smeared vaseline on the outer side of cut surfaces.

There may have been many failures in their experiments then, and probably also in Carrel's work earlier. Carrel noted with pride that in

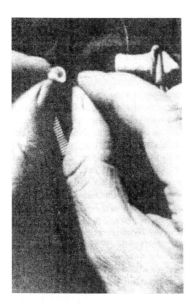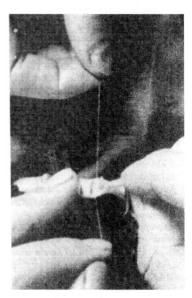

Carrel at work, without gloves, using straight needles, and now using sutures penetrating the entire wall: no 'triangulation' was needed on this occasion. (*Courtesy of the Georgetown University Library Booth Family Center for Special Collections.*)

the month of August 1905 before Guthrie's St. Louis visit started, they did '13 arterio-venous anastomosis without one failure'. But in a letter to the absent Guthrie in November that year, he wrote that 'after one month of hard work I have only two good results'. Carrel blamed the failures on Wilson, his medical student assistant, who, he said was 'mediocre like 95% of the medical men'.[22] Guthrie, later estranged from Carrel, wrote darkly of his 'high regard for Dr. Carrel's earlier [Lyon] persistence in the face of a long series of unsuccessful operations'.[23]

Results

The Carrel–Guthrie work was the first sustained study of blood vessel surgery. Their attention to detail and perseverance with a single surgical technique was unusual, and they were rewarded with increasing success in procedures which others had dropped after discouraging short-term involvement. Constant practice of one skill had its rewards. Faster and more skilful accomplishment of their blood vessel anastomoses meant less chance of blood clotting in the vessels, which many thought was unavoidable. The *mentalité* in the surgical world was that a broad range of surgical research topics was desirable. Carrel was discarding this assumption: perhaps his exposure to the physiologists' world suggested to him to concentrate on one topic in depth.

With increasing experience, in the rapid series of the celebrated Carrel–Guthrie publications, they went beyond simply studying how to join blood vessels. They moved into regular replacement of segments of blood vessels and also into organ transplantation. It was a master-class which demonstrated the potential of vascular surgery.

Vessels and Organs

Carrel and Guthrie did more experiments joining the leg arteries to the adjacent leg veins, as before, exploring the Jaboulay strategy of routing

---

[22] Guthrie instead considered that the student Wilson was skilled, and Guthrie obtained a surgical job for Wilson with Murphy in Chicago; see Harbison (note 13): 412–13.
[23] Walker, *Guthrie-Carrel* (note 20): 360.

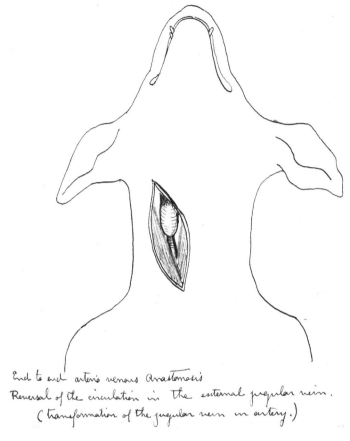

End to end arterio venous Anastomosis
Reversal of the circulation in the external jugular vein.
(Transformation of the jugular vein in artery.)

Carrel's own sketch from 1905 showing his continuing interest in joining the carotid artery to the jugular vein, hoping to increase blood flow to the brain. (*Courtesy of the Georgetown University Library, Booth Family Center for Special Collections.*)

arterial blood into the venous system of a limb or brain, with clinical hopes of improving distal tissue vitality.[24] They cut out segments of arteries and used veins to replace the missing artery; the vein wall thickened up in the following weeks, and persisted as a successful, permanent replacement for the artery. This was to be established as a standard method in surgical practice later — much later.

---

[24] Alexis Carrel and C.C. Guthrie (1906) 'Results of the biterminal transplantation of veins' *American Journal of Medical Sciences* 132 (1906).

In organ grafting, they were more interested in doing thyroid rather than kidney transplants. The reason for this was not far to seek. Emil Kocher, the eminent Swiss surgeon, was claiming success with human thyroid gland grafts for treating thyroid deficiency. Kocher used 'homograft' tissue (i.e. taken from other humans) and used implantation of thin slices of the gland. If the whole gland, instead of slices, could be grafted using blood vessel anastomosis, then even better results might be obtained. Carrel and Guthrie's first publication in their organ graft series was on removal and re-grafting of the whole thyroid gland in the same animal.[25] They also reversed the circulation, joining a gland vein to an artery, again hoping to increase the gland's performance in the dog.

They also looked at kidney grafting. Carrel had attempted a dog kidney graft in Lyon, and in October 1905 in Chicago Carrel and Guthrie had a technical success with a dog's own kidney grafted to its neck. They noted a large dilute urine output which they pessimistically concluded was because donor kidneys lacked nervous connections and no longer had lymphatic drainage and hence would malfunction.[26] Carrel was influenced by the views of his teacher at Lyon, the distinguished physiologist Jean-Pierre Morat (1846–1920), who taught (wrongly) that a transplanted kidney would not function properly when detached from its nerve supply.

At this time in 1905, Carrel and Guthrie accordingly changed technique and instead placed the transplanted kidneys back in their usual position in the abdomen. But the organ often twisted after placing it in the kidney bed. Instead, they attempted, and eventually achieved, the much more difficult grafting of both kidneys, still attached to segments of the aorta and vena cava, into a prepared gap in

---

[25] The thyroid gland transplant work with Guthrie is 'Extirpation and reimplantation of the thyroid gland with reversal of the circulation' *Science* 22 (1905): 535.

[26] A. Carrel and C.C. Guthrie (1905) 'Functions of a transplanted kidney' *Science* 22: 473. See Jean-Pierre Morat *Physiology of the Nervous System* (Chicago: W.T. Keen, 1906, translated by H.W. Syers): 346. Later such experimental kidney grafts were better-supported when put in the pelvis, close to the bladder, the position used routinely in human kidney transplantation.

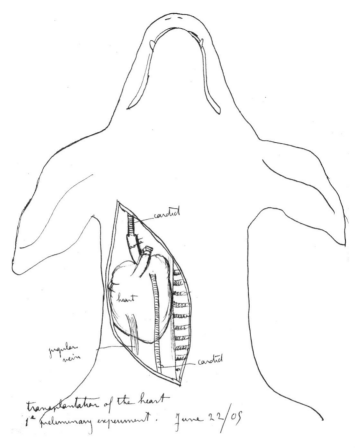

Carrel and Guthrie made attempts at heart transplantation in dogs. Placed in the neck, starting with the simple connections shown in Carrel's own sketch, only brief function could be expected from this 'accessory' heart graft. (*Courtesy of the Georgetown University Library Booth Family Center for Special Collections.*)

another dog's aorta and vena cava, replacing the host kidneys — the so-called *en masse* technique.[27] Better kidney function was achieved. They also transplanted a dog's heart to its neck with initial success, but the 'accessory' graft, in its unusual position, inevitably failed after two hours. They tried grafting both heart and lungs, but the lungs became

---

[27] A. Carrel and C.C. Guthrie (1906) 'Successful transplantation of both kidneys from a dog into a bitch with removal of both normal kidneys from the latter' *Science* 23: 394–5.

fluid overloaded. A leg graft in a dog was also carried out in 1906,[28] and an ovary graft was reported that year.[29]

The Patch

An important technical addition to their methods at this time was what is still called the 'Carrel patch'.[30] But Guthrie, while at St. Louis, may have used it first.[31] This was an important improvement, one routinely used thereafter to obtain success with organ grafts supplied by small vessels which are too small to stitch. Instead, the small vessel, such as the renal artery, is removed from the donor while still on a disc of its major vessel of origin, such as the aorta. This substantial patch (with the little artery emerging from its centre) is then easily sewn into the recipient using a similar size of opening cut in any large host vessel. This method was published by them both in 1906, with drawings by Carrel.

The Publications

The two men published at speed, usually submitting short papers reporting on only one operation of each type. Carrel, though he was still hesitant in spoken and written English, had a crisp prose style, and this may have neutralised Guthrie's own tendency to prolixity. Guthrie had never published at this speed before, nor did he thereafter: Carrel, the older of the two and perhaps the dominant partner, urged the need for

---

[28] A. Carrel and C.C. Guthrie (1906) 'Complete amputation of the thigh, with replantation' *American Journal of Medical Sciences* 131: 297–301, and a further attempt is described in *Science* 23 (1906): 393–4.

[29] A. Carrel and C.C. Guthrie (1906) 'A new method for the homoplastic transplantation of the ovary' *Science* 23: 591. See R.T. Morris (1895) 'The ovarian graft' *New York Medical Journal* 62: 436–7. For Morris's work see H.H. Simmer (1970) 'Robert Tuttle Morris (1857–1945): a pioneer in ovarian transplants' *Obstetrics and Gynecology* 35: 314–28.

[30] A. Carrel and C.C. Guthrie (1906) 'Anastomosis of blood-vessels by the Patching Method and transplantation of the kidney' *JAMA* 47: 1648–50.

[31] See the personal memo in Guthrie's archive, quoted in Stephenson and Kimpton (note 3): xvi, and also S.P. Harbison's 'Introduction' to the University of Pittsburgh's 1959 reprint of Guthrie's *Blood Vessel Surgery and Its Applications*.

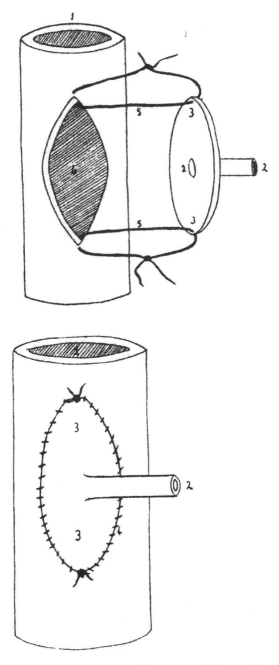

A 'patch' of an artery (3), retained on a small donor vessel (2) supplying an organ, greatly assisted stitching. (*Carrel's own drawing, from Reference 30.*)

publications.[32] One understandable reason for speedy publication at this time was that there were developments in organ transplantation in Europe. After Ullmann's technical success with a dog kidney autotransplant graft in 1902, in 1905 Floresco had obtained long-term dog kidney autotransplant survival after transplanting the animal's own organ.[33] To add to this, news would soon come from Lyon that Jaboulay had attempted the first human kidney grafts in two patients dying of renal failure.[34]

Over the time they worked together, totalling less than a year due to Guthrie's absences in St. Louis, the two men published 10 papers in American medical journals. Carrel's name was always first in these papers, and Carrel drew the useful diagrams for their publications. One article sent to the *American Journal of Physiology* was acknowledged but earned a rebuke from the editor that 'no doubt Dr. Carrel understands our rule that papers published in the journal are not to appear elsewhere'. In an unusual move, they did publish their results, in duplicate, in French fast-publication journals, notably *Presse médicale* or *Comptes rendus hebdomadaires des séances de l'Académie des sciences*. These appeared promptly in the next issue after reaching the editor. In these French-language publications, curiously Guthrie was often the first author, and in total they had 16 short French-language publications. It seems that Carrel, far from cutting himself off from France, wished to keep his name in front of French surgeons and scientists.

---

[32] American biomedical research output was increasingly competitive at this time. With rapid publication rising, the wits could remark that publications now appeared 'before the slides were dry'; see J.S. Nicholas 'Ross Granville Harrison 1870–1959' *Biographical Memoir: National Academy of Sciences* (Washington: National Academy of Sciences, 1961): 136–62.

[33] N. Floresco (1905) 'Recherches sur la transplantation du rein' *Journal de physiologie et de pathologie générale* 7: 47–59. He was the first transplanter to put the ureter into the bladder, rather than leading it onto the skin surface.

[34] M. Jaboulay (1906) 'Greffe de reins au pli du coude par sutures artérielles et veineuses' *Bulletin du Lyon Médical* 107: 575–7. This work was reviewed at length, possibly by Carrel, in the *New York Medical Journal* of 22 December 1906. Jaboulay used pig and goat kidneys, a not unreasonable donor source at the time. For joining the vessels, Jaboulay used Payr's hollow stents inside the vessels, not a stitching method, in spite of his and Carrel's experience in Lyon with stitching blood vessels.

Even so, Guthrie, like Carrel, was also getting concerned that they might be overtaken by others. From St. Louis, he wrote to Carrel about their latest paper:

> I regret that the work is so widely known at this time as our experiments are I think, in the preliminary stage as yet — comparatively speaking of course. If such men as Cushing take it up now it means that we will be 'beat out' in making human applications, as their facilities for such work are at present vastly superior to ours — you understand I mean opportunities to get and operate on suitable patients. Still I cannot believe that anyone, or set of surgeons can equal our results before they have worked much longer on the techniques that you and I have together. I think it might be a good plan to keep the important details of the actual technique to ourselves for a time — not many of them will take the time to look up your first paper and besides, I believe certain details are somewhat improved since then, are they not? A few blood clots would serve to cool their ardour.[35]

Guthrie's concern was that the American surgeons, who had patients to treat, would put their new methods to clinical use before they had any similar chance in Chicago.

First Publicity

Carrel replied promptly on 13 September, 1905, and he had more news. Reports of their work had appeared in the newspapers:

> Dear Dr. Guthrie:
> Today, a man sent me a stupid article published by a journal of New York. I saw two ridiculous articles in the newspapers of Chicago. It represents probably the opinion of the students and of the janitor about our experiments. Fortunately it is so stupid that it is not dangerous. Our technique is absolutely unknown and will remain unknown. My first paper published in French, has no importance, for the details which make the operator successful are not described.[36]

---

[35] Walker, *Carrel-Guthrie* (note 20): 360.
[36] Harbison, *Origins* (note 13): 415.

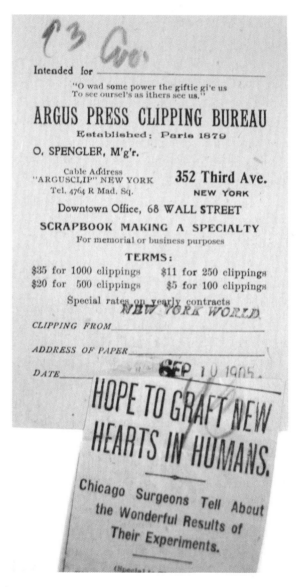

Two New York newspapers reported Carrel's work in 1905, and this clipping reached him via an agency. (*Georgetown University Library Booth Family Center for Special Collections.*)

This arrival of newspaper coverage is intriguing and was perhaps linked with a mysterious event earlier. A few months earlier, Prof. Stewart and Guthrie were astonished to see that three Chicago newspapers carried what they called a 'garbled and misleading account of certain experiments communicated by us to a meeting of physiologists of the central states'. They were taken aback, since at that time newspapers normally had little interest in their area of science and, mystified, wrote to the editors pointing out that no reporters had been invited to the meeting and added that 'we are entirely opposed to the discussion of such matters in the lay press'. The editor was also asked to reflect on 'how injurious such notices may be to the reputation of scientific investigators'.[37]

The new September stories about the Carrel–Guthrie work appeared in the *New York World* and *New York Herald*, but were credited to a Chicago source. The *Herald's* headline was 'May Replace Man's Heart With That Of A Monkey'. The articles were well-informed on the breadth of the Carrel–Guthrie experiments and included the thyroid, leg, and blood vessel graft surgery. Carrel was apparently quoted as saying, 'this work is in its infancy ... it will be of great and lasting benefit to mankind'.[38] The articles also described the dog heart transplant to the neck. Carrel, whose French army service was noted, was further quoted as pointing to the use of monkeys in the future as human heart donors.

Carrel's explanation to Guthrie, that the information came from low levels within the laboratory, possibly the porters or students, seems improbable. Instead, in Chicago, Carrel knew two journalists, the daughters of former Governor Llewellyn of Kansas, one of whom wrote for the *Chicago Inter Ocean* newspaper, and they perhaps were looking for stories.[39] If Carrel was involved, it was his first tentative contact with the newspapers since the Lourdes controversy. The New York newspaper stories reached other city papers, and a reader of the *Los Angeles Examiner*

---

[37] G.N. Stewart and C.C. Guthrie (1905) 'Science and the newspapers' *Science* 21: 667–8. This generalist journal regularly discussed the press coverage of science.
[38] Press clippings, box 39 folder 2, GULBFC (note 2). Carrel's Georgetown archives have these cuttings, sent to him by both the Argus and Henry Romeike agencies in New York. Carrel was apparently quoted, but 'invented' quotations were part of journalistic practice at the time.
[39] Theodore I. Malinin, *Surgery and Life: the Extraordinary Career of Alexis Carrel* (New York: Harcourt Brace Jovanovich, 1979): 34. Carrel's only other female acquaintance at this time was Ruth Perry, a Chicago photographer, with whom he exchanged occasional formal friendly letters.

wrote to Carrel requesting a bone graft to replace a humerus destroyed by infection.

Guthrie replied immediately to the news of the press interest:

> The newspaper notoriety is deplorable but it cannot be helped. We should, I suppose, show our animals to absolutely no one in the future. If we could maintain secrecy for say a year and write all our results in book form, it would be the ideal way, I think, but that is not possible. ... At first I lacked complete confidence in the permanency of the results, but now we have overwhelming data to my mind, to assure us on the results.

It was in Guthrie's nature to be cautious and reclusive in judging the outcome of their work, and also as regarded publication. But he seems to have agreed with Carrel, who was in no mood to wait. On 26 September Carrel wrote:

> Our only hope to be not stolen is to publish very quickly all we can. I am very sorry to be obliged to make such superficial publications, but it is absolutely necessary.[40]

American Surgeons' Interest

However, Carrel was not inclined to hide their work from the surgical world. In Guthrie's absence, shortly afterwards, in the autumn of 1905, Carrel made sure their work was known to some influential American surgeons. The occasion was the meeting in Chicago of the Society of Clinical Surgery on 5–7 October. This group consisted of the 'Young Turks' who, being dissatisfied with the format of the meetings of the well-established, restricted membership and conservative American Surgical Society, had formed this new surgical society. It was agreed that the format of their meetings would be practical demonstrations of surgical technique, rather than lectures, and that they would have a

---

[40] Harbison, *Origins* (note 13): 411.

minimal administrative structure, with no entertainment to be provided by the hosts.

At the Chicago meeting the word went round about Carrel's work and Harvey Cushing recalled an impromptu visit to meet him.[41]

> One interesting event of that last afternoon [7 October] in Chicago the "minutes" [of the society] fail to mention, for the secretary and many of the Eastern members had already left for their lunch, Matas passed the word around that in the Physiological Laboratory at the University of Chicago a young Frenchman named Alexis Carrel was doing some interesting work on anastomosing blood-vessels and transplanting organs and, were we interested, he would be glad to give us a demonstration.
>
> We certainly were interested, and though the anastomosis had to be made on a dog no longer alive for reasons that need not be gone into, it was the only original experimental work that had been shown to us for some time. ... We were to see Carrel again 2 years later at work in more elegant surroundings.[42]

Carrel gave a demonstration of dividing and re-joining a dog's carotid artery. The dog, as Cushing recalled, died under the anaesthetic because George Crile offered to be the anaesthetist and had overdosed the animal. Carrel also demonstrated four other post-operative animals, with obviously successful flow of arterial blood into veins, and he handed out reprints of his articles on the work.

It was a technique seeking a use. Crile, despite his embarrassment, was particularly impressed. He came away from Chicago enthused with a

---

[41] Matas had visited Carrel earlier during that meeting. In New Orleans he had huge clinical experience in dealing with syphilitic aneurysms: see K.R. Matas (1940) 'Personal experiences in vascular surgery. Statistical synopsis' *Annals of Surgery* 112: 802–39.

[42] H. Cushing (1969) 'The Society of Clinical Surgery in retrospect' *Annals of Surgery* 169: 1–9, at 7. Carrel's later 'more elegant surroundings' were at the Rockefeller Institute. Cushing, writing much later in 1969, had forgotten that, after reading Carrel's *American Medicine* article, he, like Matas, wrote seeking to visit Carrel's lab. The Chicago meeting, including the contact with Carrel, is reported in *Surgery, Gynecology & Obstetrics* (1905) vol. 1, p. 458. For Cushing, see Michael Bliss *Harvey Cushing: A Life in Surgery.* (Oxford: Oxford University Press 2005.)

The last Thursday, Mates introduced me to Crile, who was in Chicago. He was a nice fellow and he has been sorry not to see you.

Harvey Cushing was also in Chicago. He is a splendid fellow, very intelligent and broad minded. He told me we must make other researches very actively, for they have a great future. Saturday, Mates, Harvey Cushing and Crile came to the laboratory, but, unfortunately, about twenty other people; Morse, Lecan, Murphy, etc. came also. It was overcrowded and it was impossible to see anything. Everything must be cleaned before it be possible to operate again. We operated a day. But Crile was making the anesthesy. Within five minutes the dog was dead! It was very funny.

Now, everybody knows our experiments. It is necessary to publish very quickly, and to make new experiments as soon as possible. I have been very glad of this occasion to know there three men Cushing, Mates and Crile, for they are very good and interesting.

faithfully yours, A. Carrel

Carrel's letter to Guthrie describing the 1905 visit by the Society of Clinical Surgery. (*Courtesy of the State Historical Society of Missouri, Guthrie Papers.*)

new idea, and 10 months later he was first to employ Carrel's stitching in clinical work. At the time, blood loss and shock was treated with saline infusions, but blood transfusion would be more suitable. Attempts at transfusing human blood were thwarted by clotting in any cannulas or tubing used, and Crile used Carrel's technique to solve this old problem. He carried out the first 'direct' transfusion of human blood by joining the blood donor's wrist artery to a vein in the recipient.

After the Society's visit, Carrel wrote promptly from Chicago to the absent Guthrie.

> 9 October 1905
> Saturday, Matas, Harvey Cushing and Crile came to the laboratory, but unfortunately, about twenty other people, Monro, Lecont, Murphy, etc. came also. It was overcrowded and it was impossible to see anything. Everything must be cleaned before it would be possible to operate again. We operated a dog [sic]. Crile was making the anestheze [sic]. Within five minutes, the dog was dead! It was very funny.
>
> Now, everybody knows our experiments. It is necessary to publish very quickly and to make new experiments as soon as possible. I have been very glad of this occasion to know these three men, Cushing, Matas and Crile for they are very good and interesting.[43]

Guthrie wrote back from St. Louis on 31 October and gave Carrel some further news. The earlier Chicago newspaper story had been taken up beyond America.

> Dr. Miller is the pathologist in St. Louis and has just returned from spending the summer in England and Germany. He says we have great international reputation on having successfully transplanted the heart! Is it not ridiculous? Newspaper fame again. It is a pity for so much advertising to go to waste. It would be worth thousands to any one of dozens of 'surgeons' I could name. I have no doubt at all but that at this moment the work is being assayed in a dozen different laboratories. Our main protection is the difficulty of the technique…

Carrel replied on 6 November that he had already heard the news.

> The stupid articles of the American newspapers have been reproduced by the newspapers of London and Paris. I received a letter of a friend from London about it. Even an illustrated newspaper of Paris consecrated one page to caractures [sic] about us. … It is stupid, but is has, fortunately, no importance.

---

[43] Rutkow, *Letters* (note 20): 677.

MONKEY'S HEARTS FOR MEN.

According to experiments which have been conducted under the auspices of Chicago University by Doctors Gutherie and Carrell, a time may soon come when worn-out hearts in human beings can be replaced. In the course of experiments with dogs they learnt many important lessons on this point, and they begin their new experiments in October. " What we have learned," said Dr Carrell on Sunday, " gives us hope that some day we may replace a wounded or worn-out heart in a human being with a healthy, youthful, strong one from a living monkey."—" Daily Telegraph."

The American reports of Carrel's work spread virally, reaching London's *Daily Telegraph*, and thence north to the *Hull Daily Mail* of 11 September 1905. (*Courtesy of the British Library Newspaper Archive.*)

In London the *Daily Telegraph* had taken the story from the New York papers and from London the story spread to other British city papers. The two men were in an unusual position as regards publicity. Though doing surgical work, always of interest to the press and public, they were not constrained by the usual professional code, which was to shun personal publicity, which was seen as advertising for services. Guthrie had wryly noted how private surgeons would have welcomed their high profile, bringing in patients and fees.

Hopkins Interest

After the Chicago meeting, on returning to Baltimore, Cushing was still impressed with the visit to Carrel. Although Cushing was junior to Halsted, the celebrated Hopkins surgeon, Cushing was gaining unusual responsibilities and authority under Halsted. Halsted had a well-concealed problem with cocaine addiction and morphine supplements which made him unreliable and frequently absent.[44]

---

[44] Gerald Imber, *Genius on the Edge: the Bizarre Double Life of Dr. William Stewart Halsted* (New York: Kaplan, 2011).

Cushing wrote to Carrel from Baltimore:

7 November 1905

I told Dr. Halsted of your work yesterday, and he was very much excited over your superlatively good results, and I doubt not will correspond with you about them himself. I sent your reprints also to Prof. Kocher, my old teacher in Bern, and I hope that he will incorporate them in the new edition of his text-book.

I do wish that we had you down here. I would give you a corner in my new laboratory gladly, and all the animals and assistants that you could need. Do you suppose that anything would induce you to come down here and do your work where we can get the benefit of it at first hand?[45]

Cushing was sincere about this offer of a job to Carrel, and added diplomatically that Carrel should speak to Dr. Stewart at the Chicago Hull Laboratory 'as we do not want him to feel we are pinching you from him'. In fact, Stewart at the time was planning a move of his own, hoping to return to the chair of experimental medicine at Western Reserve University.[46] Carrel replied, dropping a hint that he was restive in Chicago, and that he was interested.

But the facilities in Baltimore which Cushing mentioned were not yet at the level he claimed. Though the Medical School was expanding steadily, Cushing's 'new lab' was evolving only slowly into what would later be the celebrated Hunterian Laboratory.[47] The 'assistants' offered to Carrel would simply be the ever-changing young residents in training. Moreover, Carrel made it clear that he wanted to concentrate on research, not patient care. This created difficulties for Cushing: there were no such posts.

---

[45] Cushing to Carrel, November 7 1905, box 2 folder 5, FA 208 Malinin Collection of the Papers of Alexis Carrel and Charles Lindbergh, RUA RAC (note 10).

[46] John F. Fulton, *Harvey Cushing: a Biography* (Springfield: Charles C. Thomas, 1946): 248. Fulton wrongly states that 'Carrel's letters of this period are uncomfortable documents.' This view, in 1946, must instead reflect the post-WWII hostility to Carrel, in which Fulton shared.

[47] The Hunterian Laboratory, developing at the time, was described with pride by Harvey Cushing in 'Instruction in operative medicine' *Bulletin of the Johns Hopkins Hospital* 17 (1906): 123–34; see also Fulton *Cushing* (note 46): 217–20.

Further Contact

Three months later, at the beginning of the new year, Cushing was still clear he wished to recruit Carrel, and he wrote:

15 February 1906

> I am anxious to get you down here [Baltimore] sometime this spring. Many of us are trying to do some work along the lines which your splendid studies have suggested, and in case you could see your way clear to come down, and have something that you would like to present before the Hospital Medical Society, I will make a date for you. ... I understand very well that you are not receiving a scholarship and that the expenses of the trip may be something to make you hesitant about coming. ... What are your plans for next year? I still hope that we may induce you down here for a year's work in Baltimore. Are you working under a Rockefeller Scholarship? If not, and if I can succeed in getting one for you, would you feel like spending your next winter here in Baltimore? Nothing would be of greater satisfaction to me than to have you do so.

This was strong support from Cushing and a firm suggestion, carefully thought out, for Carrel's immediate future. Cushing knew there was new money for support of research. The Rockefeller Institute in New York had been launched, in a small way in 1901, and initially the policy was to offer outside fellowships, rather than support a central research establishment.

Carrel accepted Cushing's idea, and Cushing put in for Rockefeller funding for Carrel to move to Baltimore for a year. The fellowship application on Carrel's behalf listed his proposed work as 'Study of the transplantation of the kidney and of the thyroid gland, from a physiological and therapeutic standpoint' and 'The study of metabolism of organs after some new operations on their vessels and nerves'. This was carefully worded, with Cushing's assistance, to engage the Institute's interest. It was prudently designed not to be a purely surgical programme. The application appealed to scientists by raising hopes of altering organ function by changing blood inflow or altering the organ's nerve supply.[48]

---

[48] See Faculty/Alexis Carrel 1906–1916, box 2 file 41, FA 231, RUA RAC (note 10).

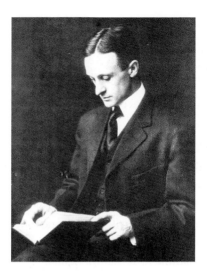

Harvey Cushing at Johns Hopkins Medical School took an early interest in Carrel's work and hoped to attract him to work in Baltimore. (*Courtesy of the National Library of Medicine.*)

Carrel had slowly warmed to the American surgeons, and with this attention from the Rockefeller Institute, Carrel changed his views about American scientists. Carrel wrote to Guthrie in 1906 that 'My opinion about American Scientists, of which I have spoken to you, is changed, for I found some really superior men'.

Meanwhile, while funding was sought, arrangements were made for Carrel to give a lecture at the Johns Hopkins Hospital Medical Society on 23 April 1906. The Society met every two weeks over the winter and heard mostly invited lectures plus presentation of one or two local cases. The proceedings were published in their hospital journal, founded in 1890.

The Baltimore Meeting

Johns Hopkins was the most prestigious medical school and hospital in America at the time, with Halsted, William Welch and William Osler leading their talented staff. Hopkins (died 1873) was a financier, and left an $8 million bequest, half to go to the University in Baltimore and half to be devoted to an Institute for the indigent sick 'without regard for sex, age or colour'. Importantly the hospital was part of the university medical school, and the 'full-time principle' had attracted talented staff who had no wish to have to earn a living through private practice. On the night, Carrel first had dinner with Halsted and then, at the evening 'dress coat' gathering, Carrel gave his lecture on 'The Surgery of Blood Vessels'.[49] Though his English was still poor, this may have added piquancy to the event. America was still in awe of European medicine and surgery, and many of the audience members had spent essential training time in Europe. Now instead they had an innovative European in their midst, a man who had chosen to settle in America.

For many in the audience, Carrel's surgical studies must have been a revelation. They went well beyond the restricted blood vessel surgery attempted at the time, namely simple attempts at vessel repair after injury, or closing down the vessels feeding an aneurysm, and Carrel's confident introductory remarks rather dismissively termed this as 'classical vascular surgery'. Carrel went over the details of his stitching technique, emphasising that strict asepsis was required, not the more casual routine in clinical surgery. He told of hopes for altering organ function by varying the blood supply. He told the audience how he could remove segments of arteries and replace the gap successfully with a length of vein. Carrel had transplanted kidneys, hearts and also thyroid glands. His audience was well aware of Emil Kocher's claims for thyroid gland slice grafts as a solution to thyroid deficiency.[50] Carrel felt instead that a whole gland graft, grafted using his methods of joining the gland's blood vessels, was a better option than using implanted slices as did Kocher. He told the audience:

> Clinical applications of the transplantation of organs are so obvious that they do not need to be described. If I were a veterinary surgeon and had to treat a myxoedematous dog, I would not hesitate to transplant into

---

[49] Alescis[sic] Carrel 'The surgery of blood vessels, etc. *Johns Hopkins Hospital Bulletin*, January 1907, No. 190: 18–28. Cushing quickly noticed this misprint, apologized and corrected it in the reprints. There was a preliminary account of Carrel's lecture in this *Bulletin*, July 1906, No. 184: 236–7, which alone reported the post-lecture discussion.
[50] See Thomas Schlich, *The Origins of Organ Transplantation: Surgery and Laboratory Science 1880–1950* (Rochester: University of Rochester Press, 2010). A thyroid extract was available from 1891 for treatment of thyroid deficiency.

its neck a thyroid gland from another dog. In a case of a dog presenting Bright's disease [chronic renal failure], it would be a rational procedure to substitute for one of his kidneys a sound kidney extirpated from some normal dog.

Carrel was confident that these homografts from another animal would survive in the short term. But, regarding long-term function, Carrel clearly had nagging doubts, and he was soon to support a major paradigm shift by accepting instead that homografts were routinely lost ('rejected' in later terminology) after a period of successful function. In his lecture there were hints of his new understanding, since in his kidney grafts from one dog to another, there was death of the organ after about a week. Carrel thought that genetic factors were involved and outlined his plans to investigate this:

> We intend very soon to perform a series of similar operations [organ grafts] on pure bred animals, preferably dogs or pigs, with a view of studying the problem of transmission of characters...

This was a remarkable statement. By 'transmission of characters', he revealed that he understood, well ahead of his time, that homograft loss might be under 'character', i.e. genetic, control.[51] He also understood, again ahead of his time, that clarification in this area would come from use of in-bred animals.[52]

His perhaps reluctant acceptance that graft rejection was a problem led him to look for ways to thwart graft loss. One way he suggested was modification of the donor organ:

> We intend to try to immunise the organs of an animal against the serum and organ extracts of another. ... The transplanted organ must be prepared to support the serum of the animal on which it is to be grafted.

---

[51] Lexer in Königsberg was also considering a genetic role in graft loss, and published his concept later in 1911; see David Hamilton, *A History of Organ Transplantation* (Pittsburgh: Pittsburgh University Press, 2012): 110–11.

[52] Inbred pigs were not created until the 1980s, and were indeed helpful in organ transplant research.

Carrel did not on this occasion propose host modification to allow graft acceptance. He would do so later. He then looked to the future of human transplantation:

> The difficulty of finding organs suitable for transplantation on man must be met. … As regards the kidneys, the thyroid and the glands in which the endothelium is easily injured by a short interruption of the circulation, the problem is more complex.[53] Then it would be extremely difficult to have an organ to transplant in good condition. In some exceptional cases it would be possible perhaps to use the kidneys of a man killed by accident or the cadaver of an executed criminal.

The alternative was to use fresh animal organs, later called xenografts. Carrel had somehow realised correctly that these cross-species grafts were immediately destroyed by an immunological reaction involving pre-existing antibodies in the recipient — which he called 'cytolysins'. He went on to state correctly that 'on account of cytolysins it seems improbable that indiscriminate heterotransplantation can be successfully performed'. To do so, he suggested neutralising the harmful antibody by use of 'anticytologic serums'. One hope was that monkey organs might not be attacked in this way, but he saw difficulties since 'anthropoid apes are very expensive, and difficult to handle. Their use would probably be impracticable'.[54] Instead he felt pigs would be a better choice:

> The ideal method would be to transplant on man organs of animals easy to secure and to operate on such as hogs, for instance. But it would

---

[53] Carrel here is using C.C. Guthrie's understanding of the differential death rates of tissues. Carrel knew that kidney function ceases quickly after death, but poignantly was unaware that the kidney could then revive well, even after many days of failure, and produce urine.

[54] In 1905 Carrel proposed 'to transplant some little slices of monkey's thyroid under the skin of an idiot and observe the results. It is not [a] dangerous operation and it will show if the thyroid of monkey is destroyed by the human serum'; see Harbison (note 13): 411. The French surgeon Serge Voronoff's use of monkey testis in humans came later in the 1920s, and by then Carrel was confident enough to dispute Voronoff's claims; see David Hamilton, *The Monkey Gland Affair* (London: Chatto & Windus, 1986): 25.

in all probability be necessary to immunise organs of the hog against the human serum. The future of transplantation of organs for therapeutic purposes depends on the feasibility of hetero-transplantation. Researches must be directed along this line.

Astonishingly, he had successfully identified the road map which was not revived until the 1960s. He had even identified the pig as the animal of choice for human xenografting; his lecture still reads well.

After the lecture, the usually less-than-gracious Halsted spoke first and said there 'was work here for an army of investigators. ... in a short time there will be great revelations. For the first time it seems necessary for surgeons to develop great manual dexterity.' William Welch, the physician and dean of the Medical School followed and spoke glowingly of the work as 'a most startling presentation of a field suggesting an entirely new line of work'.

After the lecture, Carrel visited the surgeon William Keen in Philadelphia, and then travelled to New York to be interviewed by Simon Flexner at the Rockefeller Institute regarding the fellowship. But the Institute's policy regarding outside fellowships was changing, and these were no longer being offered. The funds were being used instead to staff the new Institute, which was soon moving to its new building. Because of this, the Institute's Director, Simon Flexner, instead offered Carrel a post in New York, and he accepted.

What If?

It is of interest to speculate on what would have happened if Carrel had moved to Baltimore, as planned at first. A remarkable surgical troika would have emerged — Halsted, Cushing and Carrel. Carrel, as a committed laboratory surgical-scientist, would have used the new Hunterian Laboratory facilities for his full-time work on blood vessel and organ grafting. Baltimore's Hunterian Laboratory now had two operating theatres and facilities to hold 50 dogs for experiments.[55] It also served the surgical training of the talented young residents who, when appointed to the new research-minded medical schools then appearing elsewhere in the

---

[55] Warfield Firor (1952) 'The story of the Hunterian Laboratory' *Surgery* 32: 485–7.

U.S., would have spread the news of Carrel's methods and attempted to improve on them. Carrel's studies would have fitted well with Halsted's own vascular surgical experiments on the challenge of aneurysm surgery.[56] Halsted and Cushing as innovative clinical surgeons would have encouraged application of Carrel's methods to their patients and shielded him if there were clinical failures. At Baltimore, they might even have attempted human kidney transplants, particularly as Jaboulay in Lyon had taken the initiative with two attempts in 1906. Instead, in New York, Carrel was to be far from surgical wards and have no regular clinical links. Nor did he have surgical assistants passing through. Had Carrel moved to Hopkins, this part of the history of surgery might have been different.

With Carrel diverted to New York, Halsted still had a talented senior resident, Stephen H. Watts, doing the vascular surgery studies. Watts carefully repeated the Carrel–Guthrie findings, but he broke no new ground.[57]

More Publicity

In that summer of 1906, a New York newspaper sent a reporter to interview Carrel in Chicago, and on 2 June 1906, both the *New York Herald* and *New York Sun* carried articles describing the Carrel–Guthrie work. The *New York Times* followed next day with an editorial saying that the new blood vessel surgery 'opens up a possibility of profound significance'. These accounts had some surgical detail, and described the

---

[56] See Emil Goetsch (1952) 'Comments on Halsted's contributions to arterial surgery with particular reference to progressive occlusion of the large arteries by means of the aluminium band' *Surgery* 32: 488–92 and Daniel B. Nunn (1995) 'Halsted and "The Vibrant Domain of Surgery"' *American Journal of Surgery* 180: 356–65.

[57] Stephen H. Watts (1907) 'The suture of blood vessels. Implantation and transplantation of vessels and organs. An historical and experimental study' *Bulletin of the Johns Hopkins Hospital* 18: 153–79, a remarkable paper reflecting the high standards of scholarship, both scientific and historical, set locally by Osler and Cushing. This built upon the Carrel–Guthrie work, and is a long, detailed paper, with high-quality photographs and drawings of the operations. For Watts' career, see W. Randolph Chitwood (1976) 'Stephen H. Watts: a disciple of Halsted' *Surgery* 79: 293–98.

CAN ALTER BLOOD CURRENTS AT WILL

Chicago Surgeons Discover Method of Transposing Circulatory System.

MAY TRANSPLANT ORGAN

By Changing Veins Into Arteries Fresh Vital Fluid Can Be Sent Into Diseased Areas.

OPENS NEW SURGICAL FIELD

Hitherto Incurable Diseases of Heart, Liver and Brain Can Be Reached by New Method.

[SPECIAL DESPATCH TO THE HERALD.]
CHICAGO, Ill., Friday.—As the result of experiments which have been conducted for nearly a year by Dr. Alexis Carrel and Dr. C. C. Guthrie, in the Hall Physiological Labratory at the University of Chicago, discoveries have been made that promise to revolutionise surgery.

Further press interest in Carrel's work in the *New York Herald* of June 1906.

success with vein grafts, the plans for organ transplants and the hopes that reversed blood flow could revive failing organs. The New York papers' story was then taken up by other city newspapers throughout America. The *Washington Post* followed up the story six days later on 8 June. But *The Post* took a different line. It contacted two local surgeons and asked them about the idea of using reversed flow to deal with brain disease. One of them, Dr. L.T. MacDonald, opined that 'there is nothing in it — absolutely nothing. When the brain is diseased, a fresh supply of blood will not remedy the evil'. The second surgeon, Dr. J.R. Wellington, even scorned the use of veins for arteries. 'I don't believe the idea is practical. I think the man who wrote this story let his imagination get the better of him.' Carrel now received more letters from the public, including one from a British patient with liver cirrhosis, seeking a liver transplant.

Although the surgeons perhaps deplored Carrel's appearances in the press and studiously avoided publicity themselves, Carrel's future employer, Simon Flexner, may not have disapproved. The Rockefeller Institute was a bold new venture which had to prove itself and gain not only public approval but also please John D. Rockefeller, its single benefactor. Good news was required from the Institute, and perhaps Flexner realised that Carrel could provide it.

Before the move to New York, Carrel had a farewell dinner with his contacts at the *Chicago Inter Ocean* newspaper. He started work in the new Founder's Building of the Rockefeller Institute on 1 October 1906.

CHAPTER THREE

Early Years at the Institute

Carrel joined the Rockefeller Institute for Medical Research in the first full year at its new building. It was a new venture. Before it emerged, the American medical schools and universities rarely supported full-time bio-medical researchers, nor usually wished to. Departmental staff such as anatomists, physiologists, pathologists or bacteriologists, if motivated, might find time for research, but they were paid for their teaching or diagnostic services, and these commitments had priority. At the turn of the century, young American research-minded medical men (and it was men only) looking for further training and experience spent time at Europe's medical institutions. On their return, they regularly pointed out the need for local support of research — 'they do things better in Europe' — was the mantra. In Europe the famous university departments were added to by new, free-standing, research institutes, often aided by public funds, and often based on single talented individuals and their work. These included the Pasteur Institute in Paris, opened in 1887, the Imperial Health Office in Berlin, headed by Robert Koch from 1891 and Ehrlich's Institute for Experimental Therapy in Frankfurt starting in 1899.[1] The Lister Institute in London emerged in 1891, but it could not follow the European experimental tradition, being constrained by British public opinion, and

---

[1] The Russian Imperial Institute of Experimental Medicine in St. Petersburg (1890) had been privately funded, as was Shibasaburo Kitasato's Kitasato Institute in Tokyo, emerging later in 1914. The German government-supported Kaiser-Wilhelm-Gesellschaft, opening in 1911, used the Rockefeller Institute template; the United States National Institutes of Health did not appear until 1930.

71

the philanthropists who funded the project, were opposed to animal experimentation. It disavowed such work and devoted itself instead to other strategies in the study and prevention of disease.

There was as yet nothing comparable in America to the French and German Institutes. The best of the medical schools, such as at the University of Pennsylvania, had distinguished clinicians, but the only research facility at their medical school was the small Henry C. Lea Laboratory of Hygiene, gifted in 1889. A significant move to support research in Baltimore came when The Johns Hopkins University Medical School opened in 1893, and as described earlier, under the leadership of Dean William H. Welch (1850–1934) it set up pre-clinical departments of anatomy and physiology, with laboratories, headed by talented investigators. Added to this, Welch's talented clinician colleagues like Halsted, Cushing and Osler, accepted the 'full-time principle', and took salaries, diminishing the need to seek private practice. Research and development did flourish in Baltimore, but any suggestions to go further and support career posts in full-time medical research, without clinical work, was seen as strange, and even mistaken, by many in America.

Philanthropists

In Europe, governments had often accepted a role in funding medical research, but in the U.S. it was the philanthropists who stepped in with support at the turn of the century. At this boom time, the Gilded Era gave way to the Progressive Era, and many who had become rich in the laissez-faire business world turned in later life to philanthropy. The two richest men in America (and the world) were Andrew Carnegie (1835–1919), dominant in the steel industry, and John D. Rockefeller senior (1839–1937), who controlled the oil sector. From 1886 onwards, Carnegie had written on broader subjects, and accepted a duty, in his 'gospel of wealth', that private fortunes should not be retained in the family. Perhaps aware of the Christian teaching regarding the difficulty of rich men getting into heaven, these fortunes were to be disbursed during the owner's lifetime. Carnegie started in 1881 to offer money to cities to build and endow

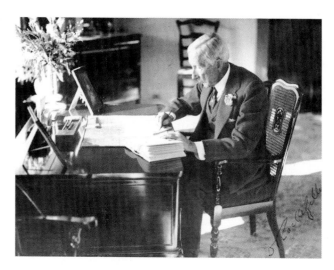

John D. Rockefeller senior, after retirement, devoted his fortune to philanthropy, including funding the Rockefeller Institute for Medical Research in New York. (*Courtesy of the National Library of Medicine.*)

public libraries and followed this with funds for public parks and concert halls. In 1901, Carnegie was bought out by John Pierpont Morgan for $225,639,000, the largest-ever personal transaction. In that year he gave $2 million for his Carnegie Institute of Technology at Pittsburgh, now known as the Carnegie Mellon University, and from 1902 he started many other academic benefactions, including $2 million for his Carnegie Institution for Science (as it is known now) at Washington. Other similar American single-philanthropist-funded institutes appeared in the early 1900s, notably the Phipps Institute for Tuberculosis in Philadelphia (Phipps being a partner in Carnegie's company), and in Chicago, where the Harold F. McCormick's Infectious Disease Institute was funded by a business man who had married into the Rockefeller family.

Rockefeller Money

John D. Rockefeller senior gained his wealth from aggressive, and at times ruthless, acquisition of companies involved in oil production, oil refining, and the transport sector, at a time of minimal regulation and low taxation of industry.[2] Amalgamating these purchases into the Standard Oil Company, he moved the company headquarters from Cleveland to New York. With his Baptist upbringing, he had from early days given the usual tithes to his church, and when he prospered, he gave out additional funds, case-by-case, favouring scattered educational and church projects. As he became richer, the increasing requests gave difficulties. Moreover, like Carnegie, he opposed purely charitable giving if no effort was required thereafter by the recipient. To assist him in allocating his funds, Rockefeller recruited an energetic and resourceful acquaintance, Frederick T. Gates (1853–1929) to review and advise him on his disbursements, and Gates moved to New York as advisor to Rockefeller. This former Baptist pastor, the son of a doctor, had gained a reputation as a shrewd businessman when dealing with the Church's affairs. Gates decided that small 'retail' gifts should cease and that instead 'wholesale' philanthropy would be offered, supporting larger initiatives whose terms could be laid down, and allowing accountability to follow. Rockefeller retired from business in 1897 and sharply increased his involvement in philanthropy.

Gates' Plan

As a pastor, Gates had visited the sick, and was sceptical about the effectiveness of both conventional (allopathic) practice and the then-popular homeopathic system. Still curious, in June 1897, Gates took away a copy of William Osler's standard *Textbook of Medicine* for a holiday read. Osler himself had become a therapeutic nihilist, and in his book he made no attempt to hide the fact that few curative medical remedies existed. This confirmed Gates' own view, and he concluded that

---

[2] Gerald Jonas, *The Circuit Riders: Rockefeller Money and the Rise of Modern Science* (New York: Horton, 1989) and E. Richard Brown, *Rockefeller Medicine Men: Medicine and Capitalism in America* (Los Angeles: University of California Press, 1979). Rockefeller's gifts to his various foundations eventually totalled about $466 million, at initial cost, exceeding those by Carnegie by $100 million.

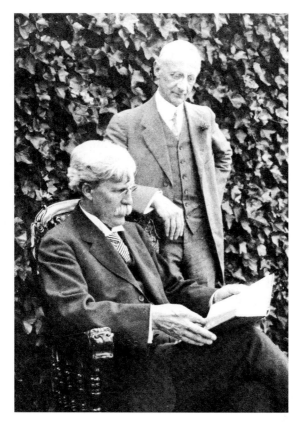

Frederick T. Gates (seated) suggested funding a medical research institute to J.D.Rockefeller. Gates is seen here with Simon Flexner, the Institute's first director. (*Courtesy of the Rockefeller University Archives.*)

the development of medical knowledge lagged behind the growth of the physical sciences. Gates' view was clear:

> Medicine could hardly hope to be a science until medical research should be endowed and qualified men could give themselves to uninterrupted study and investigation, on ample salary, entirely independent of practice.

His solution was that this situation could be improved by new arrangements. Like others, he looked to Europe for a template for a research institute since most of the discoveries about infectious diseases had been made in Europe, with notable contributions from the Koch Institute in Berlin and particularly the Pasteur Institute in Paris.[3]

Gates sent a memorandum on his ideas to Rockefeller senior. As usual the route was via Rockefeller's son, John D. Rockefeller junior (1874–1960), who did not go into business, but instead had an increasingly important role in the family's philanthropy. Gates' advocacy used the analogy with business investment, suggesting that spending on medical research would bring dividends in health. It was a shrewd approach to use with Rockefeller senior, who also knew that industrial scientific research had enabled gains in productivity in the oil sector. Eventually, the father was persuaded to allow a cautious start. This was in spite of his life-long support of homeopathy, which had the support of many wealthy Europeans and Americans at the time.

Gates went ahead and made enquiries about the structure of the existing European institutes and reported back, but even so, the Rockefellers, father and son, spent two years considering the details. It was only after the death, from scarlet fever, in December 1900, of Rockefeller's first grandson, that the family made final moves towards funding a medical research institute. The knowledge that Carnegie, Phipps and McCormick were also making similar moves helped firm up plans. Looking for an institutional base, a university connection was suggested at the outset, and the first idea was that the new institute should be linked to the University of Chicago, which had been revived with Rockefeller funds from 1889. Problems arose and Harvard University in Boston was instead briefly considered as a host, but the idea was not taken further.

In early 1901, William H. Welch of Johns Hopkins and an advisory group were asked to draw up a new plan.[4] Rockefeller and this group were

---

[3] However, both Simon Flexner and William Welch had eponymous fame through the organisms they identified — *Shigella flexneri* and *Clostridium welchii*.
[4] George W. Corner, *A History of the Rockefeller Institute 1901–1953* (New York: The Rockefeller Institute Press, 1964). Welch was to have a long influence, not only at the Institute, but at most other medical endeavours at the time, and he was also a trustee at the Carnegie Institution of Washington.

cool towards links with universities, concerned that routine teaching and other duties might intrude and divert the energies of the staff. On their part, the universities regarded full-time medical research, detached from teaching and medical practice, with suspicion. Rockefeller junior approached Carnegie, who agreed not to compete and that at Washington the emphasis would be on the physical sciences. Rockefeller got the best reward in the short term, since his Institute in New York and its work quickly received acclaim. The work of Carnegie's Washington Foundation was less prominent and had some difficulties later.

Rockefeller now cautiously launched the Rockefeller Institute for Medical Research with a grant of $20,000 annually for 10 years. Rockefeller's advisors, all distinguished medical men, became the Board of Scientific Directors, and they met for the first time on 14 June 1901.[5] They decided they would use the money for a small New York headquarters, and have a programme of external grants for individual workers. The New York newspapers were informed, and carried the story, and they added the hope that the new Institute would rival the Pasteur Institute. Applications for research support flooded in, confirming that there was an unmet need for such funding. It was America's first grant-giving body, and the Institute started cautiously in New York in November 1904 in converted residential quarters on 50th Street.[6]

Rockefeller and Gates' criteria of success were probably vague, but at all times Pasteur's high personal profile and his Paris institution seemed the model, namely success against infectious disease. Pasteur had a populist approach to science, using public lectures and public demonstration of

---

[5] Welch's advisory group became the Board and comprised William H. Welch, Theobald Smith, Christian Herter, Hermann Biggs, L. Emmett Holt and T. Mitchell Prudden, with Simon Flexner added later. All came from the east coast and all, except Smith, had studied in Germany or France. William Osler was notably absent from the group, perhaps because at that time he was cool towards full-time medical research, instead believing that science was a only a 'leaven' to be added to the mix towards obtaining progress in clinical medicine. In any case, Osler soon left for Oxford in 1904.

[6] The Rockefeller Institute evolved into the Rockefeller University in 1973. It should not be confused with The Rockefeller Foundation which, emerging in 1913, was initially involved only in educational and international projects.

vaccine efficacy, and he had involvement in tense debates at Paris scientific societies. Public expectations in New York had been raised, and Rockefeller senior and Gates were hoping for good news.

A Director Appointed

A director was sought before the occupation of the Institute's temporary home. The first choice for the post was Harvard's Theobald Smith (1859–1934), America's first internationally known 'microbe hunter', famous for showing for the first time that insects could transmit disease.[7] He had moved to Harvard in 1895 but declined the Institute post, though he was to arrive later in 1915 as director of the Institute's Animal Pathology Department. Instead, Simon Flexner (1863–1946), the distinguished pathologist at the University of Pennsylvania, agreed to take the new post, starting in summer 1903, and he first took the next year out, studying chemistry in Germany and Paris.[8]

Staff Recruitment

For his first staffing, Flexner had some refusals from established talented senior investigators, mainly bacteriologists, who were hesitant to take a step into the unknown. Flexner did not offer professorships or university links, nor was there as yet a hospital affiliated to the Institute, and the Institute's future funding was uncertain. Some of those approached had scruples about being supported by the new philanthropy, and to some, Rockefeller money was tainted. Flexner's early appointments were therefore often unusual, perhaps because his first choices were not available, but the eventual multidisciplinary composition allowed him to extend the Institute's studies beyond the traditional emphasis on

---

[7] In 1889, Theobald Smith showed that Texas Cattle Fever was transmitted by the tick-borne parasite *Babesia bigemina*.

[8] Peyton Rous 'Simon Flexner 1863–1946' *Obituary Notices of Fellows of the Royal Society* 6, (1949): 409–45. See also Darwin H. Stapleton (ed.), *Creating a Tradition of Biomedical Research: Contributions to the History of The Rockefeller University* (New York: The Rockefeller University Press, 2004).

infectious disease. He knew that a new approach was needed and that chemistry and physics might make inroads into the mysteries of the body in health and disease.

Flexner made three initial appointments to the permanent 'member' posts. The grades used in the Institute — 'member', 'associate', 'assistant' or 'fellow' — were those usual in learned societies and differed from the grades of professor and lecturer used in academia. Only the members had tenure, and the others were expected to be promoted or move on. For laboratory support, the scientists had technicians, and 'helpers'. The first members were Hideyo Noguchi, the highly productive Japanese bacteriologist who came with Flexner from Philadelphia, Phoebus Levene (1869–1940) the Russian biochemist, recruited in spite of poor health and a reputation for serious budgetary irresponsibility,[9] and Eugene L. Opie (1873–1971) who had linked sugar control to the pancreatic islets, narrowly failing to find the hormone insulin. Later, Samuel Meltzer (1851–1920), a New York Russian/German physiologist was glad to escape from the need to do private medical practice and joined the Institute, with success, at the age of 53 in 1906.

It was a polyglot group, with Opie the only American-born member, and some of the early staff would encounter New York's anti-Semitism and xenophobia. Difficulty with the English language was not a handicap, since neither teaching nor clinical work was required. Flexner appointed some women assistants, unusually for the times, and there were also junior grant holders and volunteer workers. Flexner was firmly in charge, and the senior staff had to submit regular reports to him and the Board on their work. Although his Board was consulted about new senior 'members', Flexner made all the other appointments and allocated the funds for running costs. Flexner was on the Board and was also a Trustee and thus successfully avoided being merely the Board's executive. He retained his powerful and unusual position, even when the Institute expanded greatly later.

---

[9] Levene worked steadily, identifying ribose in 1909 and deoxyribose in 1929. He showed that these were linked as nucleotides, but his bold tetranucleotide model for DNA proved incorrect.

Outside Concerns

The medical establishment in New York had not sought the project nor had it been consulted; the idea of the Institute was a lay initiative coming from Gates and the Rockefellers, and the local profession was generally cool towards it. Their view was that innovation could not be bought, and medical science instead advanced through revelations to those involved in bedside medicine. Others pointed out that talented scientists emerged rarely and randomly, and that innovators would not appear simply because an institute existed. But slowly, as part of the new Progressive Era's reverence for experts, the sceptical doctors came to realise that laboratory research was at least of assistance in elevating the status and mystique of medicine.[10]

More Funds

Rockefeller, though retired, was still under some pressure. His business methods had always had their critics, and with Theodore Roosevelt succeeding the business-friendly President William McKinlay in 1901, the mood turned against the monopolies, cartels and corporate trusts of America's laissez-faire industrial world. The Supreme Court made moves to bring in anti-trust legislation and in particular to break up the Standard Oil company. Rockefeller senior's own reputation suffered as a result of new hostile biographies, notably Ida Tarbell's 'muckraking' book, *The Rise of the Standard Oil Company* of 1904. The old 'robber barons' of old were portrayed as irresponsible, secretive, self-seeking and lacking interest in the public good. Rockefeller senior could do with more good news, and this may have spurred on his philanthropy.

Rockefeller now agreed to release more funds for purchase of land and a new building for the Institute. Farmland was bought for $175,000 between 64th and 67th Streets on the East Side waterfront, and

---

[10] For an overview, see Andrew Cunningham and Perry Williams, *The Laboratory Revolution in Medicine* (Cambridge: Cambridge University Press, 1992).

construction of a new building started in summer 1904. But the cautious elder Rockefeller still gave no guarantee of long-term support. He did not offer an endowment, but agreed that $1 million could be spent over 10 years. Carnegie in Washington had offered security to his institute, from the first, with a $10 million endowment.

The New Home

The Rockefeller Institute's Founder's Building was opened on 11 May 1906 with a ceremony for 500 guests, attended by the presidents of both Harvard and Columbia Universities. The building did not have the stately marble façade of Harvard's Medical School, since the architects were told to plan construction 'as simply as is consistent with the present purpose', a brief perhaps reflecting Rockefeller senior's own frugal attitudes. At the ceremony, Rockefeller must have been pleased when Harvard's president, Charles W. Eliot, when praising fundamental biomedical research, said it would aid American industry by diminishing losses due to illness and untimely death. Gates was happy with the event, and for an interesting reason: it was his idea. He wrote:

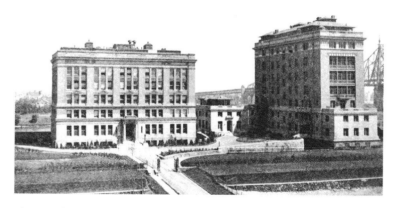

The early Founders Building of the RIMR and its Hospital (built later) were set in spacious grounds on New York's East River. (*Popular Science Monthly* April 1912.)

These doctors did not come to us. We went to them. Other people conceive schemes and come to us. ... They come to us with urgency, with zeal and in the spirit of the professional advocate to wring from us every dollar that can be got.[11]

Gates was also pleased with the simplicity of the governance, unlike many of the large charitable bodies he dealt with.[12] Rockefeller had been cautious with this further support, but continued to be pleased with the Institute, and by January 1907, he could be approached by the Board for an endowment to secure the future. A sum of $6 million was suggested, which would have considerably expanded the staff and provided each permanent member with new assistants, fellows and skilled helpers. This was a bold but reasonable request, in view of Carnegie's liberality in Washington. But again Rockefeller was cautious, and though conceding that an endowment was now appropriate, he gave only $2.6 million, and again watched events. The new funding was the income from an endowment of Rockefeller company shares and bonds, mainly railway stock, yielding between three-and-a-half to five percent.

Soon each division had a secretary. Flexner used his funds to establish an illustration department, and he employed a photographer and a librarian. The Institute inherited the *Journal of Experimental Medicine*, which had emerged at Johns Hopkins in 1896 with William Welch as editor. But, burdened with his many activities and seriously behindhand in dealing with a backlog of manuscripts, Welch successfully appealed to Flexner to take over. It became the Institute's own journal from 1905, and soon had a profitable circulation of 450 copies. Flexner was sole editor, which kept him well informed. His policy was that 'long papers were undesirable', and as editor he offered rapid acceptance and publication. In the novel *Arrowsmith*, based on the early work of the Institute, the Director tells a young scientist that he must hasten to publish his results.

---

[11] Gates to Rockefeller Jr, 7 February 1908, RU RG 526–1, box 44, Rockefeller University Archives, Rockefeller Archives Centre (RUA RAC).

[12] The Institute Trustees had control of finances and were Gates (chairman), Rockefeller junior, Starr J. Murphy (their attorney), Welch, and Simon Flexner. Flexner and his Board of Scientific Directors dealt with the science, and these Trustees were added to oversee the finances.

'Get right to it. In fact you should have done it before this. This is no longer an age of parochialism but of competition, in art and science…we can't have somebody stealing a march on us.'

The library was well stocked, since 60 journals were received in exchange for the Institute's own *Journal of Experimental Medicine*. Flexner took the view that lunchtime arrangements were important for interaction between the staff, and the subsidised meal cost 25 cents. The tables in the scientists' dining room seated eight people, encouraging group staff interaction. Women had a separate dining room, and the other grades had to eat outside at lunchtime.

Carrel Starts

Carrel started work in New York in September 1906. He was on the lowest of the Institute's grades, with a 'Fellowship in Experimental Physiology' for one year in the first instance, which gave a quite generous $1,000 per annum, paid quarterly. It was Carrel's first salary in America. The pension arrangements were generous, as Carrel was to find much later, and a two-month summer holiday was allowed to the scientists, but not to the other staff. Carrel also had support from two laboratory assistants. His laboratory was on the top floor of the Institute, and it would be modified and expanded over the years to come. He had use of the new animal house and operating suite, and an annual budget of $500 for equipment and supplies. It was impressive support for the time. Another young scientist recalled encountering the facilities available at the Institute when he arrived from Michigan:

> What a temple of science the Rockefeller Institute was! It gleamed, materially, in comparison to the department of bacteriology at Ann Arbor. That grubby den of research reeked of guinea pigs, rats, and rabbits. At the Rockefeller you did not smell the animals. They were brought to you from a beautiful animal house in the bowels of the Institute by a servant. … Lab servants washed the glassware and cooked the culture medium and if you had a well-enough trained technician, he could even do your experiments for you.[13]

---

[13] Paul de Kruif, *The Sweeping Wind* (New York: Harcourt, Brace & World, 1962): 13.

Carrel could get on with his adventurous surgery and all his needs were met. He was content to have no clinical or teaching duties. Since his work was surgical and only he could accomplish it, for many years he did not add to his small staff. Carrel's facilities were better than in Chicago. He was in touch with Guthrie, his former research partner now settled at St. Louis, and they compared notes on their new situations. Carrel wrote:

> We have two men for keeping the animals, and one of them is good. There is a man for histological sections. As personal assistants, I have one girl and one man. The girl assists me during the operations, and is in charge of the sterilisation, needles etc. The man sterilises and etherises the animals, assists me for the physiological experiments etc … I operate every day in the old operating suite.[14]

In other letters, he praised the surgical assistance from Miss Johnston, his assistant, provided she kept calm — 'une femme a beaucoup plus de qualités chirurgicales qu'un homme à condition qu'elle ne soit pas nerveuse'.

Larger animals like the monkeys for Flexner's experiments and horses for serum production were held elsewhere, and the Institute eventually purchased the 98-acre Clyde Farm near New Brunswick in New Jersey. In the year 1907, Carrel's first year, the Institute used 300 dogs, 100 monkeys, 16 horses, 10 cattle and 40 goats.

Carrel's First Year

Flexner had perhaps taken a chance with Carrel's appointment: to bring in a surgeon was a very unusual move.[15] But Flexner was proved to be right and was proud of Carrel, whose high profile and international reputation

---

[14] S.P. Harbison (1962) 'Origins of vascular surgery: the Carrel-Guthrie letters' *Surgery* 52: 406–18, at 413.

[15] There was one other surgeon at the Institute in 1906, and Joshua Edwin Sweet, on a short-term fellowship, made Eck's fistulas for Levene's studies. Sweet moved to be assistant professor of surgical research in the University of Pennsylvania.

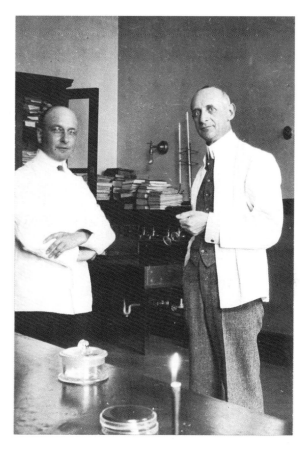

Simon Flexner never wavered in his support for Carrel. (*Courtesy of the American Philosophical Society.*)

would reward Flexner and please the Rockefellers. In one of his regular reports, Flexner even drew attention to Carrel's appointment, which he deemed as 'highly satisfactory'.[16] By April 1907, one year later, Carrel was promoted as an assistant, and his salary increased to $1,500. Later that year he was promoted to associate and named in a division of his own. Flexner and Carrel were close to each other throughout their careers, and during the difficulties later, Carrel said that 'only Flexner understood him'.

---

[16] Minutes, 12 January 1907, Scientific Directors Minutes, FA 856, box 2, RUA RAC (note 11).

Courting Publicity

As he sought to establish himself and his Institute, Flexner was not averse to any publicity about their work. Normally he and the staff might have shown the usual academic detachment, but the new 'Pasteur-on-Hudson' institute was expected to deliver. Increasingly, the American newspapers sought vivid accounts of scientific discoveries and also personal details of the savants behind these innovations.[17] Public approval would please the Institute's single benefactor, and Rockefeller might provide further

> ## Dr. Flexner Announces Discovery of Influenzal Meningitis That Follows Grip Attacks.
>
> ### FATAL IN MOST CASES
>
> **Spread of the Malady Recently Noted and Rockefeller Institute Finds a Serum for It.**
>
> Dr. Simon Flexner, Director of the Rockefeller Institute for Medical Research, announces in the current issue of The Journal of the American Medical Association that it has been discovered that cerebro-spinal meningitis, secondary to influenza or the grip, is far from uncommon and very fatal. At the same

Favourable publicity for Flexner's anti-meningitis serum in the *New York Times* in 1907.

---

[17] Bert Hansen, *Picturing Medical Progress from Pasteur to Polio* (New Brunswick: Rutgers University Press, 2009).

long-term funding if there was success with dealing with infectious disease. Arcane advances in chemistry or physiology meant little to journalists and newspaper readers. In addition, Flexner could see that Carrel's work might assist in bolstering the reputation of the Institute.

Flexner's own 'microbe-hunting' work got off to a good start. In the winter of 1905, an epidemic of meningitis killed three quarters of the 4,000 affected in New York. In response, Flexner made an anti-meningitis serum, which needed intra-spinal injection, and it was a success in the cases in 1907. Flexner's serum resulted in five supportive stories in *The New York Times*. Rockefeller senior was particularly pleased when the *New York World* of 6 August 1907 reported that 'Cure is Found for Meningitis with John D.'s Aid'. He rarely contacted the Scientific Directors, but on this occasion he sent a letter to them saying that news of Flexner's cure was 'special to him'. Rockefeller junior one year later announced approval of new funds to build a hospital at the Institute, and his formal letter said:

> My father thus enlarges the scope and possibilities of the Institute in grateful recognition of the services of Dr. Simon Flexner ... [which] led him at length to the discovery of a cure for epidemic cerebro-spinal meningitis.[18]

Favourable coverage for the Institute was gained in a number of other ways. The Institute started to send out advance copies of their *Journal of Experimental Medicine* directly to local newspapers and encouraged journalists to study the content. Initially the Associated Press was left out, and they asked to be put on Flexner's mailing list and to be given notice of 'any discoveries to be announced'. They added that 'we will be objective and accurate, if we get it before others do it badly'.[19]

---

[18] Corner, *History* (note 4): 61. There is a full account of Flexner's anti-meningitis serum in Karen D. Ross' PhD Thesis, *Making Medicine Scientific: Simon Flexner and Experimental Medicine*, University of Minnesota 2006: UMI Microform 3230247.
[19] AP to James, January 1913, 210.3(27), Business Manager Publicity File, RUA RAC (note 11).

Personal Details

Carrel did not like cities. New York was expanding and was increasingly crowded and noisy. It was very hot in summer: air conditioning was still to come. Horses were still in use in the streets, although pigs were gone. Feral cats and dogs abounded, and some ended up in the Institute captured by 'volunteer dog catchers' paid 25–50 cents per animal by the Institute. The city's health was poor, with mortality rates higher than Boston, Paris or London. There were regular epidemics of dysentery, trachoma, smallpox, cholera, typhus, meningitis and diphtheria, and polio was to arrive later.

We know a little about Carrel at this time. He was 5 feet 3¼ inches in height, 160 lb in weight, with a hat size of 7⅛. When younger, he had a beard, but this was now gone. His many portraits from this period invariably show a closely shaved head, an enigmatic smile and his iconic pince-nez Skelton or Vanderbilt Zyl eyeglasses required for his short-sightedness. His French accent was declining but was not absent. In the laboratory he wore white trousers, a short white jacket and a square white cap, a borrowing from the world of surgery. He worked late and with intensity. He spoke in crisp, short sentences and with disconcerting bluntness.

Disliking the city, Carrel soon left the apartment he rented initially and moved outside to board with a family at Larchmont on Long Island Sound, giving an hour's daily commute to the Institute via Grand Central Station. He stayed outside until 1908, when he rented a city apartment at 130 W 57th Street and bought a car — a Hupmobile 32. He was a tidy, organised man, living a bachelor life, and later joined the Century Association, a gentleman's club in New York favoured by academics and writers, where he could have had dinner in the evenings. He joined the Fencers' Club, one of a number in New York, where he had a locker. At the Club, one sparring partner and friend was the lawyer-author Arthur C. Train (1875–1945). They met when Carrel noticed Train's novel *Mortmain* of 1907, in which he depicted a skilled surgeon who could graft cat's paws and then carried out a human hand transplant. Train's inspiration had come from the operations of the New York plastic surgeon Robert Abbe, not from Carrel's work. After a robbery at his apartment later, Carrel bought and carried a Colt pistol for safety on his nocturnal journeys to and from the lab. He was later an enthusiast for law, order and punishment.

He had no obvious interest in the cultural life of the city. In his social involvement he was invited to colleagues' houses, notably that of Christian Herter and his wife, and also joined the family of the emigré French sculptor Francois Tonetti, who was engaged on decorating the Rockefeller estate at Kykuit. Carrel could be charming and attentive to women, but he had no romantic attachments in New York and remained un-married until 1913.

Summer Break

Though a hard worker, driven by his 'surgical personality', Carrel accepted the academic habit, usual at the time, of taking a long summer break. This lasted about two months, starting in July, and he increasingly used it to return by sea to Europe. In this way he escaped New York's heat and kept his links with family and European surgery. He travelled first class, again suggesting he was not short of money. In the summer months in Europe he visited hospitals and research units of interest, keeping up with any developments. He travelled to Lyon to visit his family there, notably his sister and his brother Joseph, and he continued the rent for his mother's château 'La Batie' after her death. It remained in the family until seizure during World War II. From Lyon in summer he went south to Lourdes to hear of any further unexplained cures, talking over matters with the controversial Dr. Gustave Boissarie, still in charge of the Medical Bureau.

Surgical Work

Carrel's archives have a valuable list of his day-to-day surgical work at the Institute starting in late 1906.[20] Dogs were the main experimental animals, and Carrel was the Institute's biggest user. Over his first six

---

[20] Operative Diary, October 1906–April 1907, box 1 folder 25, FA 208, Malinin Collection of the Papers of Alexis Carrel and Charles Lindbergh, RUA, RAC (note 11).

months, he carried out at least one operation each day, a workload which was only possible with skilled assistants and a helpful staff in the animal house. The commonest procedures in his first year were leg transplants (37), kidney transplants (23), abdominal aortic replacements (17), 'other' artery grafts (8), carotid artery-jugular vein anastomosis (8), wound healing studies (7) and smaller numbers of other procedures, including simple cutting of the nerves to the kidney(4).[21] The novelty of doing simple small blood vessel surgery was wearing off and aortic surgery was a new challenge. The number of kidney grafts carried out is substantial, and these will be looked at later, as will his determined, and perhaps surprising, study of leg transplantation.

Career Options

Towards the end of his first year in New York, Carrel had two interesting job offers. George Stewart, his head of department earlier in Chicago, now back as professor of experimental medicine at Western Reserve University, had not forgotten him, and he offered Carrel a post with $2,000 p.a. at Western Reserve, where George Crile also headed the surgical department. Crile made contact and assured him that 'aseptic work would be supported', knowing that Carrel wanted facilities for his animal surgery comparable to those at the Rockefeller Institute. Crile was persuasive and told him that 'sooner or later his [Carrel's] methods would transfer to clinical work and that Cleveland had this potential link, whereas the Institute did not'.[22] Crile pressed him further and tried to arrange a visit, but in the end nothing came of it. Yet again, the history of American surgery might have been different had Carrel moved to this clinically-orientated research post. Carrel was also considered for the Harvard chair of surgery that year, but Cushing in Baltimore was instead approached and accepted. The Boston view was that 'Carrel is nothing

---

[21] Carrel's less frequent operations were vein graft (3), ovary plus fallopian tube graft (1) and intestine graft (1).
[22] Crile to Carrel, 7 February 1907, box 41 folder 44, Alexis Carrel Papers, Georgetown University Library, Booth Family Center for Special Collections (GULBFC).

but a very expert sew-er'.[23] This was the verdict of others, namely that his work was of purely surgical interest, rather than having any fundamental significance. Meltzer at the Institute, never diplomatic, shared this view and had also disparaged the transplant work. This view rankled with Carrel. Carrel felt he was more than just a surgeon. He wrote to Guthrie:

> We will show Dr. Meltzer whether the work is entirely experimental surgery or whether it is at foundation a study of the elemental physiological conditions, processes and adjustments in mammals.[24]

Otherwise, Carrel seemed content in New York and was thereafter steadily promoted, reaching the grade of associate member in 1910 and the final honour of membership in 1912, giving him $5,000 per year. He had not been forgotten by the surgeons, who were increasingly curious, and wrote requesting details of his methods. Many also visited, including Halsted and other Baltimore surgeons still interested in dealing with human aneurysms, as did Emil Kocher, the Swiss thyroid transplanter, who visited in 1907; in turn Carrel visited Kocher when in Europe that summer.

Publications

Carrel continued to publish, and he now used the *Journal of Experimental Medicine*. Carrel also used the generalist journal *Science* or the *Journal of the American Medical Association* for short papers and, as before, he continued to make sure that France knew of his work, sending papers with the same results to the French rapid-publication journals. In the next four years, he published 19 English-language papers, 11 French, two German and one in a Spanish journal.[25]

---

[23] John F. Fulton, *Harvey Cushing: a Biography* (Springfield: Charles C Thomas, 1946): 335.

[24] Carrel to Guthrie, 16 November 1907: box 2 folder 13, Malinin Collection, FA 208, RUA RAC (note 11).

[25] See Sutter's excellent bibliography in Robert Soupault, *Alexis Carrel* (Paris: Libraire Plon, 1952), a list used by other biographers later. Other Rockefeller staff still published in German journals: of Levene's 21 papers in 1906, nine were in German.

Institute Projects

Flexner's appointment of Carrel had the perhaps unintended consequence that the other members of the Institute had a skilled and adventurous surgeon on hand. Human abdominal surgery had been developing, particularly in Lyon, and Carrel used these techniques experimentally to help others in the Institute with their physiological and biochemical studies. In summer 1909, he worked with Theodore C. Janeway doing the necessary surgery for him which produced a major discovery. Reducing the blood flow to the kidney created high blood pressure.[26] This finding must have encouraged Carrel's conviction, from his days in Lyon, that blood flow mattered in the routine activity of any organ. Helping others, he carried out the operation of partial stomach removal for Gustave M. Meyer and also for Phoebus Levene to assist their investigations of stomach and bowel physiology. Carrel in particular helped Christian Herter, the Institute trustee, based at the nearby College of Physicians and Surgeons. For the grateful Herter, he did various procedures to help understand the functions of the pancreas — bile duct ligation, removal of the pancreas, opening the pancreas onto the skin as a fistula, or cutting the gland's nerve supply. These impressive operations were not yet standard in human work.

Kidney Grafts

Carrel's dog kidney graft experiments, second in number to his leg grafts, made a number of issues clearer. First, cutting the nerve supply to the kidney did not affect the organ's function. Nor, strangely, was the kidney lymphatic drainage, which normally took fluid from the organ, needed for satisfactory function when grafted. Hence, perhaps surprisingly, it was clear that a kidney lacking these connections could be transplanted successfully.

---

[26]Theodore C. Janeway was later appointed professor of medicine at Johns Hopkins University in 1912. The report with Carrel is 'Note on the production of renal insufficiency' *PSEBM* (1909) 6: 107.

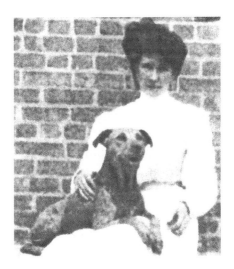

By 1907, Carrel had achieved long-term success with a re-transplantation of a dog's own kidney. (*From Reference 28.*)

In his kidney grafting work, Carrel had initially focussed on accomplishing the operation, trying to obtain blood flow through the kidney, and with urine output following. He persevered with taking out a kidney and putting it back into the same animal (an autograft), and with his skill, it now took him only about an hour for the transplant. Even his skill at the tricky insertion of the ureter into the bladder can be admired. Before grafting, Carrel flushed the removed donor kidney with Locke's saline at room temperature, but Guthrie in Minnesota was opposed to this perfusion, claiming it damaged the kidney.[27]

But Carrel retained an odd, almost mystical, belief. He was convinced that kidneys should be transplanted to their usual position in the body. It was other surgeons later who established that the pelvic position close to the bladder was much more suitable.

---

[27] C.C. Guthrie (1910) 'The effect on the kidneys of temporary anaemia, alone and accompanied by perfusion' *Archives of Internal Medicine* 5: 232–45. Curiously, Guthrie's view on the danger of organ perfusion was still accepted as late as the mid-1960s, when opinion changed to insist on perfusion with cold saline.

Post-Operative Phase

With success, Carrel's emphasis now moved to the outcome days and weeks after his dog kidney transplant operations. Daunting surgical complications were encountered — infection, bleeding and urine leakage. In particular, his hopes of fixing the kidney in its bed were thwarted, since it was free to move, and the organ often twisted on its vessels and failed. With so many deaths from these technical problems, at first he could not judge how long a dog kidney transplant of any kind would last. It was not until February 1908 that he had convincing success with an autograft (the other host kidney being removed): the dog remained well, and over the next two years bore 14 pups in two pregnancies. He now had some confidence in the operation. He noted that the good result with the autograft

> removes also, without need of further discussion, the objections of the experimenters who claimed that the section of the renal nerves, the temporary suppression of the renal circulation, or the perfusion of

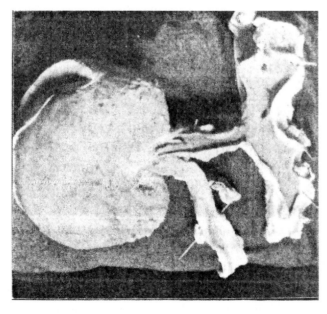

This successful single autograft dog kidney successfully sustained life. (*From Reference 28.*)

the kidneys produce necessarily dangerous and even fatal lesions of this organ. ... [But] this interactions of the host and its new organ are still practically unknown. The study of these interactions was very difficult because the complications which follow the operation were of widely different kinds. In most cases it could not be ascertained whether the cause of the accidents was biological or surgical.[28]

Though it was difficult, Carrel now proceeded with study of 'homograft' kidneys, those taken from one animal and grafted to another.[29] At the time of his Hopkins lecture in the previous year he thought that homografts might not survive. Over the next few years at the Institute it became clear to him that this was the case.

The Homograft Puzzle

The belief that homografts would survive was widespread in the surgical world, strange though it seems in retrospect. C.C. Guthrie, as late as 1915, still reported success with ovary graft work.[30] The Hopkins surgeon John Staige Davis could say of skin grafts as late as 1912 that: 'there is no doubt that iso-grafts [homografts] will give satisfactory results in a great many instances, if transplanted with the proper technique.'[31] Complicating the matter was that Carrel's own homograft blood vessel grafts survived well.[32] Bone homografts gave effective results, and most of the few small blood transfusions of the day caused no serious effects. In horticulture,

---

[28] Alexis Carrel (1910) 'Remote results of the replantation of the kidneys and the spleen' *JEM* 12: 146–50.

[29] 'Homograft' was the term used then, and is preferred here to 'allograft', the new term used from the 1960s.

[30] C.C. Guthrie and M.E. Lee (1915) 'Ovarian transplantation' *JAMA* 64: 1822–4. In this paper he again shows he was touchy about priority, in this case disputing claims from some Washington biologists.

[31] John Staige Davis (1912), *JAMA* 59: 526 [in discussion].

[32] Carrel asked a colleague called 'Wood' to study the microscopy of his blood vessel grafts, and Wood misled Carrel by saying that the muscle cells in homograft arteries and veins survived well; see Alexis Carrel (1908) 'Results of the transplantation of blood vessels, organs and limbs' *JAMA* 51: 1662–7.

hybridisation between disparate plants was a routine procedure. And above all, there was Kocher's apparent success with human thyroid homografts in treating thyroid deficiency. Kocher was awarded a Nobel Prize in 1909 for his thyroid research, and he had formidable authority.[33]

Hence in this first decade of the century, the consensus, now known to be a seriously faulty paradigm, can be called 'homograft rejection denial'. Belief in homograft survival was encouraged by the special cases of blood, bone or blood vessel grafts and optimistic observation of skin homografts. But above all, there was no biological explanation of why homografts should fail. In day-to-day surgical practice, once tissues healed in, they were expected to survive. If a graft survived and then failed, the matter was a mystery: infection or surgical incompetence could be blamed.[34]

The results of Carrel's study of dog kidney homografts at this time were difficult to interpret, since post-operative surgical complications were prominent. After a discouraging time in 1907, he turned to use the cat instead, challenging though the cat kidney surgery was, and the role of rejection was soon revealed. In the meantime, he had other projects; many were not published.

Other Projects

Carrel kept busy. Wound healing emerged as a favourite, and these experiments continued in a small way each year, in hope of increasing his understanding of the processes involved. He removed small areas of dog skin and studied the rate of wound contraction and the ingrowth of new skin. He had a scarcely hidden extra agenda. From his Lourdes experience, he accepted that unexplained, rapid healing could occur, and he told Flexner about seeing it again, even on a brief visit to Lourdes.

---

[33] Theodore Kocher (1914) 'Über die Bedingungen erfolgreicher Schilddrüsen transplantation beim Menschen' *Verhandlungen der Deutschen Gesellschaft für Chirurgie* 43: 484–566.
[34] For an analysis of 'rejection denial', see David Hamilton, *A History of Organ Transplantation* (Pittsburgh: Pittsburgh University Press, 2012): 81–5.

I was allowed to observe a few patients. On a small ulceration, I saw epithelialisation occurring in a few minutes. ... It demonstrates that my hypothesis of the enormous activation of the cicatrisation [healing] of tissues is not a dream.[35]

Carrel believed that the mechanism involved in these alleged cures was not an impenetrable mystery, and that any rapid healing worked through acceleration of normal, existing mechanisms. Accordingly, he believed that the natural processes of healing could be speeded up in a non-Lourdes setting. He constantly looked for strategies to increase this pace, but he, and all others since, have been frustrated in their search. He was pleased when Serge Voronoff, the French gland-grafting surgeon, claimed in 1909 that a thyroid gland powder would indeed accelerate wound healing. But when repeating the work in his animal model, Carrel obtained only a modest effect.

He had some clinical links in New York and joined a local surgeon when grafting a young cretinous patient with homograft thyroid slices. He skin-grafted varicose ulcers and studied their healing. He used human ovaries, blood vessels and tumours to graft to animals, including monkeys.

The Hospital

Carrel briefly considered applying for a New York licence to practise surgery, but took the matter no further. This may have been because a local opportunity for the application of his methods was likely. The early hopes for adding a hospital to the Institute were finally realised in 1910, and Flexner wanted it to be a place where the insights gained in the Institute's labs would be applied to human patients. But when Rufus Cole was appointed as Hospital director, he resisted this 'translational' flow format. Instead, Cole

---

[35] Carrel to Flexner, 3 September 1909, box 2, FA 231, Faculty/Alexis Carrel, RUA RAC (note 11).

wanted to be able to hire talented clinical staff that would have freedom to work full-time on their own research agenda. One of the staff recalled:

> Cole made it clear that the hospital was not going to be a handmaiden to the laboratories and that he and his boys were not going to test Noguchi's ideas, Meltzer's ideas or Levene's ideas…

This meant that Carrel's ideas could not be tested immediately nearby. Had Flexner's initial template for the Hospital been used, surgical staff might have been appointed and Carrel's surgical ideas used by Carrel himself in the Hospital, or under his guidance.[36]

Transplants in Cats

Discouraged by the difficulties with dog kidney transplants, notably the difficulty in fixing the donor organs in place, Carrel turned again during 1907 to experiment with cats and use the double kidney transplants he had described with Guthrie in 1906. This involved transplanting both kidneys still attached to segments of the aorta and vena cava. This gave him larger vessels to join, and although there were four tricky anastomoses to be done, Carrel was up to it. Both ureters were on a patch, which was joined to the bladder. This approach, which he again descriptively called 'transplantation *en masse*', gave better fixation of the kidneys than in the dog work.[37]

There were many complications, and many immediate deaths, but he was getting urine production and some reasonable post-operative survivals. After a while, kidney function deteriorated and there was protein in the urine. Microscopic examination of the kidneys of the two longest survivors showed 'nephritis', with a marked cellular infiltrate in one. He was describing rejection, and was slowly becoming aware that he was encountering a new phenomenon, not an infection,

---

[36] Saul Benison, *Tom Rivers — Reflections on a Life in Medicine and Science* (Cambridge: Massachusetts Institute of Technology, 1967): 70. Corner History (note 4), says of the original plans for the Hospital, that among the Institute staff 'at least two — Meltzer and Carrel — looked forward to testing and applying their ideas clinically'.

[37] This long, detailed paper is A. Carrel (1908) 'Transplantation in mass of the kidneys' *JEM* 10: 98–140. The illustrations are by the Institute's artist F.S. Lockwood.

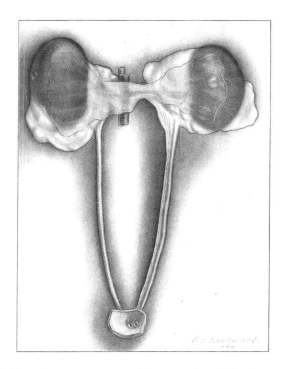

Carrel's remarkable achievement successfully transplanted both cat donor kidneys attached to the aorta and vena cava. (*From Reference 37.*)

but something else which was a barrier to organ transplantation. At this time he also made an unusual observation in one of the homografted cats, namely that the cat had developed marked calcification throughout its arterial blood vessels, though the vessels in the graft remained normal. He raised the possibility that a foreign graft might affect the host; yet again, he was right.[38]

The Cat Story Breaks

That year, Flexner was vice-president of the section on Physiology and Medicine of the American Association for the Advancement of Science,

---

[38] Alexis Carrel (1908) 'Calcification of the arterial system in a cat with transplanted kidneys' *JEM* 10: 276–82. Recently, Prof. Jon McAnulty at the University of Wisconsin in his remarkable series of over 100 cat allografts, has never encountered any such recipient calcification (personal communication). It might, however, occur in the absence of immunosuppression.

and he spoke at their Chicago meeting in late December 1907. In his address, given out ahead to the local press, he alluded to the Institute's work and in particular to Carrel's new success with cat kidney transplants. A *Chicago Tribune* journalist picked up the story, and on 2 January 1908 the *New York Tribune* also reported on Flexner's lecture, describing how kidneys could be transplanted between cats and survive well. The paper commented that it is 'not now a far cry to the time when it may be possible to transplant the vital organs from an animal body to that of a human'. These articles were then syndicated widely to newspapers throughout the country. Philadelphia's *The World* had a two-page spread entitled 'Lower animals may save men and women', using invented quotations from Flexner and Carrel, and it was accompanied by portraits of them both.

Public Concern

The cat kidney story gained traction. The *Washington Post* took it up on 11 January, but took a different line. It was able to add more detail to Flexner's short account of the cat transplants because Carrel's detailed account had just become available, as usual, in advance copies of the January issue of the *Journal of Experimental Medicine*.[39] Carrel's unusually long article was full of surgical detail: it was aimed at a professional audience.

The contrarian *Post* was in no mood to join the chorus of praise. In his paper, Carrel had given full details of all his cat grafts, listing the many early deaths and early failure in all but two attempts. The daily observations of the suffering of each of the cats towards the day of death made melancholy reading. The *Post* alleged that even the survivors were in agony, as victims of 'the horrors of vivisection'. Referring to the Rockefeller Institute, it claimed 'the gossip of the East Side [of New York] gives the mysterious pile a hundred horrors'. Agreeing with the *Post*, the

[39] This *JEM* issue with the cat graft data was dated 1 January 1908. Flexner's published lecture has only a brief allusion to Carrel; see Simon Flexner (1908) 'Tendencies in Pathology' *Science* 27: 128–36.

New York Herald also attacked the Institute, and for the next four years it would assist the New York antivivisectionist's cause.

With the controversy continuing, Carrel was alarmed and received unpleasant anonymous letters. On 12 January he wrote to Guthrie:

> Will you go next summer to the meeting of the American Medical Association? I shall go very probably. But I hesitate very much on account

TELLS OF VIVISECTIONS

Practitioner of Art Depicts Agonies of Subjects.

CATS' KIDNEYS TRANSPLANTED

Surgeon in Rockefeller Institute Records "Success" in Proving Organs "Can Resume Functions Efficiently"—Some Animals Suffer for Weeks, but All Ultimately Die from Operation.

New York, Jan. 10.—Vivisection as practiced in New York City to-day is fully explained and its cruelties are set forth thoroughly in an article just written by one of the leading vivisectionists of the Rockefeller Institute for Medical Research, Dr. Alexis Carrel. Dr. Carrel's

The *Washington Post* on 11 January 1908 supported critics of animal experimentation.

of the Chicagoan newspapers. We have just now had a very bad time. The address of Dr. Flexner in Chicago has been published in the daily press and the newspapers of New York have published the most unpleasant articles about vivisection. Two days ago the *Herald* presented me to the public as a monster, a kind of low criminal, just fitted for the electric chair.[40]

There was a further setback for Carrel, and the Institute, with *Life* magazine's coverage on 5 March:

Carrel is having fun while cats die in agony. Mr. Rockefeller's doctors are certainly making things lively for the animals. Livelier than Mr. Rockefeller made things for his competitors in the oil business. And that is saying a good deal.

New York Antivivisectionists

At the time, the New York antivivisectionists were increasingly organised and active, and publication of the details of the cat transplants gave them ammunition. American libertarian culture meant that animal experimentation was tolerated, unlike in Britain. Although antivivisection bills had been presented in the District of Columbia in 1896, and similar proposals appeared in Congress in 1897, they were headed off, largely through the influential opposition organised by William H. Welch.[41] Other attempts followed, and in 1907, one year before the cat kidney controversy, a bill in the New York State legislature was accepted but defeated in committee.

Following shortly after the publicity about Carrel's work, a public meeting of the New York Anti-Vivisection Society was held in February at the Carnegic Lyceum, organised by Mrs. Diana Belais, a tireless critic of animal use, and it attracted clergy, politicians and celebrities. The meeting carried by acclamation a resolution urging John D. Rockefeller and the Rockefeller Institute to take steps to restrict their animal

---

[40] S.P. Harbison, *Carrel-Guthrie letters* (note 14): 416.
[41] One medical man, Albert Leffingwell (1845–1916), campaigned tirelessly against animal experiments in America from the 1890s, not seeking outright abolition, but merely control of animal use.

experiments. The Society then set up a booth near the Institute and invited local citizens to take direct action, urging them to rescue animals from the Institute.[42]

These early months of 1908 following Flexner's lecture and the disclosures about the cat surgery were an uncertain period for the Institute. While the scientists could dismiss the views of the antivivisectionists camped outside and ridicule the activists, Flexner and the Rockefellers were ruffled, particularly by losing the support of the *Washington Post* and the *Herald*. Moreover, in New York, hearings were imminent on new legislation on animal experimentation. This Davis–Lee Bill was sponsored by the moderate Brooklyn Society for Prevention of Abuse in Animal Experiments and it obtained 700 doctors' signatures as sponsors.

Carrel's experiments had aroused public hostility. But soon after, it was another Carrel venture that won back public approval.

---

[42] Corner, *History* (note 4): 85, and for the New York antivivisection activity and the effects on the Institute, see Bernard Unti 'The doctors are so sure that they only are right' in Stapleton, *Tradition* (note 8): 175–89.

CHAPTER FOUR

Carrel Established

Public opinion changed in the Institute's favour when they had a stroke of luck. On 18 March 1908, Carrel was consulted urgently late at night by Adrian V.S. Lambert, a New York surgeon. Their five-day-old baby daughter was affected by melaena neonatorum, a serious blood disorder of the new-born in which the blood does not clot, and gives a potentially fatal diffuse gastro-intestinal bleeding.[1] Blood transfusion was not routinely attempted at that time, since fresh blood clotted in any tubing used for donation, and there were no methods of blood storage. The significance of the blood groups described by Landsteiner in 1901 was, perhaps surprisingly, still to be realised; when William Moss at Baltimore announced his own blood grouping system in 1910, he could only add cautiously that 'it may have practical application in the transfusion of blood from one individual to another'.[2]

The first successful attempts at direct human transfusion prior to Carrel's night-time consultation had been by George Crile in Cleveland

---

[1] Melaena neonatorum is now easily prevented by giving Vitamin K, but there was a high death rate at that time. Carrel's unmatched random blood transfusion from father to child had about a one in three risk of a serious reaction.

[2] New York's Mount Sinai Hospital did pioneering work in this heroic age of blood transfusion. By 1912, they were using syringes for blood transfusion, including the first direct matches, and these creditable local events are described in Richard Lewisohn (1943–44) 'The development of the technique of blood transfusion since 1907' *Journal of the Mount Sinai Hospital* 10, 605–22. The story of the Mount Sinai pioneering blood matching is told by R. Ottenberg and David Kaliski (1913) 'Accidents in transfusion' *JAMA*, 61, 2138–40.

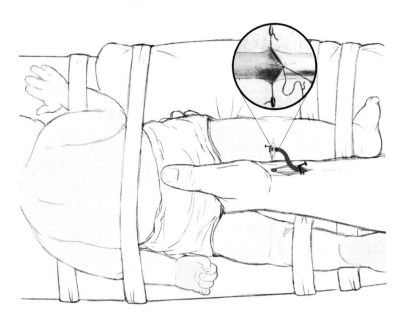

Carrel used Crile's method of direct blood transfusion in an infant, obtaining arterial blood from an adult donor. (*Courtesy of James G. Chandler, J. Vasc. Surg. 56 (2012): 1173–77.*)

three years earlier.[3] Crile was one of the admiring surgical group who visited Carrel's lab in Chicago in 1905 and, having seen Carrel's method of joining blood vessels, Crile realised that the method could be used for person-to-person blood transfusion, thus avoiding the clotting of blood during transfer. He promptly tried it in December 1905, but had poor results with his first two attempts.

The New York doctors who called in Carrel knew that human transfusion was possible in this way, as shown by Crile, and that Carrel could do it routinely in animals. Carrel normally had little interest in doing

---

[3] See N. Nathoo (2009) 'The first direct blood transfusion: the forgotten legacy of George W. Crile' *Operative Neurosurgery* 64, 20–27. In a further four attempts at direct human transfusion, Crile instead connected the donor and recipient vessels over a short connecting tube. Watts at Hopkins in February 1907 made four attempts with direct vessel stitching, obtaining good flow in two cases. See Stephen H. Watts (1907) 'The suture of blood vessels. Implantation and transplantation of vessels and organs. An historical and experimental study' *Bulletin of the Johns Hopkins Hospital* 18, 153–79.

human surgery, and was not licensed to operate in New York, but in this serious situation, he agreed to attempt the operation on the baby. On this occasion, the legal niceties were partly dealt with, since George E. Brewer, surgeon to Roosevelt Hospital, was present and did the preparatory surgical dissection of the two vessels for Carrel to use. Father Lambert was to be the blood donor, and Lambert's brothers Samuel and Alexander were present, as was Tom Painter, the obstetrician involved. With the father resting on the dining room table, the flaccid baby was placed close by on an ironing board and, though lightly secured, required no anaesthetic. An artery at Dr. Lambert's left wrist was mobilised under local anaesthetic and divided, using his left arm in case the hand was endangered. The popliteal vein behind the child's knee was mobilised and divided — said by a witness, to be 'like a match stick and the texture of wet cigarette paper'. Carrel then took over the challenge of joining the two blood vessels. It was a tricky task to carry out in a fraught atmosphere in the crowded room with poor lighting. But Carrel successfully joined the artery and the vein, at the third attempt.[4]

With the clamps released, blood flowed, the baby's colour quickly improved and she began to struggle. In awe of the achievement and unable to gauge how much blood had been given, the group were a little late in clamping and tying off the vessels. The blood in the surgical wound of the baby's leg began to clot and the bowel bleeding stopped. Dr. Lambert's hand also survived.[5]

---

[4] The events were related by the baby's uncle in Samuel W. Lambert (1908) 'Melaena neonatorum with report of a case cured by transfusion' *Medical Record* 73, 885–7. Carrel published a personal account of the transfusion of the baby later in a Lyon journal — 'La transfusion direct du sang (Méthode de Crile) *Lyon Chirurgical* 1, (1908): 13–19. See also J.G. Walker (1973) 'Carrel's transfusion of a five day old infant' *Surgery, Gynecology & Obstetrics* 137, 494–6 and T.W. Clark (1949) 'The birth of transfusion' *Journal of the History of Medicine* 4, 337–8.

[5] Adrian Lambert remained a friend of Carrel, and in 1917 translated, from the French, a short book co-authored by Mme Anne Carrel on the Carrel-Dakin method of managing war wounds. Lambert soon after was appointed as attending surgeon to Carrel's War Demonstration Hospital in 1918 — see Chapter 9.

Word Spreads

The story reached the newspapers immediately and the *New York World* on 20 March 1908 reported on the operation of two nights previously.

> Physicians and surgeons are discussing with keenest interest an operation recently performed by Dr. Alexis Carrel, head of the Rockefeller Institute, on the little daughter of Dr. Adrian V.S. Lambert, of Number 29 West Thirty-sixth street, which they regarded as most convincing proof of the value of vivisection. Antivivisectionists are centring their attack on the Rockefeller Institute and the fact that the operation was performed by one of the leading surgeons connected with it gives it a peculiar significance. …
>
> Dr. Carrel was called in when the life of the child was despaired of. The only possible hope lay in transfusion of blood. Dr. Lambert, the child's father, volunteered to give all of his own blood that was necessary to save the child's life and Dr. Carrel undertook the operation in spite of the slight chance there appeared to be of success.
>
> Friends of Dr. Carrel, who declined with some abruptness to discuss the case, say that the operation would have been out of the question except for the skill gained from many similar operations on the lower animals.

Doubtless, the 'friends' who spoke with such authority and detail to the newspaper were Carrel or Flexner, who shrewdly used this chance to brief the newspaper and make the case for animal experiments. Even the *Washington Post* was impressed. Their article was headlined 'Father's Blood Saves Baby: Vivisectionists Point With Pride To Rare Operation', and the paper accepted that since the child was little bigger than a cat, the necessary human surgery needed practice on the cats.

This episode gave Carrel and the Institute favourable exposure and some relief from the antivivisectionists who were pursuing them. It also gave Carrel the admiration of Rockefeller senior, who received a memorandum on the events from Gates and a picture of the thriving baby from Mrs. Lambert. Next year, Rockefeller's reminiscences included a tribute to Carrel's achievement.[6]

---

[6] John D. Rockefeller, *Random Reminiscences of Men and Events* (New York: Doubleday Page, 1909): 149–51.

The nocturnal triumph was timely. The Rockefellers, father and son, perhaps concerned at the time that the Institute was getting a bad press, were reassured. Nor were the lessons lost on the politicians in New York, then under pressure to bring in legislation to limit surgical operations on animals. The rescue of the Lambert baby changed the issues in the debate.[7]

Legislation Stalls

In the week following the baby's transfusion, on 28 March, the New York state legislature committee had before it the Davis–Lee bills which would have placed limits on animal experiments in New York State. Adrian Lambert, the baby's father, testified to this Albany committee and told the now well-known story of Carrel's remarkable operation. Lambert stressed that it had only been possible using skills gained from animal experiments. Flexner and others testified to the Committee and added that animal use was essential for vaccine and antitoxin production to control the major infectious diseases of the day. In spite of this impressive attack on the Bill, it did progress towards consideration, but ran out of time.

When it returned, next year, it failed to pass the Committee stage. In summer 1909, there was an arson attack on the Institute's New Jersey farm which killed many animals. Those involved were never traced, and antivivisectionist action thereafter faded for a while.

Lectures and Leg Grafts

With his high profile, Carrel was now increasingly invited to speak at medical and scientific meetings. In this year of 1908, he spoke at the American Medical Association in Chicago in June, and at the Clinical Congress of Surgeons of North America at Philadelphia in autumn. In Philadelphia, he also addressed the American Philosophical Society in November.

---

[7] Carrel carried out a similar operation on another doctor's baby in 1909, and the surgeon Dr. Roy McClure, from Hopkins, visiting for a year in 1908, did other similar transfusions in New York for Carrel.

At the June 1908 meeting of the AMA he gave a wide-ranging lecture, including an account of new experiments on storing tissue in the cold.[8] He also described transplants of spleen and intestine and, in a bit of surgical showmanship, he described an ear transplant in a dog comprising the ear, scalp and other tissue supplied from the external carotid artery.[9]

But Carrel had even more startling news for the meeting. He announced that he had successfully grafted legs between dogs. In a confident mood, he said limb grafts were 'much simpler than the transplantation of a gland, since the structures were less delicate'. He told the delegates that there was 'no reason why the leg or arm of an animal or human being could not be transplanted successfully on another animal of the same species or another human being'. Carrel had made a considerable effort with leg grafting over the last three years, and it was his favourite procedure in this period. He was skilled at joining the blood vessels, but there were other hurdles. Uniting the femurs of the graft and host had been difficult, and he eventually used a nail within the bone marrow cavity.[10] In May 1907 he had written from the Institute to Guthrie:

> The technique of the transplantation of the thigh from dog to another is very nearly perfect. I found a simple manner to fix the thigh. But the suture of the bone is not yet strong enough. Nevertheless, I was able lately to keep a white dog with a black thigh alive for ten days with an excellent circulation.[11]

But one discouragement would be concealed from non-medical audiences. The biggest hurdle, obvious to surgeons, was that the divided

---

[8] His lecture was published on 14 November 1908 as Alexis Carrel (1908) 'Results of transplantation of blood vessels, organs and limbs' *JAMA* 51, 1662–7, plus a discussion on p. 1676. He also gave the leg graft results briefly in two French journals at this time.
[9] A picture of the ear-grafted dog is found in the article in *McClure's Magazine* (note 17).
[10] He used an 'Elsberg's aluminium splint' inside the bone, an idea from Charles A. Elsberg, a young local New York surgeon, later a neurosurgeon. It is usually said that such intra-medullary nailing did not enter human or veterinary practice until introduced by Gerald Küntscher in Germany in 1942.
[11] S.P. Harbison (1962) 'Origins of vascular surgery: the Carrel-Guthrie letters' *Surgery* 52: 406–18.

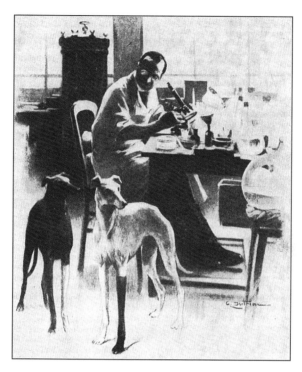

Carrel's leg transplants in dogs were failures, but caught the public imagination. (*Lectures pour tous, 1913.*)

nerves in the dog's leg, even though joined to the corresponding cut nerves in the graft, would re-grow only slowly or poorly into the new leg, at about only 1 mm a day. No muscle function or sensation would exist after operation, and the leg would be useless and certainly unable to bear weight. Added to this, management of the dogs after the surgery was difficult. The disabled dog, fretting about the useless leg, had to be nursed and restrained in a special hammock, holding it off the ground in the post-operative period.

The Washington Post somehow got hold of the text of his AMA presentation, and now supported Carrel — 'Grafted New Leg On Dog' ran the headline on 4 June 1908. The story was syndicated widely from Washington, appearing, for instance, in Ohio's *Hamilton Telegraph*, the *San Antonio Light* and California's *Woodland Daily Democrat*.

In the autumn, Carrel's address to the meeting of the American Philosophical Society was at the invitation of William Keen, the Philadelphia surgeon, who was president of the Society that year, and one of Carrel's admirers. Carrel's presentations that year were illustrated with lantern slides, a novelty at the time, reflecting Carrel's interest in photography from his Lyon days. In Philadelphia, he went over much the same ground as in the AMA lecture, and showed these pictures of the leg grafts in the dogs.[12] Next day, his address was given in some detail in the *New York Times*, with approval.

Shortly after the meeting, Keen was taken aback to hear that British newspapers had reported on the meeting at Philadelphia saying that Carrel 'had carried out new astonishing operations'. The London medical journal *The Lancet* was curious and, wishing to have the medical details, wrote to Keen, asking what had actually been said. Keen was embarrassed at this international press attention and wrote to Carrel advising him to discuss such publicity with Flexner. Flexner, unlike the surgeon, was unconcerned.

Further Publicity

The New York Times decided that the time had come for a full account of America's new surgical hero. On Sunday 15 November 1908, one week after their coverage of the Philadelphia meeting, the *Times* magazine section carried a long article headed 'The Marvels Wrought By Plastic Surgery'. It spoke of Carrel as 'assailed in vain by the most bitter of the anti-vivisectionists' but 'avoiding publicity and appearing at only rare intervals before some ultra-scientific body … the world hears little of his work'.

In the article, Flexner's work on meningitis was also highlighted and the case for use of animals in research was made again. The two-page spread read like an interview with Flexner and Carrel, but instead used quotes from Carrel's articles, or from the now-growing newspaper

---

[12] Alexis Carrel (1908) 'Further studies on transplantation of vessels and organs' *Proceedings of the American Philosophical Society* 47, 677–98. This is the only description of his leg grafting method, and Carrel never published the results in full. The *NYT* carried the story on this Philadelphia talk on 8 November 1908.

clippings file on Carrel. The American press now knew that they had a star, a man who could transplant organs, glands and even legs, and one who offered good news about the new and exciting possibilities of medical science.[13] The populist *The American* could announce that 'at the Rockefeller Institute they cut off a leg, put it in cold storage for a week and then sew it on again, and it knits, and heals, and is alive'.[14]

It was unusual for a surgeon to have such a high profile. Medical practitioners' strict professional code on advertising and publicity obliged them to shun the press. When the *New York Herald* correctly reported in 1912 that Cushing had done a pituitary gland transplant, Johns Hopkins firmly denied that the operation had been carried out. But the same restrictions did not apply to Carrel. He was a scientist doing surgery rather than a practising surgeon doing research. With the newspapers tapping into the view that scientists were an important source of new knowledge and power, a surgical scientist like Carrel was seen by the press as doubly blessed. Carrel was useful to them. Moreover, the dark, irresponsible side of transplantation, as seen in H.G. Wells' 1896 novel *The Island of Dr. Moreau*, seemed absent. Carrel might be wizard, but he was not seen as a latter-day Frankenstein.

Carrel now had the ultimate stamp of a celebrity: he was increasingly known only by his surname. He seems to have enjoyed the exposure, which other scientists chose to avoid. He employed a press cutting agency in both New York and Paris and regularly had personal studio photographic portraits taken.[15] One surgeon noticed Carrel's increasingly high profile, but approved. George Crile, who had pioneered the direct transfusion

---

[13] Carrel still had a lowly place in the Institute hierarchy; the salaries in 1908 were Flexner ($10,000), Opie ($5,000), Levene ($4,000), Meltzer ($3,500), Jobling ($2,000), Noguchi ($2,000), Auer ($2,000) and Carrel ($1,800). Carrel's salary as an associate was raised to $2,500 in 1908, to $3,000 next April and to $5,000 in June of 1910. He still had only a staff of two nurses and two skilled attendants.

[14] *The American* quoted in the *Washington Post*, 2 December 1910.

[15] Carrel collected his press cuttings using these agencies from 1908 onwards, and his archives show six press stories in that year, rising sharply to 96 in 1909, of which three-quarters were from French newspapers, falling next year, but rising sharply in his Nobel Prize year of 1912.

method, wrote in 1908 to Carrel supporting him, and, hinting that there was criticism, reassured him that 'men of prominence like you have to pay the penalty of celebrity. What is the art of writing for, if not to approach men with ideas?'[16]

Institute Action

After this favourable autumn of 1908, early in 1909 the Institute felt that the pressure on them was lifting, and decided to be proactive and provide some favourable coverage for the public. The Institute make themselves available to the serious-minded *McClure's Magazine*. It was a curious choice, because this journal had been first to use investigative 'muckraking' journalism, and had serialised Ida Tarbell's hostile account of Rockefeller's businesses. But the Institute clearly controlled the content of the article and had provided illustrations and portraits. The 16-page scholarly article by Burton J. Hendrick, normally a sceptical investigative journalist, shows Flexner's influence. Entitled 'Work at the Rockefeller Institute', it was sub-titled 'The Transplanting of Organs'.[17] The article starts with a detailed insider history of the Institute, with details of the founders and trustees. Carrel's experiments, including his blood vessel, kidney and leg grafts occupy most of the text, with only brief accounts of the work of others. A portrait was provided of Carrel, plus an image of his female assistant holding the kidney-grafted dog and a picture of a black donor leg grafted onto a pale dog. For those aware of surgical history, this recalled the miraculous grafting in mediaeval times, of a black human leg to a white recipient, carried out with the posthumous assistance of Saints Cosmas and Damian.[18] The article shows that while Flexner had been prominent as America's own microbe hunter, Carrel was now being put forward as the public face of the Rockefeller Institute.

---

[16] Crile to Carrel, 1 December 1908, Malinin Collection of the Papers of Alexis Carrel and Charles Lindbergh, box 1 folder 4, FA 208, Rockefeller University Archives Centre (RUA RAC).

[17] *McClure's Magazine*, February 1909, vol. 32, 367–83.

[18] See *Lectures pour tous* 1913, and for a full account of the leg graft miracle see David Hamilton, *A History of Organ Transplantation* (Pittsburgh: Pittsburgh University Press, 2012): 5–6.

The magazine supported the need for animal experimentation and Flexner dealt with the sensitive matter of where the Institute obtained experimental dogs and cats. For the Rockefeller dogs, it was a good death, Flexner said, ending a miserable life since they were 'half-starved, homeless, marauding animals given a good home and terminated eventually with chloroform, not suffocated as in the public pounds'.

The content of the *McClure's* article soon reached the pages of many city and small town newspapers throughout America.

Public Involved

Because of the publicity, Carrel increasingly received letters from the American public, including enquiries about limb transplants. Letters also

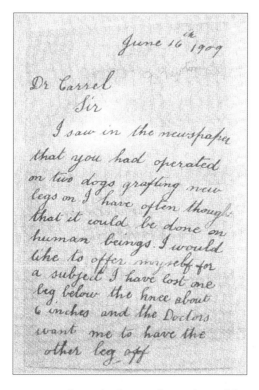

Carrel's public prominence brought letters from the public requesting leg or organ grafts. (*Courtesy of the Georgetown University Library, Booth Family Center for Special Collections.*)

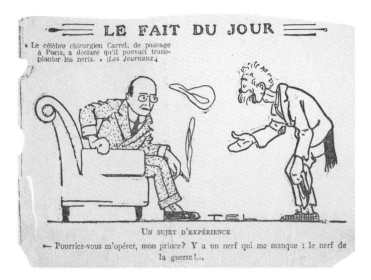

French newspapers followed Carrel's work closely, and liked his proposals for nerve grafting. (*Courtesy of the Georgetown University Library, Booth Family Center for Special Collections.*)

came from France, Germany, Spain and even New Zealand, and by 1914, his archives show about 200 enquiries about limb transplants. In addition, his mail increasingly included enquiries on other medical matters, and there were offers of blood donation or offers of the writer's body after death, and some correspondents offered kidneys for sale. Brain transplants were requested to treat mental deficiencies, and new eyes or enlargement of sexual organs might be sought. He and his secretary patiently dealt with the letters, using a standard reply, reasonably declining to help on the grounds that Carrel was not a licensed surgeon, and that the work was as yet experimental. Occasionally he offered to send word if there were any helpful developments. Other approaches came from cranks and disturbed persons who might call in looking for Carrel. One asked for Carrel at the Institute, and before the request could be dealt with, he committed suicide with cyanide in the Institute's entrance hall.

In France, Carrel was now well enough known for his work to be included in Maurice Renard's novel *Le Docteur Lerne* of 1908, in which a skilled Paris surgeon works in a secretive establishment where animal parts, including brains, are transplanted to humans and vice versa. Renard took his task seriously when producing his 'scientific-marvellous' novels, which he proposed should be 'forcefully convincing by their very rationality'. Carrel would appear more explicitly in Renard's later highly successful novel *Les Mains d'Orlac* of 1921, involving hand grafting.[19]

Caution Required

Flexner had used Carrel's work to boost the Institute and was pleased with the credit Carrel brought in. But he now feared an overkill, aware of the fickleness of the press. He wrote privately to the editor of the *New York Times* on 24 June 1909 saying:

> Dr. Carrel's work has been sufficiently presented in popular literature in this country to satisfy all reasonable demands and interest concerning it, and I do not therefore approve of any further publication at present in the press of his work.[20]

Shortly after, when travelling in Europe as usual in the summer of 1909, Carrel survived what might have been a public relations disaster. That summer, he commented in Paris on the new French Cala Law, which proposed that criminals facing the death penalty should, instead of execution, be handed over to doctors for risky human experiments. Approving of this, Carrel told the papers that he hoped that some American states might follow and meet the needs of surgeons by providing doomed human subjects for experiments. This use-of-prisoners story went no further.[21]

Flexner had another reason to clamp down on Institute stories, since his own high profile had caused local annoyance. Flexner was seen as the

---

[19] Carrel's fencing partner Arthur Train was displeased to see that this novel borrowed heavily from his novel *Mortmain* of 1907.

[20] Flexner to *New York Times*, 24 June 1909, Flexner Administrative Correspondence, box 43 folder 39, FA 138, RUA RAC (note 16).

[21] 'Would Experiment On Condemned Men' *NYT,* 25 July 1909.

man with the cure for meningitis, but there was an effective serum available in New York, prepared earlier in the public health laboratory headed by the talented Dr. William Hallock Park. Park had responsibility for New York's health, which was not Flexner's role. About this time there was a stormy meeting between Park and Flexner, and Park later went public with a complaint in the *New York Evening Post* about the 'so-called Flexner serum', detailing a 'Rockefeller campaign of publicity' which had marginalised Park's contribution.[22]

Flexner would vary in his attitude to publicity over the coming years, but at a high level in the Institute, it was still welcomed. Frederick Gates was still keen to have the exposure, and as late as 1915, he could urge Flexner to spread the word:

> You announce a discovery here. Before night your discovery will be flashed round the world. In thirty days it will be in every college on earth. In sixty days it will be at the bedsides of the best hospitals, and from these hospitals it will work its way to every sickroom.[23]

Institute Visitors

Carrel had many followers, and was a welcome addition to the American surgical community. He had many letters requesting details of his methods and particularly about the needles and thread he used. Visitors were made welcome, and he enjoyed showing his surgical operations to surgeons like J.B. Murphy, Rudolf Matas, Cushing, and Crile. Walter B. Cannon at Harvard sent a staff member to learn Carrel's blood vessel suturing methods, and Halsted sent Roy McClure from Baltimore to be trained. But few thereafter persevered with his techniques, either losing interest or having no suitable human cases to operate on. However, when

---

[22] Park and Flexner correspondence, Confidential Papers, FA 913, box 2 folder 11, RUA RAC (note 16). For the long-running tension between Flexner and Park, see Wade W. Oliver, *The Man Who Lived for Tomorrow: A Biography of William Hallock Park M.D.* (New York: E.P. Dutton & Co, 1941): 298–304.

[23] George W. Corner, *A History of the Rockefeller Institute 1901–1953: Origins and Growth* (New York: Rockefeller Institute Press, 1964): 159.

back in Baltimore, McClure eventually convinced Cushing to use a vein graft to by-pass the block in a hydrocephalic patient.

Surgeons from Europe were made welcome, and in this age of sea travel, New York was the portal of entry and even those heading elsewhere in America would call in to the nearby Institute. There was an important visit by Emil Kocher's surgeon son in May 1907, just before Carrel started to question Kocher senior's claims for success with human thyroid homografts. Théodore Tuffier from Paris visited New York for some weeks, and he returned later to work successfully with Carrel in the Institute in 1913 on experimental heart surgery. Hogarth Pringle from Scotland arrived in 1910 and on return to Glasgow carried out a successful vein graft in the Carrel manner to replace a leg aneurysm. The arrival of the French surgeon Samuel Pozzi (1846–1918) in 1909 added a frisson to life at the Institute, since he brought along his mistress, the actress Sarah Bernhardt (1844–1923), still glamorous at the age of 65. She toured holding the arm of Simon Flexner with her dog held on the other arm, and with Noguchi following carrying her feather boa. Sarah was impressed with Carrel and told the press afterwards that he was 'A charming man … the vivacity of his movements, the fire of youth in his quick glance, his penetrating voice … the apostle of 'everything is possible''.[24] Lyon's Mathieu Jaboulay, his mentor earlier, came to the Institute in 1908, and in Lyon he had attempted the first-ever human kidney transplants two years earlier, in January and April 1906; doubtless they discussed these cases in detail.[25]

These visits also gave surgical opportunities. With Jaboulay in New York, the two surgeons 'together examined a human ateriovenous anastomosis', suggesting that they or someone else in New York had tried this operation, probably joining the femoral artery to the femoral vein hoping to increase blood flow to a leg — the strategy long favoured by Jaboulay. There was a similar event when René Leriche, Carrel's old pupil,

---

[24] Press cutting, box 72 folder 119, Alexis Carrel Papers, Georgetown University Library, Booth Family Center for Special Collections (GULBFC).

[25] For Jaboulay's visit, see the Scientific Reports to the Corporation and the Board of Scientific Directors of the Rockefeller Institute for Medical Research, April 1909, box 1 vol. 2 p. 45, FA 145, RUA RAC (note 16).

now well established in Lyon, visited in 1909, and they did 'an arteriotomy in a case of acute arteritis', probably exploration of a blocked artery with removal of clot.

A similar consultation came when Carrel visited Lyon in 1908. He and Leriche tried to deal with an urgent vascular problem, with Poncet and Jaboulay watching and Léon Berard assisting them. The patient was a young woman with a gangrenous leg caused by taking ergot to cause an abortion. The main artery was explored behind the knee and clot removed with initial good return of pulsation. Two days later they removed further clot at three levels, but amputation had to follow. The procedure was carefully described in a Lyon journal. Berard added a commentary about his own experience in 10 similar cases, reporting poor results. He suggested that Carrel's use of a vein graft was the best solution if the position of the block could be found.[26]

Guthrie in St. Louis

By 1909, Carrel's increasingly high profile did not please some, and one man in particular, and he soon said so publically. Charles C. Guthrie, who had been close to Carrel in Chicago earlier, had moved to St. Louis, and had continued with vascular surgery projects, publishing in a low-profile manner and eventually producing his substantial work *Blood-Vessel Surgery and Its Applications* in 1912.[27] He and Carrel kept in touch

[26]This article by Leon Bérard and J. Arnaud appeared in '*Theses de Lyon*' December 1909, p. 80: there is a translation in Angelo M. May and Alice G. May, *The Two Lions of Lyons* (Rockville MD: Kabel Publishing, 1994): 105–7.

[27]Charles Claude Guthrie, *Blood-Vessel Surgery and Its Applications* (London: Edward Arnold, 1912). This book was in the series 'International Medical Monographs', edited by the British physiologists Leonard Hill and William Bulloch, who asked Guthrie, now in Pittsburgh, to write this volume for the series. It is curious that Guthrie rather than Carrel was chosen. Guthrie's text showed some disdain by playing down Carrel's original Lyon method. He even attributes the triangulation method to 'Frovin', i.e. the Paris surgeon Frouin, who described the method to a Brussels meeting in 1904. Guthrie ignored Carrel's famous paper and its illustration published two years earlier. Guthrie's

INTERNATIONAL MEDICAL MONOGRAPHS
General Editors { LEONARD HILL, M.B., F.R.S.
{ W. BULLOCH, M D.

BLOOD-VESSEL SURGERY
AND ITS APPLICATIONS

BY

CHARLES CLAUDE GUTHRIE, M.D., PH.D.

PROFESSOR OF PHYSIOLOGY AND PHARMACOLOGY, UNIVERSITY OF PITTSBURGH; FORMER
PROFESSOR OF PHYSIOLOGY AND PHARMACOLOGY, WASHINGTON UNIVERSITY; INSTRUCTOR
IN PHYSIOLOGY, UNIVERSITY OF CHICAGO; DEMONSTRATOR OF PHYSIOLOGY,
WESTERN RESERVE UNIVERSITY, ETC.

ILLUSTRATED

LONDON
EDWARD ARNOLD
NEW YORK: LONGMANS, GREEN & CO.
1912
[All rights reserved]

Charles Guthrie continued his experimental blood vessel surgery studies in an unostentatious way in Pittsburgh.

initially. But Guthrie did not have Carrel's unerring sense of the way forward, as judged by later events, and began to lose his way. Guthrie was convinced that homografts did survive, and soon was into deep water, claiming that ovaries transplanted from one animal to another would not only survive, but support pregnancies. This was a serious claim, which opened up important vistas, not least in dealing with human infertility, but his experiments were flawed and criticised.[28] In other homograft

book was reprinted in 1959 with an added commentary by the editors Samuel P. Harbison and Bernard Fisher.

[28] Guthrie was rebuked at a meeting at Yale in 1910; see C.B. Davenport (1910) 'Inheritance of plumage colour in poultry' *PSEBM* 7, 168. Guthrie's unfortunate claims for ovary homograft survival in chickens were either the result of incomplete removal of

work, Guthrie also described a tasteless experiment in which he grafted a dog's head and neck onto another dog, with apparent short-term success.[29] It is a tribute to Guthrie that this operation was concealed from journalists; it is also a tribute to Carrel that he did not follow this unfortunate lead.

Nevertheless, in 1907 it was Guthrie who helped unravel the mystery about the fate of homografts. Homograft blood vessels from one animal to another seemed to survive well, and this suggested that other homografts would also do so. Guthrie now showed that if artery homografts were treated with formaldehyde before grafting — a treatment which completely 'fixed' and destroyed the cells — the vessel grafts were still as successful.[30] The homograft vessels were not homografts at all: they were simply useful inert tubes.

Guthrie Takes Offence

By this time, Guthrie was again nursing some resentment towards Carrel, dating back to their earlier joint Chicago work. After Guthrie left for St. Louis, Carrel had published his important 1906 Johns Hopkins lecture alone, and this added to Guthrie's hurt. Carrel's increasingly high public profile now offended Guthrie, and he wrote to Carrel in 1908 making the slightly ambiguous comment that 'your name rivals the President'.[31] Guthrie then noticed that in Carrel's American Medical Association lecture published on 14 November 1908, Carrel credited a paper by New

---

all recipient ovarian tissue, or faulty in-breeding of the experimental animals; see Hamilton *Transplantation* (note 18): 85.

[29] For an account of Guthrie's two-headed dog and the similar much-publicised experiments by Vladimir Demikhov in Moscow in 1959, see Blair O. Rogers (1959) 'Charles Claude Guthrie, M.D. PhD: a remarkable pioneer in tissue and organ transplantation' *Plastic and Reconstructive Surgery* 24, 380–3.

[30] Guthrie announced in September 1907 that arteries rendered cell-free by formalin treatment could be successful grafts. See C.C. Guthrie (1907) 'Heterotransplantation of blood vessels' *American Journal of Physiology* 19, 482–7 and C.C. Guthrie (1908) 'Transplantation of formaldehyde-fixed blood vessels' *Science* 27, 473, an article published on 20 March 1908.

[31] Guthrie to Carrel, 15 January 1908, Malinin Collection, folder 18 box 2, FA 208, RUA RAC (note 16).

York's Levin and Larkin with showing that formalin-treated vessels would serve well as grafts. The last straw for Guthrie was that Levin and Larkin said their successful surgery was due to the 'fine technique elaborated by Carrel'.[32]

Guthrie, always touchy, was looking for a fight. He now made a public complaint early in 1909 in the journal *Science*. He said that Carrel had ignored his crucial earlier success with formaldehyde-treated grafts. Moreover, Levin and Larkin were also wrong, Guthrie said, to credit Carrel with developing successful blood vessel surgery methods, since he, Guthrie, had made a vital contribution. Guthrie then added this stinging rebuke:

> The dubious distinction of *priority* which it would appear is the goal sought by some of our contemporaries, presents slight attraction to the sincere investigator whose reward largely is the consciousness that his labors may in the end add a line to the encyclopaedia of science.[33]

Guthrie had not yet gained a line in the encyclopaedia of science. Though he would gain some later, Guthrie correctly sensed that, at the time, he was being written out of the story of early blood vessel surgery. Carrel had to respond and wrote privately to Guthrie:

> 8 January 1909
> My dear Dr. Guthrie:
> I am very sorry that you feel so badly about the part of my [*JAMA*] article which deals with yours and Dr. Levin's experiments on the transplantation of devitalised vessels. While writing these lines, I was more interested by the histological than by the clinical side of the question, and therefore I gave more importance to the work of Dr. Levin, whose histological sections I had carefully examined. But if I had supposed that you considered that questions of formalised vessels as so important I would have taken more care of the ordinance of my sentences....

---

[32] Isaac Levin and John H. Larkin (1907–8) 'Transplantation of devitalised arterial segments' *PSEBM* 5, 109–11.

[33] See C.C. Guthrie (1909) 'On misleading statements' *Science* 29, 29–31. The editor's acceptance of this unusual personal complaint suggests that Carrel had other critics.

I hope that you shall recover soon. I remain very sincerely yours,
Alexis Carrel.

Their contact ceased; Guthrie did not 'recover'. Years later, Guthrie was unrepentant and remarked that Carrel's 'pre-eminence in publicity and personal promotion attributes have been widely internationally demonstrated'.[34]

Homograft Failure Recognised

Guthrie's findings on the success of the formalin-treated 'dead' blood vessels were crucial for Carrel in resolving the homograft puzzle. Carrel increasingly considered that the failure of his grafted homograft cat kidneys and the leg grafts after two weeks was not from infection or technical problems but was to be expected and was a biological mechanism not previously described. Carrel's perceptiveness was taking him towards a crucial new paradigm, later accepted — that all homografts are rejected. A constraint had been that blood vessel homografts seem to survive; this finding was no longer relevant. One remaining problem was Emil Kocher's claims for successful thyroid homografting in human patients. Carrel no longer believed the results from the eminent Swiss surgeon. At a symposium in Pittsburgh in 1909, Carrel was increasingly confident and boldly criticised Kocher, saying that his method 'had given few successes and many failures in Europe and in America'. Carrel explained that the thyroid homografts were destroyed through 'the action of the organism on the graft'.[35]

But it would be a long journey for Carrel. Not until 1911 was he confident that he had been looking at a new biological phenomenon. The teaching and textbooks of the day were of no assistance, nor was there a

---

[34] Hugh E. Stephenson Jr and Robert S. Kimpton, *America's First Nobel Prize in Medicine or Physiology: The Story of Guthrie and Carrel* (Boston: Midwestern Vascular Surgery Society, 2001): 158–64. In 1935, Guthrie was asked to make nominations for the Nobel Prize, and he took this opportunity to make further detailed complaints about Carrel.

[35] Proceedings of the Pittsburgh Academy of Medicine: Symposium on the Thyroid Gland, 9 February 1909, *Surgery Gynecology & Obstetrics* 8, (1909): 606–12.

word for this homograft loss. 'Rejection' was the neologism to be used later, much later, in the 1950s. But others in Europe were also reaching this position, as were some journalists. The populist *Munsey's Magazine* in October 1911 was not impressed with Carrel's leg and organ grafts:

> The leg has never been shown to be more than a worthless appendage. He transplants kidney, spleens and other organs. He has never proved that they ever resumed normal function. Spectacular, Yes? Practical, No.

Carrel by this time may have privately agreed with this verdict.

Whatever the reason, Carrel now moved into other projects. He did no more such leg grafts after 1908 nor ever gave a full account of the work. Perhaps, following this slow and discouraging epiphany regarding graft loss, the idea of regrouping and studying this powerful, fundamental and mysterious mechanism did not attract him. His hazy ideas of 'immunising' animals to provide acceptable organs to use for human organ grafting, as suggested in his Hopkins lecture, might have been revived, but he did not make moves to consider this strategy.

Further Antivivisectionist Pressure

Early in 1910, there was a further brief controversy involving Carrel and animal experiments at the Institute. The pressure this time came from *The New York Herald*, now regularly supporting Mrs. Belais and the antivivisectionists. The *Herald's* owner, a dog-lover who brought his dogs to work, also had a grudge against the medical profession in New York, since they had successfully prevented his and other local newspapers carrying the advertisements for quack medicines which gave a steady source of revenue for his paper. The *Herald* revived the earlier claims of cruelty to animals at the Institute when it published allegations made by three former Institute animal house workers. Carrel's work figured prominently in the story.[36]

One complainant was a former animal house porter who alleged that he tried to rescue the dogs brought into the Institute by seeking their

---

[36] Corner *History* (note 23): 84.

owners before the dogs were used. The other witnesses alleged that living dogs were put into a refrigerator, that dogs were hit with fists, that scalding water was poured on the animals, and that animal experiments might be done solely as demonstrations for visitors. The newspaper's witnesses also claimed that the dog leg grafts never functioned properly.

The Institute was alarmed, and turned to Starr Murphy, Rockefeller senior's own attorney, for professional support. Murphy took formal statements from Institute staff, including Carrel, and they drew up a strong defence. In it they stated that stray dogs were indeed purchased and brought in, but the animal house staff were instructed to watch the 'Lost and Found' columns in the New York newspapers, and in this way many animals were returned to their owners. Cold (not hot) water was indeed splashed on dogs in the animal house, but as the usual strategy to separate fighting animals. Blows with the fist were used in theatre as the standard first step in resuscitation after cardiac arrest due to ether over-dosage. It was denied that there were demonstrations of animal surgery to visitors, who only witnessed routine experiments. The bodies of dead animals were indeed moved at night to a refrigerator.[37]

Flexner issued a carefully-worded statement on 17 January 1910 and went on the offensive to discredit the witnesses. Two of the complainants had been dismissed earlier from the Institute for 'good reason' and the *Herald*, they discovered, had paid for the witness's stories. Flexner added that one of the witnesses, while employed earlier, had even attempted to sell her neighbour's cat to the Institute. With this impressive rebuttal, there the matter ended, or almost ended. While the antivivisectionists did not pursue the complaints, the journal *Town Topics* of 24 February 1910 took a parting shot at Carrel, saying that:

> Grafting the ears of a donkey and the tail of a monkey upon Dr. Alexis Carrel would inflict unnecessary pain upon the other animals and would not make Dr. Carrel any more contemptible.

---

[37] These detailed witness statements are in Confidential Papers: Anti-vivisection, box 2 folder 1, FA 913, RUA, RAC (note 16).

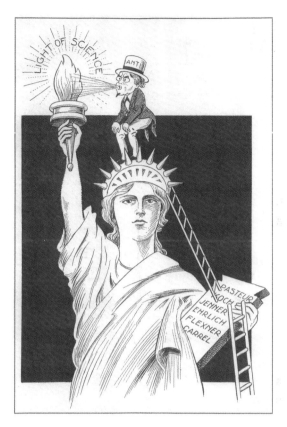

Many American newspapers had supported animal experimentation, and with Carrel's successes, now felt vindicated. (*From Medical Pickwick c1907.*)

Carrel's lawyer-author friend and fencing partner Arthur Train (now in practice as the firm of Train and Olney), advised him to sue — 'it costs nothing, give the damages to charity' — but Carrel did not do so. The outside pressure to limit animal experiments had lifted, and did not revive again for decades. Public opinion had rallied to the experts of the Progressive Era and it was assumed they could be trusted. The last public attack came at the International Antivivisection Congress held in Washington in December 1913, where a speaker attacked the 'Rockefeller jugglers with organs'.

New Directions

Perhaps daunted by finding that graft rejection was an almost universal mechanism, Carrel ceased his organ transplant experiments and in 1909–10 moved into a number of other projects. The year 1909 was not particularly productive, but he embarked on experiments on cold storage of tissues, particularly of blood vessels. This showed that 'tissue banking' was possible, and he made a short-lived effort to store and offer tissue for others to use.[38] Wound healing studies continued, and there was always surgery to do for the other staff. He started corneal grafting in April 1909, but then and later, infection was a problem, and despite his skill, the technique was taken little further. After his 1909 summer break, from autumn into 1910, Carrel energetically carried out a short, adventurous and visionary series of operations on the heart, which he revived in 1914, and these ventures are described together later.

One finding from the leg grafting difficulties still presented itself. Could divided nerves be encouraged to grow back faster? In spring 1910, he had sent a young man to another laboratory to study the growth of nerves when separated from the body. Carrel was soon off, as usual, to Europe, and may have planned to resume this work on nerve regeneration on his return. But when they met up in the autumn, his assistant had some dramatic news, namely that he could grow other kinds of cells outside the body. Carrel sensed the possibilities of this new venture. In a sudden change of direction, he largely left behind his vascular and transplant work. The new venture, soon called 'tissue culture', quickly attracted additional fame for Carrel, and, as always, involved him in new controversy.

Carrel's first moves had been made one year earlier.

---

[38] Alexis Carrel (1910) 'Latent life of arteries' *JEM* 12, 460–65. Soon after, this work encouraged the important development, at the Institute, of methods for cold storage of blood.

CHAPTER FIVE

The Birth of Tissue Culture

In autumn 1909, pondering the challenge of the 'dead leg' in his leg-grafted, disabled dogs, Carrel had decided to move into a study of nerve regeneration. After a nerve in the body is cut, the nerve fibres beyond the damage degenerate, since they are no longer connected to the nerve cell of origin in the spinal cord or brain. If accurate surgery is carried out, some re-growth of the nerve fibre down the old track may follow, slowly. On 2 September, Carrel wrote down his plan. He would try to speed up re-growth of cut nerves by applying various substances — enzymes, chemicals, extracts from young embryos or from glands or from 'rapidly growing tumours'. He then added that 'experiments *in vitro* can be performed by using the Harrison method'.[1]

He was referring to the work of Ross Harrison (1870–1959), the Yale biologist and embryologist, who in the previous year had given New York's annual prestigious Harvey Lecture. Harrison was involved in the important debate on how nerve fibres develop during foetal life in the tissues outside the spinal cord.[2] Some investigators thought that these peripheral nerve fibres arose first in the tissues and then connected up in both directions to join central cells in the spinal cord to the distant muscles and organs. Others considered instead that nerve fibres sprouted from cells in the cord

---

[1] Carrel note, 2 September 1909, Alexis Carrel Papers, box 89 folder 2, Georgetown University Library, Booth Family Center for Special Collections (GULBFC).
[2] See M. Abercrombie (1961) 'Ross Granville Harrison, 1870–1959' *Biographical Memoirs of Fellows of the Royal Society* 7: 111–26 and J.S. Nicholas (1961) 'Ross Granville Harrison 1870–1959: biographical memoir' (Washington: National Academy Sciences 35: 132–61).

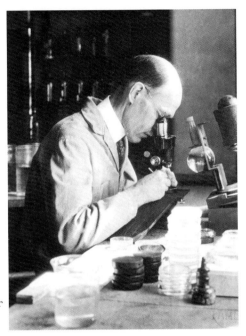

Ross Harrison at the Yale University Department of Biology. (*Courtesy of the National Library of Medicine.*)

and grew out to reach the target tissues. These earlier studies had been purely morphological, using only the microscopic appearances of the nerve fibres at various stages of development.

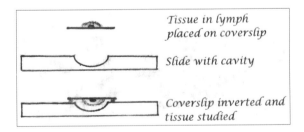

Tissue in lymph placed on coverslip

Slide with cavity

Coverslip inverted and tissue studied

Harrison's 'hanging drop' method used tissue fragments nourished by lymph on a cover slip inverted over a well in a microscope slide.

Harrison broke with this tradition, taking, for the first time, an experimental approach. He put a tiny piece of frog spinal cord into a drop of clotted frog tissue fluid (lymph) on a microscope slide's cover-slip, and,

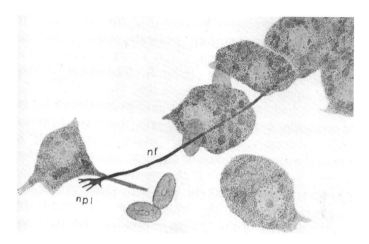

Harrison revolutionised biology by demonstrating new nerve fibres sprouting in culture from frog spinal cord cells. (From *Journal of Experimental Zoology 9, (1910), 787–846.*)

turning it over, placed the lymph drop over a hollow in a glass slide — his 'hanging drop' method. The cells within the lymph could be studied by microscopy over some days. He was rewarded by seeing outgrowth of fibres from the spinal cord fragment into the nutritive fluid. Harrison had settled the dispute on neural development, but he also offered a powerful new methodology for looking at cells. This shift was initially resisted by the criticism that tissues removed from their normal locus might behave in a different way and mislead the investigator. Harrison however won the argument, and his findings were deemed sufficiently important for him to be nominated for a Nobel Prize in 1917.[3]

Carrel's Interest

Harrison's technique for growing nerves outside the body was of interest to Carrel, since he was interested in factors which might speed up nerve regeneration. He arranged with Flexner that Montrose T. Burrows

---

[3] No award was made during WWI: Harrison was nominated again for a Nobel Prize in 1933 for his work in the field of 'asymmetry', but was again unsuccessful.

(1884–1947), a new arrival at the Institute, should go to work for a short time in the summer with Harrison. In Carrel's laboratory, Burrows had already started to look at degeneration of cut nerves and the effect of treatment of these nerves by possible stimulating substances.

Burrows, when he reached Yale, imaginatively improved on Harrison's method. Using frog tissues at first, he grew cells in serum separated from blood instead of lymph. With this change to a more easily obtained culture fluid, he switched to look at tissue taken from warm-blooded animals, and chose the chicken. He used chicken embryos taken from the egg and looked for nerve growth in his cultures. He wrote to Flexner asking for more time, since he had promised to return to finish up the study of the specimens resulting from the nerve stimulating studies. In spite of then being off work with a bad back for a while, at the end of August he reported good news to Flexner. 'All things hoped for came at the last minute. The [embryo] heart grew well, but no nerves seen.'[4] Burrows though initially disappointed had made a crucial observation. He had failed to grow nerves, but the chicken embryo heart cells continued to beat in hanging drops of serum. It was commonly supposed that heart cells were driven by their nerve supply; it was now clear that the heart cells instead had their own intrinsic ability to beat. This was a biological revelation of considerable importance.[5] And other cells might also survive.

Back to the Institute

Burrows brought his new skills and insights back to Carrel's laboratory. Carrel immediately put aside any plans for study of nerve regeneration and repair in his animals and promptly started to explore the other possibilities raised by Burrows' news. A spur to the work was that the 'microbe hunters' around Carrel at the Institute routinely grew and kept

---

[4] Burrows to Flexner, 23 August 1910, reel 19, Flexner American Philosophical Society, FA 746, Rockefeller Archives Centre (RUA RAC).

[5] For a detailed account, see the 'Historical Review' in Albert Fischer, *Tissue Culture: Studies in Experimental Morphology and General Physiology* (Copenhagen: Levin & Muksgaard, 1925): 19–33 which in turn credits Oppel's 'dramatic' account in *Gewebekulturen Sammlung Vieweg* (1914) heft 12.

pure strains of micro-organisms. If cells could be cultivated *in vitro* and kept for study like bacteria, important possibilities opened up. Carrel had pioneered the storage and preservation of tissues in latent life at low temperatures; cell cultivation seemed another approach to keeping tissue alive, but at normal temperatures. Added to this, the cell clumps perhaps offered a miniature test bed for seeking Lourdes-like acceleration of wound healing. Another factor may have been Carrel's old sensitivity to the jibe by Melzer at the Institute that he was merely an 'expert sew-er'. Burrows on his return had unexpectedly opened up a new prospect for Carrel on understanding cellular life and death. Carrel was also heeding the advice of the distinguished biologist Jacques Loeb, who had been appointed to the Institute at a senior level in that year, and who urged all biological phenomena should be reduced to the simplest systems of study, the 'reductionist' strategy.[6]

Carrel and Burrows moved with energy into attempts to grow a variety of tissues for extended periods. They quickly used the routine sub-culturing strategy of the Institute's bacteriologists, taking cells from the edge of the first growth and moving them in to fresh culture fluid; Carrel now made the dramatic claim that 'the cultivation of normal cells would appear to be no more difficult than the cultivation of many microbes'. Initially Carrel used the accurate word 'culture of' or 'cultivation of' cells, and only later did the inaccurate phrase 'tissue culture' gain acceptance. It was Burrows who first used this enduring phrase.[7]

---

[6] Jacques Loeb published his *Mechanistic Theory of Life* in 1912. His powerful reductionistic stance is portrayed in Sinclair Lewis's novel *Arrowsmith* (1925), and Loeb was famous for inducing unfertilised sea urchin eggs to develop by chemical means. Carrel, in his tissue culture papers, mentions Loeb's influence.

[7] For general accounts of tissue culture, see Hannah Landecker, *Culturing Life: How Cells Became Technologies* (Cambridge: Harvard University Press, 2010): 48; Frederick B. Bang (1977), 'History of tissue culture at Johns Hopkins' *Bulletin of the History of Medicine* 51: 516–37; and Hannah Landecker 'Building "A new type of body in which to grow a cell": Tissue culture at the Rockefeller Institute, 1910–1914' in Darwin H. Stapleton (ed.), *Creating a Tradition of Biomedical Research: Contributions to the History of The Rockefeller University* (New York: The Rockefeller University Press, 2004): 151–74.

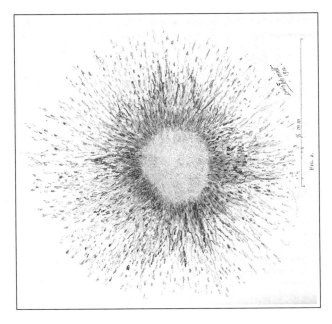

Carrel observed growth of cells from explants of tissue placed on silk gauze in hanging drops of culture medium. (*From Reference 32.*)

New Vistas

Carrel had a small laboratory staff available to move onto the new project, and new data emerged quickly. As when working with Guthrie years before, Carrel chose to publish rapidly on the new findings and offered the drafts of their articles to Harrison at Yale, telling him to telegraph back any corrections. But Harrison seemed to disapprove and did not cooperate. Later, Flexner wrote apologising to Harrison about the unseemly haste, excusing and explaining it by 'Carrel's exalted state of mind'.

Starting within weeks of Burrows' return to the Institute at the end of September, over the next two months, they sent off four short papers to the *Journal of the American Medical Association*, starting on 15 October, with Carrel as first author.[8] Carrel, as always, made Europeans aware of

---

[8]The Carrel and Burrows series of papers total only seven pages and were *JAMA* 55 (1910): 1379–81, *JAMA* 55 (1910): 1554, *JAMA* 55 (1910): 1732, *JAMA* 56 (1911): 32–3, with Carrel publishing alone in *JAMA* 57 (1911): 1611. Their first paper in 1911

his work and sent off the same data immediately to journals in France. In their first *JAMA* paper, they claimed not only success with cultivating thyroid cells, but also that organised thyroid gland structures appeared in these culture clumps. They also described cultivated kidney cells re-forming into kidney-like tubules. In their second paper two weeks later, on 29 October, they said that the Peyton Rous sarcoma, the famous chicken tumour studied at the Institute, would grow outside the body using their method. In a no-less dramatic claim two weeks later, they reported they had grown the cells of a human sarcoma.

But Carrel's confidence that routine long-term cell culture had arrived was premature: he had achieved only short periods of apparent survival of some cells. It was decades before thyroid, kidney or tumour cells were successfully cultivated for reasonable periods, and they never reorganised during culture as an organ. A later commentary on these events said Carrel's accounts of his experiments were 'dramatic and couched in such a way as to attract the maximum attention. ... In Carrel's case the drama is associated with a great deal of over-optimistic inaccuracy'.[9]

The newspapers picked up the cell cultivation story immediately, or were alerted to it. The first mention came in the *New York Times* of 20 October 1910, only five days after Carrel and Burrows' first published paper in *JAMA*. The *Times* reported enthusiastically 'Rockefeller Institute Announces Success Of Experiments Which May Revolutionise Surgery' and added a further subtitle 'May Bring A Cancer Cure'. The *Washington Post* carried the story one day earlier as 'Tissues Live In Jars', noting in passing Harrison's contribution and that, though working at Yale, he was originally from Baltimore nearby. The *Washington Post* carried a further story saying that the method would 'make possible to grow young men and create new forms of animal life'. The story spread to other city papers throughout America. As always, nothing was done by Carrel to discourage the coverage, and there were never any denials.

---

reported that plasma taken from chickens bearing the Rous sarcoma would prevent the growth of the sarcoma cells in culture; this important claim was never confirmed.
[9] Henry Harris, *The Cells of the Body* (Cold Spring Harbor: Cold Spring Harbor Press, 1995): 35.

For Ross Harrison, the pioneer, simply obtaining long survival of cells was of no interest. Carrel was opening up a quite different and important endeavour. Harrison understandably did not follow Carrel's lead in looking for prolonged survival, and was amused at the involvement of the press.

> The fact that tissues of the higher animals may be cultivated outside the body has been heralded in the newspapers and magazines as a notable, if not a revolutionary discovery. When we pause to consider this claim in the light of what has actually been accomplished, we find there is danger. ...[10]

Later Harrison called it the 'gold rush' to grow cells.[11]

Professional Tensions

The relationship between the work of Carrel, Burrows and Harrison is of interest, then and since. Because of its high profile, there were immediate allegations that Carrel failed to acknowledge Harrison's lead at Yale. Added to this was the New York gossip of the day that, when Burrows moved to Cornell University soon after, he had been encouraged to move out from the Institute to leave Carrel clearly in sole charge of the new important venture.[12]

On the question of priority, one of Harrison's colleagues immediately felt aggrieved and said so. Three days after Carrel and Burrows' first paper appeared in *JAMA*, Yale's Prof. Yandell Henderson, a senior figure in Harrison's university, wrote bluntly to Carrel about his concerns:

> I have seen the notices in the newspapers of your and Burrows' tissue culture. I followed Burrows work here [at Yale] last summer with

---

[10] Ross G. Harrison (1912) 'The cultivation of tissues in extraneous media' *Anatomical Record* 6: 181–93, at 181, Ross G. Harrison (1913) 'The life of tissues outside the organism from the embryological standpoint' *Transactions of the Congress of American Physicians and Surgeons* 9: 63–75 and Ross G. Harrison (1912) 'The cultivation of tissues in extraneous media' *Anatomical Record* 6: 181–93.
[11] See the lively account in 'Ross Granville Harrison' *Biographical Memoirs of Fellows of the Royal Society* 7 (1961): 110–26.
[12] Merrill Chase, later working at the Institute, told of this widely-held view of Carrel's actions (personal communication to the author).

interest. This morning I read your paper in the *Journal of the American Medical Association*. I am very much upset and distressed by it. It seems to me that an immense injustice is being done to Harrison, and that the Rockefeller Institute is claiming the credit for something that belongs to Harrison's department of this University. Now I cannot believe for an instant that you realise this. ... everyone (unless you correct the idea) will think that you supplied the brains and that Burrows did his part under your guidance, and this great thing will always in future be spoken of as <u>Carrel's</u> <u>discovery</u> [sic] ...[13]

Carrel replied stating in his defence that Harrison's work had been well known for five years and that he had carefully acknowledged it in their first paper. Carrel added disingenuously that he had been cultivating tissue within the whole body for years. But Henderson's premonition that Harrison would be written out of the story was correct. Soon after, Carrel's further public claims for the success of the method and his rapidly enlarging experience did indeed link his name firmly and forever with the technique. The controversy would linger on and was known abroad. A British surgeon noted the rumours saying that 'Carrel has ignored the many scurrilous attacks which have been made upon him personally and on his methods by the ignorant and timid'.[14]

An editorial in the *New York Times* two years later alluded to the criticism, but exonerated Carrel:

The honors which have been thrust upon him [Carrel] because of his marvellous accomplishments in surgery have awakened some professional jealousies both here and abroad, with the usual intimation that he has decked himself in others' feathers. In his published reports, Doctor Carrel has acknowledged the work of Leo Loeb of St. Louis, of Dr. Harrison of Yale. ... In this work Dr. Carrel owes much to his predecessors and contemporaries, but the broadening impetus imparted

---

[13] David Le Vay, *Alexis Carrel: The Perfectibility of Man* (Rockville MD: Kabel Publishing, 1996): 102. Henderson's use of 'tissue culture' suggests that the phrase was in common use at Yale.

[14] W. Arbuthnot Lane 'The award of the Nobel Prize to Dr Alexis Carrel' *The Lancet*, 12 October 1912, 1103.

to it by his original efforts, his genius, and his enthusiasm will not in any quarter be denied.[15]

Much later, Harrison's biographer alluded to these murmurings and said that 'Harrison himself did everything he could to correct the invidious rumours which accused Carrel of capitalising on his work'.[16]

Carrel's new method and the direction of his work were quite different from that of Harrison. Carrel's offence in the eyes of his scientist colleagues was different. His vigorous promotion of his work, the brevity of his publications and his public profile as a celebrity — a 'visible' scientist — were judged to be professionally unseemly.[17]

Technique Improves

Carrel's early method used fragments of tissue on silk discs in 'hanging drops' of plasma from which cells grew out as a widening clump into the nutritive fluid. It was not a culture of separated-out cells, as later. After a few days, the clump was subdivided and, freed from the old plasma, was moved to fresh plasma. He tried to irrigate the cultures to save the laborious sub-culturing, but had no success at this time. The area of growth could be traced and measured by microscopy, but quantification was awkward, and observer error was possible. Carrel's surgical training led him naturally to use scrupulously aseptic techniques, but infection of

---

[15] This curious *New York Times* editorial, supportive of Carrel, was clearly assisted by briefing from inside the Institute, and it has Simon Flexner's prose style. The occasion of the editorial was publication of *The American Yearbook* for 1912, which had an article on 'cultivating tissues' written by the Institute's Samuel Meltzer. He disloyally downplayed Carrel's work and instead emphasised the contributions earlier of Leo Loeb and Harrison, again suggesting personal tension within the Institute.

[16] Nicholas, *Harrison* (note 2): 149.

[17] The 'visible scientists' in favour later in the century with the media were characterised by being relevant, articulate, controversial, colourful, photogenic and quotable. Though criticised, they seldom retracted any pronouncements; see Rae Goodell, *The Visible Scientists* (Boston: Little, Brown and Company, 1975). Goodell thought that scientific 'visibility' was a post-WWII phenomenon only.

the cultures was an ever-present problem and was not solved until antibiotics were added 40 years later. His growing staff moved over from the surgical projects and worked in sparsely-furnished, isolated rooms, attentive to Carrel's almost military discipline. These rituals gave a mystique to Carrel's work in the early days, and those who could not repeat his work, which was a frequent occurrence, were told or concluded, not always wrongly, that their *méthode* was faulty.

French Reaction

As ever, Carrel also published his new findings in France. Carrel's French language versions of the new data appeared in seven short communications sent to *Comptes Rendus*, the rapid publication journal of the Société de Biologie in Paris. These brief papers appeared quickly, starting one week after the first American papers. The 22 October issue of the French journal had three Carrel papers, plus one by Burrows alone. But this formidable display, clearly designed to impress and inform the French scientists, was met with disbelief.[18]

The criticism came immediately from Justin Marie Jolly (1870–1935), the distinguished haematologist, who was head of the laboratories at the Hôtel-Dieu de Paris. He was also a prominent member of the Société, and on its general committee. Jolly not only knew about cells; he had made earlier attempts to grow cells outside the body, but failed.[19] His view was that Carrel's cultures were merely dying cells migrating out of the clump,

---

[18] Carrel biographers have said that he attended and spoke at the 'séances' — the meetings — of that Société, but instead Carrel used the journal for rapid publication. The series of Carrel papers, with or without Burrows, are *Comptes Rendus des Séances et Mémoires de la Société de Biologie* (1910) vol. 69: 293–4, 298–9, 299–01, 328–31, 332–4, and 356–66.

[19] Justin Jolly (1903) 'Sur la durée de la vie…' *CRSB* 55: 1266. Jolly is remembered for noting the Howell–Jolly body in newly-formed red cells and he made early micro-cinematographic films of dividing cells. He should also be celebrated for his important discovery, in this same year of 1911, of the role of the Bursa of Fabricius in lymphocyte production — see David Hamilton, *A History of Organ Transplantation* (Pittsburgh: Pittsburgh University Press, 2012): 115.

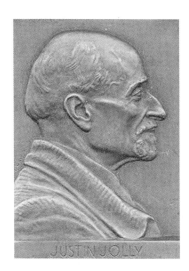

Justin Jolly, the famous Paris haematologist, severely criticised Carrel's early claims for tissue culture. (*fr.wikipedia.org.*)

and that the alleged survival was simply an end-of-life event. He attacked Carrel's findings in the Société's journal in the 5 November issue. Using the declamatory discourse of French scientific debate, he stated that Carrel's use of the phrase 'culture des tissus' was an 'abuse of language'. To prove real cellular survival, Jolly wanted evidence of mitosis — i.e. cells obviously dividing.[20] Carrel hit back, sending photographs to Paris of dividing cells, and these were on display at the Société on 7 January 1911.[21] Jolly commented immediately that these were merely dying dividing cells and dismissed them as 'moins importante'.[22] Jolly was not Carrel's only French critic. Dr. R. Legendre, a physiologist from the Paris Musée, soon also jousted with Carrel. Legendre again disputed that

---

[20] In Harrison, *Life of Tissues* (note 10) p. 70, he pointed out that both Loeb and Burrows had seen mitosis in their earlier cell culture attempts.

[21] Alexis Carrel and Montrose Burrows (1911) 'A propos des cultures «in vitro» des tissus de mammifères' *CRSB* 70: 3–4.

[22] J. Jolly (1911) 'A propos des cultures *in vitro* des tissus mammifères. Observations à l'occasion de la communication de MM Carrel et Burrows' *CRSB* 70: 4.

cellular survival had been achieved and added the cutting comment that Carrel's pictures were poor and that Carrel's published papers were unacceptably brief.[23]

Carrel's cool reception in France is easily explained. These Paris *savants* were well aware of Carrel's now regular criticism of his native France and of French medicine, which dated back to his rebuff in Lyon. The Paris academics were in no mood to accept extravagant, well-publicised claims from an unpatriotic expatriate.

Rebuttal in America

In New York, Carrel was initially on the defensive. Further work on the cultured cells was disappointing, and culture of thyroid and kidney cells did not, on closer study, produce thyroid gland structures or the organised kidney tissue he thought he saw earlier. The Rous sarcoma and human tumour cells also obstinately died out quickly in culture. Six months later, in the summer of 1911, in his regular Scientific Report to Flexner, he gloomily recorded that cells could not be kept alive beyond one month.[24] It seemed that Jolly and his French critics were perhaps right, after all. The failure to grow cells taken from his colleague Rous's famous chicken sarcoma was particularly disappointing. These cancer cells survived indefinitely when passed from chicken to chicken as tissue grafts. Others, like Leo Loeb in St. Louis (Jacques Loeb's brother), had managed to passage some tumour grafts from animal to animal indefinitely from 1901 onwards, and from 1905, the Institute had its own transplantable Flexner–Jobling rat tumour.

---

[23] R. Legendre (1911) 'Les recherches récentes sur la survie des cellules, des tissus et des organes isolés de l'organisme' *Biologica* 1: 357–65. The French complaints continued, and Legendre later returned to grumble about the quality of Carrel's work at the time of Carrel's Nobel Prize — see R. Legendre (1912) 'La survie des organs et la "culture" des tissus vivants" *La Nature* 40: 359–63.

[24] Scientific Reports of the Laboratories presented to the Corporation and to the Board of Scientific Directors vol. 2, June 1911 p. 196, FA 145, RUA RAC (note 4).

But, wounded, Carrel persevered with his cultures, convinced that events would prove him correct. He now had a new technician, Albert (Albert-Henry) Ebeling, appointed in November 1911, and their publications show that Ebeling took over the tissue culture project in June 1912. He did all the day-to-day tissue culture work in its early years, and he was to work under Carrel until Carrel's retirement. Promoted to assistant in 1919, but no higher, his long tenure was unusual: Carrel needed him and Flexner agreed to keep him.[25]

The Paris Meeting

In the summer of 1911, as always, Carrel returned to Europe. For the transatlantic voyage, he took one of the liners on the competitive 'four funnel' fashionable Atlantic route, which had a club-like atmosphere and a following among the wealthy. The passenger list was available ahead to the press, and as Carrel's fame grew, his embarkation and arrival were noticed by journalists, and Carrel might oblige the press with a quote or even a photograph. Reaching Paris in July, he gave a lecture, but perhaps because it was in a hospital setting, he emphasised that his cellular studies might allow understanding of healing and even, as he originally hoped, assist with promoting regeneration of nerves. No awkward questions were raised on this occasion. The *New York Times*, attentive as ever, said that the Paris physicians were 'greatly interested' in Carrel's studies.[26] During the visit he caught up with his surgeon friend Théodore Tuffier, with whom, as described later, he now shared an interest in experimental heart surgery. Tuffier did his research in Albert Dastre's physiology department at the Sorbonne, and Tuffier had copied Carrel in storing simple tissues in the cold for grafting later. Through Tuffier, Carrel was introduced to a widowed aristocratic lady who was working as a volunteer in the Paris surgeon's laboratory. He first proposed marriage to her that year, but she declined. They would be married two years later.

---

[25] Another tissue culture laboratory was set up at the nearby New York Lying-In Hospital involving Drs. J.W. Markoe and Joseph R. Losee. This assisted access to human tissue.
[26] 'Made Tissues Grow, Carrel Tells Paris' *NYT*, 16 July 1911.

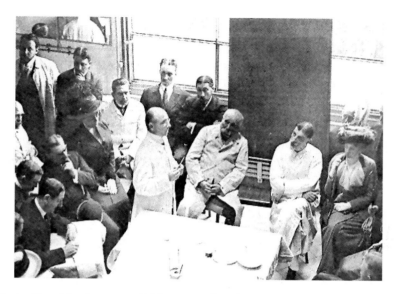

In Paris, Carrel had a respectful hearing when he spoke, with reporters present, at the surgical department at the Hôpital Broca. (*Courtesy of Project Gutenberg.*)

New Evidence

Returning home in the fall of 1911, having this time avoided French criticism, Carrel cast about for other evidence that his cultured cells were alive. Rather than just looking at them, he sought evidence that they showed function. He now produced one of the most remarkable claims of his career. Carrel now had Ragnvald Ingebrigtsen (1882–1975), from the Institute of Pathology of Oslo's University of Christiania, working as a volunteer with a scholarship of his own, and who then joined the staff for two more years.[27] Ingebrigtsen started work on nerve grafting, but Carrel put the Norwegian onto a tissue culture project in late 1911.[28] It

---

[27] Ingebrigtsen took the place of Edward Ruth who had worked from March 1911 for a year and attempted to make cultures of frog skin, i.e. an organ, albeit a thin one: see *JEM* 13 (1911): 422–24 and *JEM* 13 (1911): 559–61.

[28] Before returning home, Ingebrigtsen did research in Paris and published two papers in 1913 in the *JEM* on nerve grafting experiments and a similar one in the *Lyon Chirugicale*

was whether or not cultured white cells could make and secrete antibodies into the culture fluid. If they did, then the cells were indeed alive. Ingebrigtsen immunised guinea pigs against goat cells, cultured these guinea pig white cells and then added goat red cells. He reported that these red cells were destroyed in a few days, suggesting that the white cells were able to make antibodies against the goat cells.[29] This important experiment was repeated thereafter many times by others, usually with negative results.[30]

Successful Growth

With this major effort going on in his laboratory, and encouraged that their cultured cells seemed alive, Carrel, or rather Ebeling, tried culturing all types of cell using empirical, iterative testing of every variant in the conditions of culture. Hopes of random success were rewarded when, starting on 17 January 1912, culture No. 725 of embryonic chicken heart cells survived well, and after 14 subcultures, pulsating cells were still seen. One new addition to the culture medium had done the trick. It was first added on 1 February, and was a seriously empirical cellular extract — a 'soup' — of mixed chicken embryo tissue. The pulsating cells, disappointingly, then died out in April, but

---

in 1916. At home he was professor of surgery at Oslo from 1928, and Ingebrigtsen emphasised the lymphocyte's role in graft rejection. He was one of the first to look for anti-graft antibodies; see Hamilton, *Transplantation* (note 19): 103–4.

[29] The *in vitro* antibody production paper is Alexis Carrel and Ragnvald Ingebrigtsen (1912) 'The production of antibodies by tissues living outside of the organism' *JEM* 15: 287–91, with rapid-publication versions in *JAMA* 8 (1912): 477–478 and *CRSB* 72 (1912): 220.

[30] See A.J. Salle and W.A. McOmie (1937) 'Immunological responses of tissue cultivated *in vitro*' *Journal of Immunology* 32: 157–170. This careful study from Berkeley did not confirm Ingebrigtsen's report and reviewed 12 other attempts, of which only four, including one from Carrel's colleague Parker, reported low titres of *in vitro* antibody production. Undoubted antibody production by cultured white cells had to await the technology of fusion with tumour cells as 'hybridomas' in 1975.

HEART TISSUE BEATS LONG AFTER DEATH

Dr. Carrel Announces Startling
Results of His Experiments
with Cultures.

"PERMANENT LIFE" POSSIBLE

Fragments of a Chick's Heart Pulsated Rhythmically Two Months
After Removal.

Dr. Alexis Carrel of the Rockefeller
Institute for Medical Research, whose
surgical discoveries and innovations in
operative procedure have amazed the

The *New York Times* followed Carrel's new tissue culture announcements with enthusiasm.

instead robust connective tissue fibroblasts took over and continued to
thrive and divide.[31]

Carrel announced on 12 April 1912 in a paper in the *Journal of
Experimental Medicine* that he had produced a long-lived cell culture.[32]
The *New York Times* took the news from the *Journal* and was impressed
with these 'immortal cells'.[33] But not everyone joined the chorus of praise,

---

[31] Carrel later told a local biologist about the preparation of the embryonic juice and
said, perhaps surprisingly, that he had not previously given out details; the recipe may
also have varied from time to time. See Carrel to Kopeloff, 26 April 1927, box 4 folder
20, Malinin Collection, FA 208, RUA RAC (note 4) and p. 320.

[32] Alexis Carrel (1912) 'On the permanent life of tissue outside of the organism' *JEM* 15:
516–28.

[33] 'Heart Tissue Beats Long After Death' *NYT*, 2 May 1912. The first use of 'immortal'
came in a *NYT* headline on 10 June 1914.

and *Life* magazine, still thinking the cells were beating, was prepared to grumble: 'It is a pity these super-scientific men have no time or energy to study how to keep the whole heart pulsating in the animal body.'[34]

This cell line, called 'the old strain' by Carrel, was to be famous during its 34 years of life. Little was done to discourage the idea that the cells were still beating. These humble non-beating fibroblasts allegedly first outlived a normal chicken life-span and then outlived Carrel. The 'immortal cells' would also soon define Carrel's place in popular culture as a celebrity scientist.[35]

Cell Senescence

Carrel was not slow to draw a very serious inference from the existence of these long-lived cells. If cells were immortal, this overturned the major biological tenet of the day that all cells died off after a finite life span. If cells were immortal, something else was causing ageing. And if this factor could be found, then aging might be prevented, even reversed. Carrel started to use 'rejuvenation' — another evocative term — in this discussion, saying grandly that senility and death were not necessary but merely 'a contingent phenomenon'. The newspapers spread the word that Carrel's findings meant that men had the potential to live longer, and the papers vied with each other in their estimates of the new life span. The *Kansas Star* felt a 100-year life span was a modest target and raised their estimate to 200 years.

If the culture fluid was not refreshed, the cells died. In most of his publications, Carrel emphasised the need for nutriment in the medium as essential for growth, but occasionally wrote that the change of fluid also removed inhibitory toxic substances which could destroy cells. These are two quite different matters. He soon wrote that:

> Senility and death of tissues are not a necessary phenomenon and they result merely from accidental causes, such as accumulation of catabolic

---

[34] *Life*, 29 August 1912.
[35] The date of arrival of the cells was judged to be 17 January 1912, and the *New York World Telegram* thereafter was particularly attentive to this birthday.

substances … The rejuvenation consists in removing from the culture substances that inhibit growth …[36]

This was welcome news to Sir Arbuthnot Lane, the London surgeon famous for advocating that human ill health came from toxins absorbed from a sluggish colon. He visited Carrel in New York and wrote:

It was a great joy to see Carrel at work, his wonderful dexterity attracted me and held one's attention during his several operations. … I saw many specimens [of tissue culture] and realised the importance of his work as bearing upon chronic intestinal stasis. He showed so clearly the vital importance of drainage of tissues, and of removal of the evacuations of the cells from contact with them. … with suitable food and perfect drainage cells will live forever.[37]

Carrel remained equivocal, and was attracted to the idea that in old-age there was an accumulation of poisons. He bled a dog as fully as possible and replaced it with young blood, and considered that the old dog was revived. For once, Flexner was not impressed and advised against publication.[38] Flexner at this time was editor of the *Journal of Experimental Medicine* and accepted a speculative paper by Carrel on the power of his mysterious 'soup'. It stated that since his cultured cells were now growing at 40 times their normal speed, perhaps wound healing could also be activated in this way and that 'skin could heal in twenty-four hours and a leg fracture in four or five days'.[39] In an immediate response, a seven-column *New York Times* article was published with the headline 'Dr. Carrel's Newest Miracle — Healing In A Day'. The paper reasonably

---

[36] Carrel's view was repeated many times starting in 1912 [note 32].

[37] For Lane and his visit, see Ann Dally, *Fantasy Surgery, 1880–1930: With Special Reference to Sir William Arbuthnot Lane:* Clio Medica 38 (Amsterdam-Atlanta, Georgia: Rodopi, 1996): 350 and J. Lacey Smith (1982) 'Sir Arbuthnot Lane, chronic intestinal stasis, and autointoxication' *Annals of Internal Medicine* 96: 365–69.

[38] Scientific Reports, April 1914, vol. 3 p. 311, FA 145, RUA RAC (note 4). The idea of rejuvenation by transfusing young blood was an old one and is not yet dead: North Korea's leader Kim Jong-Il was said to be thus treated and died in 1994 age 82.

[39] Alexis Carrel (1913) 'Artificial activation of the growth *in vitro* of connective tissue' *JEM* 17: 14–19.

assumed he now had the power to summon up speedy, Lourdes-like healing.

Carrel's links with the press and journalists increased at this time. He was friendly with Norman Hapgood, the respected editor of *Harper's Weekly*, and they were members of a dining club organised by John D. Rockefeller junior which met on the third Tuesday of the month. At this time, Carrel assisted one journalist in particular — Mrs. Genevieve Grandecourt — and encouraged her work in *Harper's*, suggesting topics to her and lending books. She also hoped to write a novel on brain transplantation and transfer of memory, but nothing came of it. They exchanged friendly letters, but the salutation and signatures were always formal. Her reports on Carrel's work appeared in the *Scientific American* in 1912 and 1913.[40]

Back to Paris

In summer 1912, Carrel was back in Europe with renewed confidence. He now had the 'old strain' connective tissue cells from the chicken embryo heart surviving after five months, and he could confront the French critics he had encountered in the winter of 1910–11. Entitled to some *schadenfreude*, he first spoke in Paris at the Hôpital Broca, at a meeting organised by his friend Samuel Pozzi, the Paris surgeon, and he had a respectful hearing. Pozzi, an innovative surgeon and expert on cancer fulguration, was an imposing elder statesman in French medicine at the time.[41] His text *Traité de gynécologie clinique et opératoire* (Paris 1890) was in its fourth edition by this time. Concerned at the hostile treatment of his friend Carrel, Pozzi set up a laboratory in his Gynaecology Clinic at the Hôpital Broca, where Christian Champy (1885–1962), using Carrel's methods, published 10 articles on tissue culture between 1913 and 1921.

---

[40] Genevieve Grandecourt (1912) 'The 'immortality' of tissues' *Scientific American*, 107, October 12: 344 and 354–5 and *Scientific American* November 1913, 400 and 420. Their letters are in Alexis Carrel Papers, box 45 folder 11 and 12, GULBFC (note 1).
[41] *NYT*, 23 June 1912. See Claude Vanderpooten, *Samuel Pozzi, chirurgien et ami des femmes* (Paris: V&O, 1992).

But Carrel's critics were in attendance shortly after, when his new findings about the long-lived cells were given to the Academy of Medicine. Pozzi gave the presentation because Carrel was not a member, but with Carrel present. Carrel or Pozzi made sure that the *New York Times* correspondent in Paris had the story of Carrel's triumphant return.[42] But after the meeting, the *Times* correspondent was taken aside by critics of Carrel, doubtless including Jolly or Legendre, who were still hostile. The *Times* newspaper then carried the views of these sceptics three days later, and the new headline was 'Paris Doctors Seek Proof Of Carrel'. The article reported that Prof. Chantemesse was dubious and Prof. Pouchet was quoted as 'personally unable to believe in them [the surviving cells] without having actually seen them'. It was proposed that French biologists should visit the Rockefeller Institute to see the work with their own eyes. The *Times* journalist contacted Carrel, who responded by deploring the attitude of those who 'attacked his competence as a director of medical research'. Carrel was entitled to be annoyed.

Carrel returned to New York in the autumn of 1912, still smarting from this further hostile reception at the hands of his countrymen in Paris. But shortly after, a high honour came his way. On 13 October came the announcement that Carrel had won that year's Nobel Prize for 'Physiology or Medicine'. Curiously, it was for his transplantation and blood vessel surgery work, not for his recent tissue culture studies.

---

[42] 'Heart Tissue Grows And Beats 120 Days' *NYT*, 20 June 1912.

CHAPTER SIX

The Nobel Prize

T he Prize was set up in 1895 by Alfred Nobel, the Swedish industrialist, who grew rich as a result of his discovery of dynamite and, wishing to ensure a more attractive legacy, left substantial funds for international prizes in a range of categories. These prestigious annual awards, which also come with a substantial cheque, are judged by Swedish institutions, after seeking names of possible candidates.

```
                                        Gr. VII.  8.
            1909 - 1910.
                        N:o 10. Ink. d. 6 febr. 1909.
                             January 15th 1909.
     The Medical Nobel Committee
          Royal Caroline Institute, Stockholm.
Gentlemen
     Thanking you for the honor conferred upon me I beg to sub-
mit the name of  A l e x i s   C a r r e l   of the Rockefeller
Institute of New York for his work on Surgery of the bloodvessels.
                                        Yours truly
                                        Carl Beck.


                        N:o 11. Ink. 6 febr. 1909.
                             Chicago, Jan. 22nd, 1909.
     To The Medical Nobel-Committee,
          The Royal Caroline Institute,
```

Karl Beck continued to support Carrel by nominating him, though unsuccessfully, for the Nobel Prize in 1909. (*Courtesy of the Nobel Prize Organisation.*)

151

Carrel had already been nominated for a Nobel Prize in 'Physiology or Medicine' in 1909 by Chicago's Carl Beck, his former mentor, and this had been for his blood vessel studies.[1] Meanwhile, Carrel had moved into tissue culture, from 1910, but was nominated again in 1912 by Charles Bouchard in Paris, this time for his tissue culture work. Jules Åkerman, professor of surgery at Sweden's Karolinska Institute, was asked to make the usual assessment of possible winners from the 10 candidates nominated that year. The list included the physiologists J.N. Langley and C.S. Sherrington, and the French immunologist Charles Richet. Åkerman reviewed Carrel's tissue culture work and found that it was impressive. However, Carrel's culture methods had clearly developed from Harrison's technique, and Åkerman would learn from insiders that the matter of priority in this case was sensitive. Joint awards were not made at the time. This led Åkerman to look again at Carrel's earlier transplant and blood vessel surgery. A surgeon himself, Åkerman was convinced that both Carrel's transplant work and the development of tissue culture together merited a Prize. Guided by Åkerman, the committee unanimously chose Carrel for the 1912 award for Physiology or Medicine. At the Faculty stage, a higher level, the tissue culture component was dropped from the citation.

The Winner

Carrel was not yet 40 years old, and he was the youngest recipient in this category thus far.[2] He was also the first American-based winner of this category of award, and it was also a triumph for the Rockefeller Institute and a welcome acknowledgement of Flexner's aspirations. Phoebus Levene later recalled 'the early difficult days when your [Prize] success

---

[1] See Erling Norrby, *Nobel Prizes and Life Sciences* (London: World Scientific Press, 2010): 150–1.

[2] Carrel's Prize awarded him $39,000. Earlier Nobel Prizes going to America were the Peace Prize awarded to President Theodore Roosevelt in 1906 for brokering a cease-fire between Russia and Japan, and the Physics Prize of 1907, which went to A.A. Michelson of Chicago.

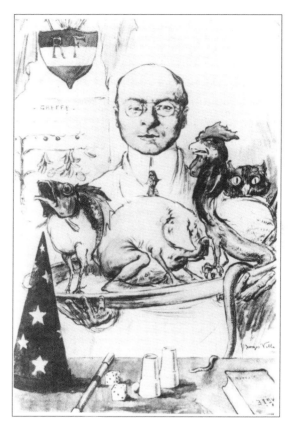

Carrel portrayed as a magician in the French journal *Chanticlair* in 1913.

meant a lot to us'. Flexner might have been personally disappointed: he had been nominated unsuccessfully for the Prize in earlier years. Carrel was not the first surgeon honoured in this way, since Theodor Kocher won the Prize three years earlier for his work on the functions and diseases of the thyroid gland.

Carrel was again a local hero, and *The New York Times* carried a major story about 'Dr. Carrel's Miracles in Surgery'.[3] The newspaper was confused over what the Prize was awarded for, instead highlighting his long-lasting chicken heart cells. American and French newspapers heaped new praise on Carrel, and cartoonists showed him backed by hybrid

---

[3] 'Dr. Carrel's Miracles in Surgery' *NYT*, 13 October 1912.

animals with transferred heads.[4] *The Independent* named him as the sixth most useful man in America, and many of the major American magazines sought an interview. The American poet Percy MacKaye composed 'A Meditation on the Nobel Prize' entitled 'The Heart in Jar', thinking the award was for tissue culture.[5] The British journal *The Lancet* praised Carrel in a reflective editorial on the past and future of vascular surgery:

> None who have followed with interest these new advances in surgery can doubt that they contain immense possibilities, and the application to man of these methods learned in animals cannot be long delayed. What are the limits of the surgery of the vascular system no one can say.[6]

Congratulations came in from many sources. Walter Cannon, the Harvard physiologist, mentioned the 'years of detraction and incredulity, and in some quarters ridicule'. Even the gruff J.B. Murphy in Chicago

S T A G E

RECEPTION TO

THE PRESIDENT OF THE UNITED STATES

AND ASSEMBLY IN HONOR OF

DR. CARREL

(RECENT RECIPIENT OF THE NOBEL PRIZE)

THE GREAT HALL

OF

THE COLLEGE OF THE CITY OF NEW YORK

SATURDAY NOVEMBER 16 AT 10:30 A. M.

ADMIT ONE

The city of New York's celebration for Carrel's Nobel Prize. (*Courtesy of the Georgetown University Library, Booth Family Center for Special Collections.*)

---

[4] His newspaper clippings file for 1912 has 705 items.
[5] Percy MacKaye, *Poems and Plays* (New York: Macmillan, 1916).
[6] 'The work of Alexis Carrel' *The Lancet*, 19 October 1912: 1091–2.

was gracious in his praise. The Prize brought Carrel a flood of new letters from admirers, including some in Europe, and with his transplant work again highlighted, many patients again sought his surgical help, looking for grafts of limbs, ovaries, uterus, eyes and other tissues. These writers often accepted that such surgery was experimental and were prepared to take the risk. To meet their need, a living donor was occasionally identified, or they suggested that tissue from executed criminals be used. Others offered their own body for medical research after death. Dealing with more conventional requests for medical assistance, Carrel might suggest a particular specialist's name. There were requests for his autograph or a signed portrait and there were begging letters. Many invitations came in, and with his confirmed celebrity status, he was offered free tickets to opening nights on Broadway. New York marked the occasion with an impressive celebration held in the Great Hall of the College of the City of New York on 16 November, which brought in an audience of 5,000.[7] President Taft attended, as did the French ambassador, who said:

> Dr. Carrel has shown that which has been dead can live again: the dead heart beats again: a lung that was dead breathes again. When you do honor to Carrel you do honor to France.

Difficulties Emerge

But Carrel was in no mood to share the honour with France in this way. It was only a few months since he had encountered embarrassing hostility to his work when he spoke in Paris. The circumstances of his earlier departure from Lyon still rankled with him, and these were now raised again in the French newspapers. One French newspaper took the view that Carrel had been driven out of Lyon and, doubtless briefed by Carrel himself, the journalist singled out Lyon's professor of medicine and mayor of Lyon, Victor Augagneur, as responsible for blocking Carrel's career. Augagneur was now an easy target since, when he moved

---

[7] 'Noted Men Praise Work Of Alexis Carrel' *NYT*, 11 November 1912.

in 1905 to be governor of the French colony of Madagascar, he had not done well.

To add to this, the Nobel ceremony in Stockholm required the winner to be introduced by their national ambassador, and Carrel was still a Frenchman. Carrel was prepared to be difficult about this, and he told the organisers that he did not wish to be linked to the French nation in this way. He even hesitated to go. The matter was tactfully dealt with, and a formula found: Carrel was represented at the ceremony on 11 December 1912 by the U.S. ambassador to Denmark.[8]

The Nobel Lecture

In Stockholm, the orator, perhaps choosing his words carefully, said of Carrel 'The clear, bright intelligence which was the patrimony you received from your country — from France — was allied to the bold resolve and energy of your adopted country.'

Carrel then gave his lecture and, not mentioning these matters nor his tissue culture work, he gave a masterly lecture on organ transplantation, one which still reads well.[9] Although it was two years since he last did any regular experimental graft work, he clearly had been keeping an eye on the literature, and in particular, thinking about the issues, homograft non-survival. The survival of his arterial homografts had misled him, and he now accepted that they survived only as a tube without cells. He now accepted that graft loss was the usual outcome when attempting homografting, and with clarity and precision, he set out his new understanding of graft failure, even correctly describing the destructive changes prior to homograft loss.

Afterwards he visited Berlin, and joined his family in Lyon. On reaching Paris he made it plain to the press that he had expected some

---

[8] See David Le Vay, *Alexis Carrel: The Perfectibility of Man* (Rockville: Kabel Publishing, 1996): 93, but no source is given.

[9] Alexis Carrel 'Suture of Blood Vessels and Transplantation of Organs' *Nobel Lectures, Physiology or Medicine 1901–1921* (Amsterdam: Elsevier Publishing Company, 1967): 437–66.

French government honour, but this had not yet been offered.[10] His mood did not improve when, arriving at the New York docks, he was not waved through Customs as usual, and had to pay duty on some items, including new instruments. Annoyed, he gave the story to the *New York Times*.

Publicity Concerns

In 1913, the Institute now decided, not for the first or last time, to be more cautious with their involvement with the public. Having a Nobel Prize winner perhaps gave the Institute enough status, and there was no need to add to it. Carrel's Prize again seemed to justify animal experimentation, but even so, the Institute took steps to prevent the antivivisectionists gaining damaging information, notably through careful sub-editing of the Institute's *The Journal of Experimental Medicine*.[11] And there were a number of other reasons to seek a lower profile. In 1912 there was public interest when Meltzer announced (wrongly) that he had discovered a third form of circulation in addition to the blood circulation and lymphatic system. To add to this, Flexner probably regretted telling the *New York Times* in 1911 that a cure for poliomyelitis was 'not far distant'. To add to this, there were increasing concerns at the Institute over the research studies of Hideyo Noguchi in Flexner's group. Prominent newspaper coverage of his 'microbe-hunting' was bringing risky publicity to the Institute.

---

[10] 'France Neglects Carrel' *NYT*, 22 December 1912. He was appointed Chevalier de la Légion d'honneur in 1913, upgraded to 'Officier' in 1915.
[11] Susan Eyrich Lederer (1985) 'Hideyo Noguchi's luetin experiment and the antivivisectionists' *Isis* 76: 31–48. The American Medical Association also produced guidelines for editors entitled 'Protecting Medical Research' to use when describing experimental animal work; see *JAMA* 63 (1914): 94.

Noguchi's Work

Hideyo Noguchi (1876–1928) was now rivalling Carrel as a Rockefeller Institute celebrity.[12] The Japanese researcher joined Flexner's laboratory in Philadelphia in 1899 and had moved to New York with him, continuing to show energy and accomplishment. In 1911 Noguchi claimed, wrongly as it turned out, that he had cultured the spirochete organism of syphilis, and also that year he announced a simple skin test for syphilis, using his 'luetin' extract; this test eventually proved to be unhelpful. The antivivisectionists in New York were by then mounting a new and slightly different campaign, contending that when scientists became accustomed to doing animal experiments, it blunted the moral sense and led on to unethical human experimentation. They highlighted Noguchi's syphilis test of 1911, since for his 'controls' — namely skin testing of disease-free persons — he had used some institutionalised orphan children. In May 1912 the New York Society for the Prevention of Cruelty to Children lodged a complaint of assault against Noguchi, but the Manhattan district attorney declined to prosecute.[13]

However, the year 1913 was Noguchi's *annus mirabilis*, and started with his crucial and correct demonstration of the organism of syphilis in the brains of those dying in the general paralysis stage. He further announced identification of the organisms causing trachoma and rabies and, more importantly, that he had grown the polio organism. These findings could not be replicated by others, and his work was increasingly erratic that year, though still admired by the press.[14] In summer 1913, Noguchi travelled in Europe and was the guest of honour at medical

---

[12] Paul Franklin Clark (1959) 'Hideyo Noguchi, 1876–1928' *Bulletin of the History of Medicine* 33: 1–20.

[13] Lederer, *Noguchi* (note 11).

[14] In 1913, there were seven *New York Times* stories describing Noguchi's work. Noguchi was repeatedly nominated unsuccessfully for a Nobel Prize, and Norrby *Nobel Prizes* (note 1): 152 concluded that Noguchi 'holds a record for non-reproducible claims'. Noguchi's reputation survived, and after his heroic death at work in Africa, his memory was much honoured.

meetings. The public took to him, and a crowd of 4,000 turned out to meet him on arrival at the Vienna rail station.

On reaching home in New York, matters were rather different. With increasing disquiet within the Institute over his work, others were asked to check his findings.

Lowering the Profile

Flexner decided to limit the exposure of the Institute. He now sought a lower profile and took the view that the Institute's regular coverage in the newspapers was counter-productive, and that it was time for some dignified detachment. Dealing with this matter was now the responsibility of a new business manager, Henry James Jr, nephew of the writer Henry James, and James, doubtless with Flexner's encouragement, now took a firm line on newspaper coverage.[15] James announced that it was 'not our policy to address the popular reader nor explain our work.... We are happy to escape notice from the daily papers'. This was a new attitude. Other exposure was discouraged. In early 1913, the philosopher Bergson was to arrive in the New York docks and a public welcome was organised. Carrel was invited to go out with reporters to meet the philosopher, but thought it wise to decline.

There was perhaps a new sensitivity about press coverage of medical science, and the Progressive Era's attitude that the public were entitled to prompt news of these advances was now in question. Dr. Harry Plotz, a young intern at Mount Sinai Hospital in New York, isolated the organism of typhus in early 1914 and was due to speak on his discovery at the American Association of Physicians meeting in May. But he leaked the news to the *New York Times* ahead of the meeting. The

---

[15] Earlier, Jerome D. Greene was in post as manager from 1910–12 and, after dealing with this difficult time, moved on to be an assistant to J.D. Rockefeller junior; he was then a banker and a trustee at both the Institute and the Foundation. Later, he organised the Harvard Tercentenary Celebrations. Henry James Jr followed Greene as Business Manager and Edric Brooks Smith then served from 1920 to 1955.

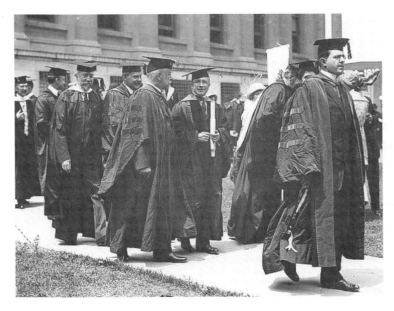

Carrel's first honorary degree, of many, came from New York's Columbia University in 1913. (*Courtesy of the Library of Congress.*)

physicians decided to act and declined to let him give his arranged paper. At this time, Carrel received a memorandum from the Congress of Surgeons of North America addressed to its members deploring the 'sensational newspaper reports which had brought discredit to the Congress'. In future, the Congress announced, it would issue its own press releases.

Carrel himself was now more cautious, and after the justifiable attention following his Nobel Prize, he withdrew a little. He had agreed to do an article for *Popular Science Monthly* but changed his mind. On 13 May 1913, van Buren Thorne of the *New York Times*, a young physician-turned-journalist with a niche interest in medical and science stories, applied to Carrel for an interview. Carrel discussed the matter with James, and James drafted a well-crafted reply for Carrel to use:

> I have recently been the victim of so much publicity — friendly and well meant — but uncomfortable and seriously inconvenient for me — that

I have had to refuse to accept any invitation whatsoever to appear in public or to appear in popular magazines or newspapers, either directly or indirectly. I have had cause to regret one or two departures from this resolution ... [16]

James noted that 'misleading reports about Dr. Carrel and fictitious interviews with him, have lately been too numerous to mention'.

Carrel was accustomed to helping journalists, and the administration's policy was now to disengage. But when another request came in, Carrel hesitated, and Henry James conceded that non-attributable briefing given to the right kind of journalist would be helpful:

I think I would reply that you [Carrel] will see him on the understanding you are not talking for publication. He is helping us in the matter of antivivisection.[17]

This *New York Times* support for animal experiments had always annoyed the antivivisection lobby, though they had the support of the *New York Herald*. The *Herald* now found that it was not getting the Institute's science stories, and softened its policy on animal experiments. Carrel's Nobel Prize had also weakened their case.

Marriage

In 1913, towards the end of the year, Carrel, now age 41, married in France. He met his future wife, Madame Anne Laura Gourlez de la Meyrie Motte, at Lourdes when she visited and assisted as a nurse on pilgrimages from her home near Anjou in Brittany. She also worked in the

[16] James to Carrel, and Carrel to Thorne, 13 May 1913, Alexis Carrel Papers, box 43 file 31, Georgetown University Library, Booth Family Center for Special Collections. See also Business Manager, Publicity File 1913–1924, 210.3(27), Rockefeller University Archives, Rockefeller Archives Centre (RUA RAC).
[17] James to Carrel, Malinin Collection of the Papers of Alexis Carrel and Charles Lindbergh, box 3 folder 4, FA 208, RUA RAC (note 16).

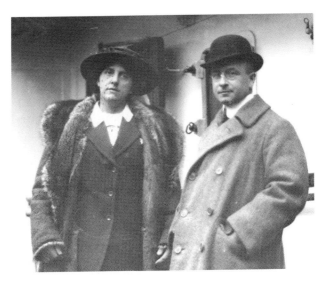

Carrel married in France at Christmas 1914 and she then settled for a time in New York. (*Courtesy of the Library of Congress.*)

Paris surgeon Théodore Tuffier's laboratory, and Carrel met her again there. Daughter of the soldier Count Alfred de la Motte, she was the widow of the Marquis de la Mairie, who died in 1909, leaving her with their five year-old son. Age 38, she was an outspoken, tall spirited lady who drove cars, and Carrel's first biographer, who met her, described her as 'grande, svelte, autoritaire, distinguée, élégante, intrepide et riche'. They had a small civil ceremony in Paris on 26 December, and those present were her parents, Carrel's brother Joseph, and his surgical friend Tuffier. Mme Carrel probably brought in an inheritance to the marriage, but it was hardly needed. Carrel already had a salary, a private income, investments in Lyon and his Nobel Prize money: the couple were not short of funds.

They sailed back to New York, and on embarkation were greeted and congratulated by journalists. Carrel was gracious and commented on some of the medical issues of the day, agreeing that the new method of 'washing the blood' showed promise for rejuvenation, but that radiation for cancer might not be affective.[18] The couple settled back in New York, living in a hotel, and until the War she assisted him in his New York laboratory. Later, she helped with this administration of his French hospital during the War.

Carrel's experiments on organ and limb transplants had slowed after 1910 as he increased his tissue culture work. But during the period 1910–1914 he periodically returned to surgical topics, and among many short-term projects, he carried out corneal grafting and surgery of major blood vessels, notably the aorta. He also made the first attempts at experimental heart surgery. Now a full 'Member' of the Institute, his small group was named 'Experimental Surgery'. These intermittent, remarkable surgical adventures can now be described together.

---

[18] 'Dr. Carrel And Bride Here' *NYT*, 4 January 1914. He was asked about J.J. Abel's dialysis of blood by a 'vividiffusion' apparatus, dubbed the 'artificial kidney' in *The Times* of London on 11 August 1913.

CHAPTER SEVEN

Heart and Blood Vessel Surgery

With the excitement over the development of tissue culture, Carrel appeared, from his publications, to spend less time on his surgical projects. Certainly, kidney grafting was put aside, and he abandoned leg transplants as impractical when his hopes for speeding up nerve regeneration were abandoned. But experimental surgery was not entirely forgotten, and with day-to-day tissue culture now in the hands of his technicians, particularly Albert Ebeling, Carrel may have returned to operating, though many projects were short-lived and publications on them were sparse. During this time he also devised a bold 'whole animal' perfusion system, attempted corneal grafting, looked at 'tissue typing' and extended his interest in arterial surgery to the abdomen and chest. Added to this, he embarked on innovative heart surgery.

'Visceral' Organism

One unpleasant project at the end of 1912 had a short life. It could be seen as tissue culture on a grand scale. Using only the animal body below the neck and ventilating the lungs via the trachea, he kept the heart, liver, kidneys and intestines alive in a temperature-controlled water bath.[1] For some hours, bowel movements were normal, food absorbed and urine produced. Carrel reported the experiments in his address to the New York Physicians Association in October 1912 just after his Nobel Prize was

---

[1] Alexis Carrel (1913) 'Concerning visceral organisms' *JEM* 18: 155–61.

announced. In spite of his heightened authority, the project caused only short-term interest. It allowed some studies of protein absorption from the intestine, and Harvey Cushing proposed to use it to study the influence of the pituitary hormones on kidney function. But the large clump of organs lasted in good condition for only a few hours before deterioration. Carrel published an account of this 'visceral organism' in 1913, and no more was heard of this awkward and unpleasant preparation.

Corneal Grafting

Carrel made a restart on corneal grafting in a joint project with New York's eye surgeon Prof. Dalen (of Dalen-Fuchs retinal nodules in uveitis, the eye disease).[2] He ordered new instruments, including a special punch to remove accurately a disc of donor and recipient corneas, purchasing the equipment from the famous Paris instrument-making firm of Charrière, Collin and Gentile, which lasted until 1978. He may have obtained finer needles and developed an almost 'monofilament' thread to go with them. His reports to Flexner suggest that corneal grafting was going well but infection was a problem. Even so, it is surprising that with his talents, nothing was achieved, and the project was eventually dropped. One factor may be that Carrel had now established with difficulty that homograft tissue would always reject, and he perhaps had no hopes for grafting corneas. Ironically, corneal grafting is an exception, and corneal homografting successfully emerged into routine human use in the 1920s.[3]

---

[2] His corneal grafts are mentioned steadily in *Scientific Reports of the Laboratories Presented to the Corporation and to the Board of Scientific Directors*, FA 145, box 1 vol. 3, 1912: 23, 40, 202, 204, 241, 286, 310, Rockefeller University Archives, Rockefeller Archives Centre (RUA RAC). Carrel's start in 1912 is described later in Albert H. Ebeling and Anne Carrel (1921) 'Remote results of complete homotransplantations of the cornea' *JEM* 34: 435–40. There had been sporadic attempts at corneal grafting in Europe from 1905, but corneal grafting did not emerge in routine clinical work until 1931.

[3] The cornea is nourished by the fluids of the eye, and lacks the blood vessels which deliver the lymphocytes necessary for rejection.

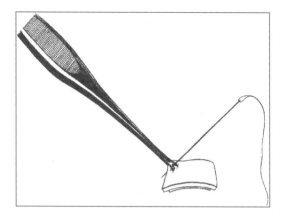

Carrel took an early interest in corneal grafting, but this was not sustained. The fine needles used had a split thread loop which minimised the tissue damage by the suture track. (*From Reference 2.*)

Developments in Transplantation

Carrel, though concentrating on his tissue culture work, continued to reflect on the mystery of tissue loss after homografting. It was clear to him that an unavoidable and powerful mechanism was involved, and others in Europe started to agree with him, although Kocher did not and this held back progress. Carrel considered that there might be occasional homograft survivals, the result of successful random matching of some kind and, if so, this would explain the conflicting verdicts and save the honour of the rejection-deniers. But Carrel had little help from current biological ideas. Karl Landsteiner had described blood 'groups' in 1900, but there was a delay in realising that they had a role in blood transfusion. Not until 1912 onwards was cross-matching taken seriously, even at the Mount Sinai, the hospital in New York which was pioneering blood transfusion at this time.[4]

---

[4] In retrospect, the first tentative use of matching had been by a young New York intern at Mount Sinai Hospital; see Reuben Ottenberg (1908) 'Transfusion and arterial anastomosis' *Annals of Surgery* 47: 486–505. His use of a cross-match is mentioned in an aside, unaware then of its significance.

Realising the significance of Landsteiner's work, Carrel decided to use cross-matching to find 'individuals between whom organs might be interchanged'. Carrel put his talented visitor, Ragnvald Ingebrigtsen, onto the study, just after Ingebrigtsen had completed the tissue culture antibody production study mentioned earlier. The visitor was to look at blood incompatibility as it affected the outcome of homografting.

Tissue Typing

Cats and dogs had not yet been blood grouped. Ingebrigtsen took 40 cats, 'grouped' them, or rather looked for cross-reactions between the serum of each cat and the cells of all the others, as Landsteiner had done in his human study earlier. From this, Ingebrigtsen found pairs of animals who were blood group compatible and pairs who were not. For homografting between the pairs chosen, cat kidney grafts would have high death rates and the many complications would obscure any role of compatibility. For a surgical procedure to test homograft survival and matching, they turned instead to a less heroic and less obvious operation, choosing to transplant small lengths of cat carotid artery. As these were only one millimetre in diameter, it was a serious technical surgical challenge. Ingebrigtsen operated and exchanged donor arteries between pairs with positive blood matches and also between those in the group of negative matches. Ingebrigtsen clearly had arrived with surgical skills, or gained them under Carrel, since three-quarters of his tiny grafts were patent immediately, and three months later, at re-operation, all these initially successful grafts were pulsating. When he removed the artery grafts for microscopy of muscle cell survival in the wall, this showed no relation to the positive or negative cross-matches.

This project, with a negative outcome, was the first attempt at 'tissue typing'.[5] Not until the late 1920s did Landsteiner, who had settled at the Rockefeller Institute, start to look for tissue groups. By then Carrel had

---

[5] R. Ingebrigtsen (1912) 'The influence of isoagglutinins on the final results of homoplastic transplantations of arteries' *JEM* 16: 169–77. Carrel curiously did not add his name to this paper.

lost interest in transplantation studies. Carrel and Ingebrigtsen's project was, as ever, on the right lines and half a century ahead of its time. On other occasions, Carrel can be faulted for wrongly claiming success; on this occasion, he resisted looking for optimistic findings in Ingebrigtsen's data. In his response to those writing to him requesting organ grafts, Carrel often replied saying that the 'problem of individuality has still to be solved'.[6]

Blood Vessel Surgery 1909–1914

Carrel and Guthrie had shown the way in 1905 when, perhaps surprisingly, they showed that vein grafts could serve well as substitutes for arteries. Others followed Carrel's lead and at Johns Hopkins, Stephen Watts, working with Harvey Cushing, also had some success with vein grafts in experimental animals. There was also news of some successful attempts with vein grafts in human cases, and José Capdevila in Madrid in 1906 was first to use a vein to successfully replace an aneurysm behind the knee; Pringle in Glasgow followed in 1913.[7] Lexer had success with a saphenous vein graft for an axillary aneurysm, but an attempt by Bernheim and Halsted failed in 1915.[8] Carrel in his papers mentions unpublished human vein graft attempts by Braun, Pierre Delbet and C. Mantelli, doubtless hearing of these cases personally on his European travels. Suitable cases for this vascular surgery were rare, and it required experience

---

[6] Alexis Carrel Papers, box 46 folder 28, Georgetown University Library, Booth Family Center for Special Collections (GULBFC).

[7] The pioneer operation is described by J. Goyanes in *El Siglo Médico* (1906) 53: 561–4 and discussed in E. Criado and F. Giron (2006) 'José Goyanes Capdevila, unsung pioneer of vascular surgery' *Annals of Vascular Surgery* 20: 422–5. For the other attempts at this time, see Emerich Ullman (1914) 'Tissue and organ transplantation' *Annals of Surgery* 60: 195–219.

[8] G. Melville Williams (1992) 'Bertram M. Bernheim: a Southern vascular surgeon' *Journal of Vascular Surgery* 16: 311–18, and I.M. Rutkow, B.G. Rutkow and C.B. Ernst (1980) 'Letters of William Halsted and René Leriche: "Our friendship seems so deep"' *Surgery* 88: 806–25. Bernheim's *Surgery of the Vascular System* (1913) was the first clinical text on the subject; see James S.T. Yao (2011) 'First textbook in vascular surgery' *Journal of Vascular Surgery* 54: 269–72.

and speed to achieve success without clotting in the vessels at the time of surgery. Moreover, simply tying off the main vessel above the aneurysm was quite effective.

Carrel now extended his ambition and started to replace larger arteries — notably the aorta. These operations were carried out intermittently from 1907 to 1914 but can be considered together here.

Aortic Surgery

Carrel transferred his experience using vein grafts placed in leg arteries to use the same strategy to replace the abdominal aorta. To get a vein of suitable diameter, a segment of the adjacent vena cava from the same animal was used. Three animals were grafted in November 1908 and there was immediate success and return of the pulses in the leg; two animals showed long-term survival. Examination of the graft wall showed, as before, that it had survived and gained strength through thickening with fibrous tissue.[9] Carrel then went further, again anticipating the events of 50 years later, and briefly considered how artificial material could be used in aortic replacement. In February 1910 he used a 5 cm length of glass tubing as a substitute for the abdominal aorta, but it clotted after six days. He then tried a simpler experiment, removing only a disc of aorta 2 cm by 1.2 cm from the wall and replacing it with a patch of thin rubber. The animal remained well, and 15 months later when the area was examined, the rubber was covered by new tissue on the outside, and there was a new smooth cellular lining inside. Carrel's three-page report on his aortic replacement operations ends prophetically by saying 'that all foreign substance, under certain conditions, does not produce an obliterative thrombosis, but can, indeed, be used in the reparation of the wall of a large artery'.[10]

---

[9] Alexis Carrel (1910) 'Graft of the vena cava on the abdominal aorta' *Annals of Surgery* 52: 462–70.

[10] Alexis Carrel (1911) 'Patching of the abdominal aorta with a piece of rubber' *JEM* 14: 126–8. He had done a similar experiment with a patch of peritoneum, a suitable biological material.

Thoracic Aorta

Using the anaesthetic technique for chest surgery described later, he could divide the aorta in the chest and re-join it, as he had done with the abdominal aorta. He found that clamping the aorta for any length of time would cause spinal cord damage, and to keep the peripheral circulation going and give himself more time, he inserted a shunt either from aorta to aorta, or from the left ventricle to aorta to allow blood to flow past the operative area. This was yet another characteristic Carrel innovation. After unsatisfactory preliminary attempts in 1909 using vein grafts to replace segments of the thoracic aorta, in January 1912 he changed strategy. He did not cut out a length of the aorta but placed tubing inside, as in the 'endoaneurysmal' surgery of almost a century later. He knew from laboratory work that tubes made of aluminium or 'paraffined' glass — glass with a thin coating of paraffin wax — where less liable to clot. He placed these as conduits inside the aorta and tied them in place. The immediate results were good, but he had only one medium-term survival, and all deaths were due to erosion of the tube through the wall of the aorta or from clotting in the lumen. He had hopes that use of other materials might be successful, such as lining these tubes with a vein, but he did not persevere with this project.

By this time he had firmly established another technique which was to be important in vascular surgery later. He had carried out a broad range of experiments showing that tissues, including blood vessels, cartilage, bone and fat stored at just above freezing point would remain useful for some time. He had no success with attempts to preserve glands or the kidney. He gave his results in a lecture to the American Medical Association meeting at Atlantic City in the summer of 1912 and announced that he could supply these stored tissues to surgeons. The *Washington Post* quoted him as saying: 'All they have to do is order them from the Institute'.[11]

---

[11] 'Tissues Of Dead Live' *Washington Post* 8 June 1912. His important lecture was 'The preservation of tissues and its applications in surgery', *JAMA* (1912) 59: 523–7. This work, from 1906 onwards, clearly influenced his colleague Rous's successful achievement of preservation of red blood cells in the cold.

The Heart

Disease of the heart valves was common at the time. It was usually caused by an earlier episode of rheumatic fever following a streptococcal sore throat or scarlet fever, and this could result in the thin leaflets of the valves, particularly the mitral valve, becoming thickened and then stuck together, giving mitral stenosis. These diseased valves might show the nodular infected 'vegetations' of bacterial endocarditis. Sometimes the valves could leak, as in mitral incompetence. There were similar afflictions of the aortic valve and, as always, many congenital abnormalities were encountered in the young, including stenosis of the pulmonary artery at its origin. Surgery on the organs within the chest was rarely attempted in humans or animals because of difficulties with anaesthesia, since when the chest cavity was opened, the lung collapsed, and oxygenation failed.

Better Anaesthesia

There had been some unsatisfactory attempts at maintaining respiration during chest surgery, and none of the strategies were routinely successful. These devices included Ferdinand Sauerbruch's chamber, which surrounded all of the body except the head and negative-pressure sucked air into the lungs. The alternative was Ludolf Brauer's method, which enclosed the head only and used positive-pressure to inflate the lungs.[12] Carrel characteristically considered that the devices used by Sauerbruch and Brauer were 'useless'. Sauerbruch had visited America in 1908, and he left behind one of his chambers in New York. It was soon rescued and used at the Institute by Samuel Meltzer, working in a laboratory adjacent to Carrel, since Meltzer and his son-in-law John Auer were looking at the treatment of tetanus, at that time an untreatable and unpleasant affliction. They treated the spasms of tetanus by giving

---

[12] For the rival respiratory ventilation methods at the time, see J.B. Brodsky and H.J.M. Lemmens (2007) 'The history of anesthesia for thoracic surgery' *Minerva Anesthesiologica* 73: 513–24.

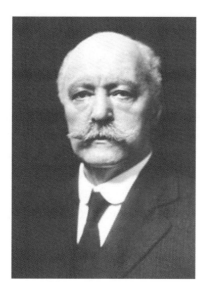

Samuel Meltzer, the talented Rockefeller Institute physiologist, devised an anaesthetic technique which permitted experimental and human intra-thoracic surgery. (*Courtesy of the National Library of Medicine.*)

muscle-paralysing chemicals.[13] If too much was given, breathing failed, and they attempted to keep respiration going, but found the Sauerbruch apparatus was difficult to use. Instead they devised their own method. In it, Meltzer and Auer passed a tube well down into the trachea (windpipe), without blocking it completely, and then continuously fed in air and anaesthetic gases. They reported their findings in 1909.[14] Similar techniques only slowly entered into the anaesthetic practice for human chest surgery from the 1920s onwards.

---

[13] For Meltzer, see A. Meltzer (1990) 'Dr. Samuel James Meltzer: Physiologist of the Rockefeller Institute' *American Jewish Archives* 42: 49–56. They used magnesium sulphate given intravenously as an effective muscle relaxant.

[14] S.J.Meltzer and John Auer (1909) 'Continuous respiration without respiratory movements' *JEM* 11: 622–5. Meltzer also used his method for experimental cardio-pulmonary resuscitation.

Into the Chest

Human heart surgery was not attempted at that time, other than during the occasional, largely unsuccessful, explorations of the chest for severe bleeding after injuries. Carrel realised that Meltzer's new system gave him the chance to operate within the chest, and from late 1909, over that winter, Carrel exploited the new possibilities with characteristic vigour. As a preliminary to operating on the heart, he did the operations on the aorta in the chest described earlier, and also carried out 12 resections of oesophagus or lobes of lung.

For his experimental heart surgery, Carrel found that more stringent aseptic techniques were needed in the chest to avoid post-operative infection. He first experimented with some procedures which did not require stopping the heart and, putting a finger into the chambers, with control of blood leakage, he noted that a mitral valve could be dilated in this way. He also tried a large encircling external suture to narrow the mitral valve as a technique for dealing with mitral incompetence. For

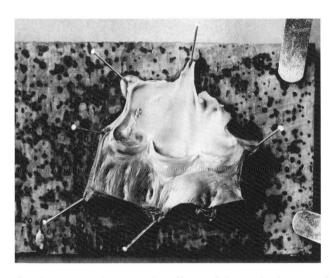

Specimen of a dog's heart showing the effects of direct diathermy of the aortic valve and the recent aortic incision used for access. (*Courtesy of the Georgetown University Library, Booth Family Center for Special Collections.*)

'open-heart' surgery, Carrel stopped the venous blood flow into the heart by clamping the major veins entering behind the heart. He then operated quickly and restored the circulation within 3–5 minutes before the brain was damaged. For valves affected by the vegetations of bacterial endocarditis, he showed he could open the aorta just above the aortic valve, quickly cauterise the edges of the valve with a heated probe, and close up. He knew that narrowing of the coronary arteries caused angina, and in a remarkable experiment, he led a graft of preserved dog carotid artery from the aorta across and joined it to a divided left coronary artery. It was the first coronary artery bypass graft (CABG). But this pioneer operation understandably took some time, and the animal died shortly afterwards from ventricular fibrillation: the *graft* may have been patent. The number of animals reported in his chest surgery series was small, but the principles established were clear, important and visionary.

As before, Carrel was not slow to publish, and there were five American publications on this work starting in 1909. Keen to have his work recognised internationally, he sent his findings to Théodore Tuffier, his French colleague and admirer, who then presented the results to a French surgical society, with publication following quickly in France in December 1909.[15] A similar paper with the same title was sent as a brief communication to a German journal and appeared early the following year.[16] Not only that, but a Spanish journal must have been surprised to get to short paper on aortic surgery submitted to them from Carrel, in Spanish.[17]

---

[15] A. Carrel 'Chirurgie expérimentale de l'aorte thoracique par la méthode de Meltzer (Rapport de Tuffier)' *Bulletin et mémoire de la Société de chirurgie de Paris* 35 (1909): 1337–40. Tuffier also transmitted Carrel's work to the French National Academy of Medicine in 1909 (note 30).

[16] A. Carrel 'Experimentelle intrathorakale Chirurgie mittels der Methode von Meltzer und Auer' *Berliner Klinische Wochenschrift* 47 (1910): 565–6.

[17] A. Carrel 'Chirurgia experimental de la aorta toracia facilitada por el metodo de Meltzer' *Clin. Mod.* (Saragosse) 9 (1910): 76–9.

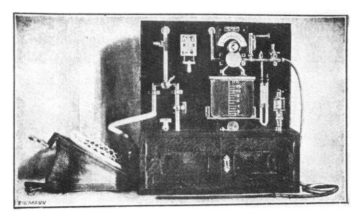

Meltzer's anaesthetic apparatus was soon modified for human chest surgery use. (*Courtesy of the American Society for Thoracic Surgery.*)

Meltzer's Studies

Meltzer also supported attempts at heart surgery in his own laboratory at the Institute. This rivalry with Carrel may or may not have been friendly. Meltzer brought in Charles A. Elsberg (1871–1948), a young surgeon from the nearby Mount Sinai Hospital, whose pioneering use of orthopaedic nails Carrel had followed in doing his leg grafts. In Meltzer's laboratory, Elsberg gained confidence with the use of the Meltzer–Auer technique and transferred it over for human use at his hospital.[18] There, in that winter of 1910, the surgeons carried out the first human thoracic operation using intra-tracheal anaesthesia given by Elsberg. At a historic meeting of the New York Academy of Medicine on 17 February 1910, Carrel and Meltzer gave papers on their surgical and anaesthetic work, and the proceedings appeared promptly in the local journal *Medical Record.*[19] The *New York Times* of 27 March enthused about the Institute operations in a long article 'Heart Surgery

---

[18] Elsberg's experimental heart surgery in Meltzer's lab was never published.
[19] Carrel and Meltzer's presentations are given in the *Medical Record (New York)* 77 (1910): 491–3. Meltzer pioneering work in anaesthesia gained the admiration of the surgical world, and in 1918 he was elected first president of the American Association for Thoracic Surgery.

Is Science's Latest Marvel'. The *Times* noted perceptively that Carrel was 'the wizard of the medical world like Luther Burbank' a reference to the botanist Luther A. Burbank (1849–1926) who pioneered plant hybridisation methods but was criticised for his rapid announcements of success, without publishing his methods fully for the scientific community. Carrel spoke at the American Surgical Association meeting in May 1910 and gave a detailed, confident account of his operations on the heart and aorta, which was admired in the discussion which followed.[20] As always, the press publicity brought in more letters to Carrel, and these now requested heart surgery.

With Carrel's work now well known outside America, at this time a *British Medical Journal* editorial commended his methods to the cautious surgical world. The journal's editorial added a poignant note about experimental surgery in general:

A great debt is owing to the many operators who have perfected their technique, and demonstrated the feasibility of extensive plastic repair on animals.[21]

This was a coded lament. Because of the strength of the British antivivisection sentiment, Britain's animal experimentation was limited. The 'operators' admired were American and European surgeons.[22]

This remarkable six months of major aortic and heart surgery for Carrel lasted from late 1909 to May 1910. Carrel went off to Europe as usual, shortly after his successful appearance at the American Surgical Association. He perhaps intended to resume his surgical work on return

---

[20] Alexis Carrel (1910) 'On the experimental surgery of the thoracic aorta and heart' *Transactions of the American Surgical Association* 28: 243–54 and *Annals of Surgery* (1910) 52: 83–95.

[21] Editorial, *BMJ*, 28 May 1910, 1309.

[22] Harvey Cushing made this point in a memorable and much-discussed lecture in London in 1913 saying that British surgery, formerly made famous by experimentalists like William Hunter, Charles Bell and Joseph Lister, was now in the doldrums and that the initiative had passed to America and Europe; see Harvey Cushing (1913) 'Address in Surgery' *BMJ* 9 August, 290–7.

in autumn 1910. Instead, as described earlier, Burrows had come back from Yale bringing the tissue culture technique, and Carrel was immediately diverted to the new venture. As described below, he would return to heart surgery for a time in late 1913, during the visit of the French surgeon Théodore Tuffier.

Attempts by Others

Carrel was not alone in looking at the possibilities for the surgery of heart valvular disease. At the Hunterian Laboratory in Baltimore, where Carrel might have been appointed in 1906, the professor of medicine William Sydney Thayer and the Hospital pathologist William G. MacCallum were planning for experimental cardiac surgery, but unlike Carrel's decisive moves to reach and explore the heart successfully, they delayed making direct attempts by first trying to create animal models of valve disease.[23] Their colleagues Harvey Cushing and J.R.B. Branch also took this up but hardly built upon the idea. Nor did Cushing use the new anaesthetic methods, but instead used a temporary tracheostomy for direct ventilation.[24] In the same laboratory, Halsted's interest in aneurysm surgery continued, and his strategy to deal with them was to constrict the arterial inflow with a metal collar to encourage alternative co-lateral flow through the adjacent smaller arteries. Halsted's work, like that of Carrel on the aorta, was plagued by erosion of the vessels by the metal device.

Heart Surgery Resumed

In October 1913, three years after his first period of study, Carrel resumed his heart surgery when his Parisian surgeon friend Tuffier visited him

---

[23] See Saul Jarcho (1974) 'Experimental production of cardiac murmurs (Thayer and MacCallum)' *American Journal of Cardiology* 34: 834–7. These were non-recovery experiments.

[24] Harvey Cushing and J.R.B. Branch (1908) 'Experimental and clinical notes on chronic valvular lesions in the dog' *Journal of Medical Research* 17: 471–86. Cushing gives a useful review of the few earlier attempts to deal with human heart injuries; see also Saul Jarcho (1975) 'Experiments on heart valves (1908) by Harvey Cushing and J.R.B. Branch' *American Journal of Cardiology* 35: 506–8.

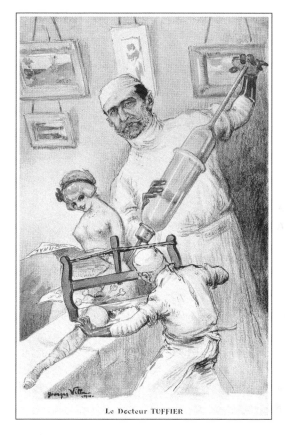

Le Docteur TUFFIER

Théodore Tuffier, the Paris surgeon, depicted in the Paris journal *Chanticlair* in 1910 using a spinal anaesthetic. He collaborated closely with Carrel in experimental heart surgery.

while on a tour of American surgical departments. The two ambitious Frenchmen admired each other's work and had similar personalities.[25] Shortly afterwards, during World War I, Tuffier would support Carrel in his disagreements with other French surgeons. Tuffier stayed for a while in New York, and they did their heart surgery together at the Institute.[26] Tuffier was interested in the possibilities of open thoracic surgery, having

[25] A heartfelt tribute to Tuffier by Carrel in the *Revue de Paris* September 1932 is translated in Joseph T. Durkin, *Hope for Our Time: Alexis Carrel on Man and Society* (New York: Harper and Row, 1965): 102–10. See also *Collectif Le Docteur Tuffier 1857–1929* (1935).
[26] Saul Jarco (1975) 'Carrel and Tuffier (1914) on experimental surgery of the cardiac orifices' *The American Journal of Cardiology* 36: 954–6.

already attempted human heart and lung surgery in Paris.[27] They worked together from 23 October to 2 December and devised an elegant method of approaching the pulmonary artery valve, which Tuffier hoped to use in patients.[28] After Tuffier left, Carrel carried on with further heart operations until the following April. In addition to repeating the techniques he reported in 1910 for operations on the heart valves, including cautery, Carrel now rehearsed operations for human congenital defects, notably defects in the internal walls between the heart chambers. As a model of one of these common abnormalities, he opened the left atrium, made a hole through the septum into the right atrium, and then rapidly closed the defect with sutures.

Carrel again described his results to a surgical audience, speaking at the American Surgical Association meeting in April 1914. The *New York Times* devoted two columns to his address and an editorial added that:

> The time is not distant, perhaps, when the lives of antivivisectionists afflicted with heart disease will be saved by the surgeons they are now attacking.[29]

Shortly after, just before the War started, Tuffier gave news of their methods and results to the French National Academy of Medicine.[30] Carrel and Tuffier also published a remarkable paper simultaneously in two generalist journals, the British weekly journal *Medical Press and*

---

[27] Tuffier had his own technique for anaesthesia for chest surgery using a cuffed tracheal tube and ventilation; see Tuffier (with Hallion 1906) 'L'Ouverture de la plèvre sans pneumothorax' *Presse médicale* 14: 57–9. This has a helpful illustrated review of the rival methods of ventilation for chest surgery. Tuffier had successfully partly dilated a narrowed human aortic valve in 1912 by invaginating a finger from outside the wall of the aorta.

[28] Theodore Tuffier and Alexis Carrel (1914) 'Patching and section of the pulmonary orifice of the heart' *JEM* 20: 3–8 describes their October to December 1913 series. Carrel's paper in *JEM* 20: 9–18, giving his January to April work on the pulmonary artery alone, has useful illustrations.

[29] 'Carrel's Surgery Amazes Experts' *NYT*, 11 April 1914 and 'Dr Carrel's Heart Surgery' *NYT*, 12 April 1914.

[30] A. Carrel and T. Tuffier (1914) *Bulletin de l' Académie nationale de Médecine* 71: 293, and a fuller account in 'Chirugie des orifices du coeur' *Presse médicale* 22 (1914): 173–7.

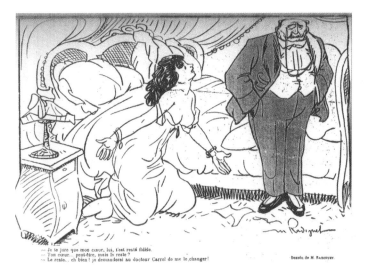

— Je te jure que mon cœur, lui, t'est resté fidèle.
— Ton cœur... peut-être, mais le reste ?
— Le reste... eh bien ! je demanderai au docteur Carrel de me le changer !

Dessin de M. Radiguet

A French cartoon acknowledging Carrel's authority in organ transplantation of all kinds. (*Courtesy of Georgetown University Library, Booth Family Center for Special Collections.*)

Circular and the *Presse médicale*.[31] They gave details of their surgical and anesthetic methods but also, aiming at a general medical audience, dealt with the case against heart surgery made by conservative physicians. The surgeons had shown that the heart muscle was robust, if the 'danger areas' were avoided, and could be touched, incised and would heal promptly. They pointed out that while in the advanced valvular disease seen at post-mortem, weak cardiac muscle was also seen, this was a secondary result of the long-standing valve defect. They predicted correctly that in cases operated on early, the heart muscle would be found to be unaffected.[32]

---

[31] A. Carrel and T. Tuffier (1914) 'Anatomico-pathological study of the surgery of the orifices of the heart' *Medical Press and Circular* 539–42 and 566–9, and *Presse médicale* 22 (1914): 173–7.

[32] The pathology of the heart was well described at the time and one of the best collections of specimens was held by Carrel's friend Emanuel Libman, the physician at Mount Sinai Hospital, New York.

It was a busy time for Carrel in early 1914. After his success at the American surgeons' conference, an important international surgical meeting was coming up shortly in New York. He was on the program to give an important lecture, not on heart surgery, but on organ transplantation. And he had some interesting news for the assembled surgeons.

Murphy's Insight

Towards the end of 1913, Carrel heard from a colleague working one floor below him at the Institute that rejection of grafts could be prevented. James Baumgarten Murphy (1884–1950) had arrived from Baltimore in 1910 to work with Peyton Rous, and in the following year, Rous had made a famous discovery, which gained him a Nobel Prize later. He found that a chicken sarcoma, a malignant tumour, was caused by a virus. Murphy extended the work and quickly found that the tumour would grow easily in the embryo sac within chicken's eggs. Murphy wondered why the chicken egg lacked the power to reject this aggressive homograft, and he found that if adult chicken lymph nodes or spleen were also added to the sac, it gave adult capability to the embryo, and the tumour would fail to grow. Murphy had crucially demonstrated that lymph node or spleen cells — the lymphocytes — were involved in tumour graft rejection. Moreover, if lymphocytes were reduced in the adult body, tumour homografts would survive. To reduce lymphocytes, he used radiation or the toxic chemical benzol.[33]

Flexner's summary report of Murphy's work by 1914 was quite clear:

> By damaging the lymphoid tissue of rats and lessening the number of lymphocytes in the circulating blood he [Murphy] has been able to grow

---

[33] James B. Murphy and Arthur W.M. Ellis (1914) 'Experiments on the role of lymphoid tissue in the resistance to experimental tuberculosis in mice' *JEM* 20: 397–403. Much later, Murphy's contributions were at last recognised by Arthur M. Silverstein (2001) 'The lymphocyte in immunology: from James B. Murphy to James Gowans, *Nature Immunology* 2: 569–71, but Silverstein missed Murphy's important use of benzol.

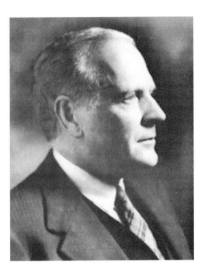

James B. Murphy gave Carrel the vital information that radiation or the use of benzol would allow foreign tissue grafts to survive. (*Courtesy of the Rockefeller University Archives.*)

mouse tumours in these animals for a considerable time, and even transplant them successfully to other rats treated in the same way. Injection of benzol, ablation of the spleen, and irradiation with x-rays have been the means employed to affect the lymphoid tissue.[34]

Flexner already knew about benzol and radiation's action on immunity to infection, but the finding of benzol's ability to prolong grafts was new. As director, he applauded Murphy's findings, commenting that: 'It is needless to say that these results have a fundamental bearing on the problem of transplantation'.

The New York Meeting

The International Surgical Congress (formally named La Société Internationale de Chirurgie), gathered in New York in spring 1914.

---

[34] 'Dr Murphy's Report on Cancer' *Scientific Reports*, April 1914, box 1 vol. 3 p. 322, FA 145, RUA RAC (note 2).

Belgian surgeons had taken the initiative in 1905 in setting up this Society, and the headquarters remained in Brussels, as a 'neutral' nation at a time of European rivalry. The Germans, although giving some of the invited lectures in 1914, did not otherwise participate in any numbers, perhaps because the prestigious German society, the Deutsche Gesellschaft für Chirurgie, met in Berlin in the same week as the New York meeting, and attracted 2263 attendees.[35]

The major themes of the New York conference were amputation, abdominal surgery and transplantation. The five speakers in the transplantation session were Carrel, Emerich Ullmann from Vienna, Hippolyte Morestin of Paris (the 'father of plastic surgery'), Erich Lexer from Jena and Eugène Villard of Lyon, one of Carrel's rivals for promotion 12 years earlier. Those who spoke on homografting agreed that these grafts did not survive. Although this seemed an emphatic international verdict, at the Berlin meeting, the speakers at a similar session on the long-term results of human thyroid homografting still showed some support for this treatment.[36] Emil Kocher spoke first and chaired the session, but Erwin Payr and Anton von Eiselsberg, whose presentations followed, were having doubts about their earlier support of Kocher in the enthusiasm for thyroid homografting.[37] Various explanations of why thyroid slice homografts might on occasions fail were offered — too little graft used, the wrong place used for insertion, delay in insertion, bleeding round the graft, or that there was lack of surgical skill or infection occurred later.

---

[35] After WWI, the German surgeons were excluded from the International Society, but were re-admitted in 1932.

[36] See the proceedings of the Deutsche Gesellschaft für Chirurgie Conference in *Verhandlungen der Deutschen Gesellschaft für Chirurgie* 43 (1914): 74–8 and the summary in Schlich, *Origins* (note 37): 57. Other speakers during the human thyroid transplantation session were Schaack (St Petersburg), Wilhelm Müller (Rostock) and Eugen Enderlen (Würzburg).

[37] For Kocher's involvement in thyroid grafting, see the account in Thomas Schlich, *The Origins of Organ Transplantation: Surgery and Laboratory Science 1880–1930* (Rochester: University of Rochester Press, 2010).

But in New York, there was harmony. Ullmann, who had been first with experimental kidney transplants, agreed that homografts regularly failed and that this was caused by 'anaphylaxis' — a word used at that time for any immunological response.[38] Erich Lexer, was critical of much previous surgical work on homografting, concluding that

> the reports in the literature of fortunate healing of transplanted skin or epidermis by homoplastie [homografting] … are the results of erroneous observation.[39]

He also suggested that Kocher's human thyroid gland grafts were failures. Carrel spoke and, having taken years to accept this great simplification, supported it again at the conference, and that

> homoplastic transplantations, though the immediate results maybe excellent, are nearly always ultimately unsuccessful, and that hetero-plastic transplantations are always unsuccessful.

Carrel then reflected on the way ahead and suggested that grafting within the family might have advantages. He then added Murphy's new findings, which took up more than half his address. He knew that Murphy had identified the lymphocyte as responsible for graft rejection, and that Murphy had gone further:

> He [Murphy] studied the effect of benzol, which has the power of diminishing the activity of leucocytes. In rats injected with benzol he found that the duration of the life of the mouse tumor [grafted to a rat] was longer. … it is certain that a very important point has been acquired with Murphy's discovery that the power of the organism to

---

[38] Ullman's lecture is given in full as 'Tissue and organ transplantation' *Annals of Surgery* 60 (1914): 195–219.

[39] Erich Lexer (1914) 'Free transplantation' *Annals of Surgery* 60: 166–95, at 172. For his earlier work see E. Lexer (1911) 'Über freie Transplantationen' *Archiv für Klinsche Chirurgie* 95: 827–51.

eliminate foreign tissue was due to organs such as the spleen or bone marrow.

It would be 55 years before immunosuppression with irradiation or chemicals was introduced with similar success into organ transplantation.

The proceedings at the meeting were widely reported, and detailed reports appeared in the *Journal of the American Medical Association*, the *British Medical Journal* and *The Lancet*. Carrel characteristically also published his paper promptly in the local *New York Medical Journal*.[40] The *New York Times* of 17 April carried the same story in full, with added material from an interview with Carrel. The *Times* editorial on 'Transplanting Organs' emphasised Murphy's discoveries, and that tissues of lower animals 'might be made serviceable in the bodily economy of man'.

After the conference, Carrel was in touch with Kocher regarding thyroid homograft transplants. In a courteous but sceptical letter to Kocher, after regretting that he was not at the conference, Carrel said: 'Concerning the homoplastic transplantation of organs such as the kidney into animals, I have never found positive results to continue after a few months'.

Carrel then told Kocher how to get prolongation of graft life:

> We must find out ways by what means to prevent the reaction of the organism against new organ, but I will send you some articles of James Murphy.[41]

He also enclosed a copy of his conference speech. It had been a remarkable two weeks for Carrel. His heart surgery paper had been praised by the American surgeons and following this came the successful International meeting.

---

[40] Alexis Carrel (1914) 'The transplantation of organs' *New York Medical Journal* 99: 839–40.

[41] Carrel to Kocher, 8 May 1914, Malinin Collection of the Papers of Alexis Carrel and Charles Lindbergh, box 15 folder 19, FA 208, RUA RAC (note 2).

Outbreak of War

Carrel sailed for France as usual on 3 June 1914 on the *La Lorraine*, and he was there when war broke out in Europe on 28 July. As a French citizen, he was drafted into the army medical service, but he joined willingly, as a patriotic duty, in spite of his criticisms of his country. As an inventive man interested in military affairs, he also knew that military surgery could offer scientific and clinical opportunities.

But at first, he was in the wrong job.

CHAPTER EIGHT

War in France

G ermany declared war on France on 3 August 1914, and the German army advanced immediately into and through Belgium in an attempt to reach Paris. The French army countered the attack and held the line. A counter-attack elsewhere was ready, and the French made their long-planned contingency move into the contested Alsace region to the north and east of Lyon, held by the Germans since the war of 1871, and formerly a part of France.

Carrel, in France for the summer, was drafted as a medical officer, and given the fairly lowly rank of aide-major second-class. He had earlier been attracted toward a military career, and joined willingly, leaving behind the many active and important research developments in his laboratory. In spite of Carrel's well-known antipathy towards his own nation, there was also an underlying patriotism, and he also believed that the discipline of a war was just what France needed.[1] Writing from France he said:

> Suddenly the spirit of France has changed. It is almost unbelievable. Our men are in splendid moral condition. We must thank Germany, which will be responsible for the resurrection of France. I believe that the young generation will come out of this war completely revirilised.[2]

---

[1] The scientists were not detached from the politics of the war, and a group of senior German scientists issued a statement declaring that Germany deserved an expansion of its national boundaries. A rebuttal by British and American scientists followed. Simon Flexner at the Rockefeller Institute declined to sign this response, and this action cost him a nomination to the French Academy of Sciences.

[2] Carrel to Coudert, in Angelo M. May and Alice G. May, *The Two Lions of Lyons* (Rockville, MD: Kabel Publishing, 1994): 152.

CARREL SEES A NEW FRANCE.

An Unconquerable Spirit, Surgeon
Says, Now Prevails Everywhere.

PARIS, Aug. 24.—Dr. Alexis Carrel of
the Rockefeller Institute for Medical
Research of New York was about to
leave for the United States, but at the
outbreak of war he canceled his departure, and is now in charge of a big
hospital where the French wounded are
treated. Writing to a friend of the war,
he says:
"France has been transformed in
miraculous fashion. Individuals themselves have changed. I could never have
believed it had I not seen it with my
own eyes. Most perfect order prevails
and enthusiasm grows daily. I am more
and more convinced that the men are
animated with the spirit that can never
be vanquished.
"I am seeking men ready literally to
give their blood for transfusions to
wounded soldiers. Already I have found
a doctor and an attorney and hope
soon to have several others."

Carrel's move to join the French army was announced in the *New York Times*.

Carrel felt that France, his France, needed a wake-up call, and this was his oft-repeated view later.

Carrel's own work in his Experimental Surgery Division was necessarily interrupted, but did not cease. In Carrel's absence, Albert Ebeling was in charge of the tissue culture work, notably maintaining the precious, long-lived 'old strain' chicken cell culture. Ebeling had picked up some of Carrel's difficult surgical techniques and continued to assist others in the Institute when these were required. But at his request, Ebeling was given regular leave to attend medical school at Yale, where he graduated later as a doctor in 1919, in spite of periods of illness. Care of the 'immortal' old strain cells was therefore in others' hands for long periods; there were no publications on tissue culture from Carrel's laboratory during the War.

Flexner, supportive as always, was sorry to lose Carrel and reported to the Board that he would retain Carrel's staff and that:

> The work of Carrel has not entirely ceased, as his assistants have been engaged in keeping up the culture of tissues and in performing [surgical] operations for other members of staff. We have in mind to keep the staff which Dr. Carrel has spent so much time in training, so that when he returns, he may resume work without losing time or energy.

Back to Lyon

In France, Carrel was posted to his home city of Lyon. Although Lyon was far from the now-static war in the far north and west, the Lyon hospitals were immediately involved in treating casualties resulting from the battles in Alsace-Lorraine closer by. Carrel was at first given a fairly humble post at the Lyon railway reception centre which triaged the injured sent back to the city, but he soon got a more appropriate move to do some surgical work at the Des Genette's military hospital and at the famous Hôtel Dieu, where Mme Carrel was made head nurse of a 50-bed ward. Characteristically, he let the *New York Times* know of his arrival. The newspaper said he was in charge of a big Lyon hospital, and Carrel gave a confident account, praising the French surgeons and that 'he saw a new France'.[3] However, as always, he was less diplomatic in private: he wrote to Flexner complaining that 'the hospital is old, the people ignorant'. He mentioned in a casual aside that his wife had lost her unborn baby after a reaction to a bee sting.[4]

Though in a more suitable hospital post, there were frustrations for Carrel. He had been out of routine clinical surgery for nine years, and had not been licensed to practise in New York, nor had he wished to be. He was junior in rank to the local surgeon Léon Berard, who had been promoted ahead of him in Lyon back in 1901, and Carrel was allowed to do only a limited amount of surgery, usually operating with Berard.

---

[3] 'Carrel Sees A New France' *NYT*, 25 August 1914. This was one of seven *NYT* stories from Lyon about Carrel in the next six months.
[4] Carrel letters to Flexner are in RGI 100N, box 64 folder 632, Rockefeller University Archives, Rockefeller Archives Centre (RUA RAC).

PRAISES FRENCH SURGEONS.

Dr. Carrel Says Americans Could Not Better the Field Service.

Special Cable to THE NEW YORK TIMES.

PARIS, Sept. 19.—The Journal gives details about modern bullet wounds gleaned from an interview with Dr. Alexis Carrel, formerly of the Rockefeller Institute in New York, now Second Assistant Surgeon Major at the Lyons Hospital. "The sanitary department," he said, "is doing wonders. Americans could not improve it. Infection is prevented by temporary bandaging on the battlefield. Then the wounded are removed to the hospital with amazing celerity which saves thousands. At Des Genettes Hospital here we have not lost one man in five hundred; at the Hotel Dieu, twenty at most of two thousand. Heavy artillery produces horrible wounds, while ricocheting pieces of shrapnel sometimes cause infection, but they represent only a trifling proportion. As for Mauser mitrailleuse wounds, I do not pretend that they are actually healthful; but I know soldiers who have absorbed six without being in a very bad state. In fact, unless they strike an essential organ, only a slight scar remains after a fortnight to warrant the bearer to declare proudly: 'You see, I was there.'"

Carrel updated the *New York Times* in September 1914 on his Lyon war surgery.

Although he had little desire to do routine surgical work, his position must have rankled. Carrel was a proud man, a recent Nobel Prize winner and a famous scientist, and he was well-known in France. This humble posting might even have been a reprisal by the authorities for his well-known criticisms of French medicine.

At this time there was some good news from New York. Carrel had been elected as an honorary life member at his Piping Rock country club, a rare honour which he shared with ex-President Roosevelt.

Local Action

Within a week of the War starting, north of Lyon the French army had moved into Alsace-Lorraine on 9 August 1914. At the Battle of Mulhouse, they captured the former French town in an important strategic and symbolic national victory, but after much rejoicing in France, the troops were forced to withdraw on 24 August. Fighting continued thereafter in this region, with mobile attack and counter-attack in which bullet and bayonet wounds predominated, and the casualties were evacuated south to Lyon. Carrel told the *British Medical Journal* about his work:

> I am in my own city. Mobilised, naturally. I am in the Hôtel Dieu in the Department of Surgery. I have more than 1,000 wounded to look after. My patients are the first who came under fire. They are those who in Haute Alsace completed with the bayonet the work of the mitrailleuse [machine guns]. Fortunately the wounds are not very serious. In all, the wounded in Lyon are about 12,000 distributed among 42 hospitals: in the district 25,000 more. ... The mortality is very low. In my hospital of 2,500 men hardly 20 have died of the wounds. Besides, our wounded go back in great numbers to the front.[5]

The military life clearly suited him. Much later he confided to his nephew, 'Why do people fear war? A violent death is a sweet thing when it is compared to death by degenerative disease'.[6]

As part of the war effort in Lyon, Carrel naturally looked for any surgical opportunities. His letters mention use of an ice box for preservation of skin, fat and blood vessels for grafting, but although he and Tuffier in Paris, now assisting the Minister of War, were the pioneers in tissue banking, Carrel seems to have had little opportunity to use such tissues. He did mention using a human foetal pulmonary artery to repair a soldier's damaged femoral artery, but the result is unknown. Carrel doubtless shared the caution of other surgeons who knew of his technique. A young Hopkins military surgeon, keen to try the newer methods, held back because

> the teachings of Carrel, together with the laboratory experiences of his followers, have so effectually demonstrated the futility of attempted blood vessels suturing in any but a non-infected field that it needed but

[5] *BMJ*, 17 October 1914, 689. This article ostensibly was a letter from Carrel 'to a friend', and he gave similar news to the *NYT* of 20 September 1914.
[6] Carrel to Gigou, 19 April 1938, FA 208, Malinin Collection of the Papers of Alexis Carrel and Charles Lindbergh, box 14 folder 6, RUA RAC (note 4).

a glance at the type of [war] wounds to be dealt with to realise from the outset the hopelessness of finer blood vessel surgery. Excision and ligation were the rule and this was rather distressing... when the continuity could have been re-established by simple end to end suture. It required a high order of self-restraint to forgo some of these cases.[7]

Carrel also carried out a small number of blood transfusions, and, after appealing for human volunteers to help with a particular case, 120 potential donors came up to the hospital. This means that direct matching was done to choose a suitable donor. The transfusion which followed would either be by joining the donor and recipient vessels directly in some way or using syringes for rapid transfer. Perhaps surprisingly, Carrel and the Allied military surgeons made no more attempts at blood transfusion until the last months of the war.

But one project presented itself daily, and it was Carrel's old favourite — the healing of wounds. In civilian life, fresh skin wounds, large and small, were cleaned with antiseptic, and could usually be safely closed immediately with stitches — the usual approach called 'primary closure'. In larger wounds, if infection was present, after cleansing with antiseptic, the skin might still be closed, and a drain left in the wound beneath the closed skin. Carrel's letter had suggested that the Lyon military casualties were untroubled by serious infection, and in another letter he made a claim, one which was odd in the light of later events. When he did have infected wounds to deal with, the usual drainage tubes displeased him, and he had introduced a new design of drain, one with multiple branches, spreading like the arms of an octopus. These he inserted into infected wounds and then closed the skin over the drain, sealing the area further with rubber sheets and a form of glue. He then applied negative pressure to the tube — the strategy used in the suction drains favoured later. He said in a letter to Flexner that using his method, 'it is surprising to observe the wonderful results in open [compound] fractures, infected joints and large abscesses'.[8]

---

[7] Bernheim quoted in Steven G. Friedman, *A History of Vascular Surgery* (Malden: Blackwell Futura, 2005): xx.
[8] Carrel to Flexner, 17 October 1914, FA 208 Malinin Collection box 2 folder 1, RUA RAC (note 4).

Carrel's enthusiasm for primary closure plus drainage was short-lived. He would soon become a celebrated advocate of the alternative, namely the 'open' strategy in wound management, leaving the wound open with delayed 'secondary closure' later.

War Moves North

After the cessation of fighting in Alsace-Lorraine, the action moved further north and to the west. Carrel had little to do in Lyon. Major battles were now fought on the flat terrain near the Belgian border, and in the Battle of Mons starting on 23 August 1914, cavalry were in action for the last time. As the battles moved nearer to Paris, there was heroic fighting by the French at the Marne from 5–12 September, when nearly 250,000 French were wounded or killed, as were 13,000 of the British Expeditionary Force which had recently joined the war. The French military surgeons in Paris obtained huge experience in dealing with these mass casualties, and the Allies eventually repulsed the German attack. The Germans fell back and dug defensive trenches, waiting to launch or endure major assaults.

During this engagement north of Paris, help for the French army medical services came from the new 570-bed Ambulance [i.e. Hospital] américaine which had been organised by American ex-pats and New York philanthropy. They sought volunteer units to come from America and senior staff from famous units soon responded.[9] George Crile at Cleveland had been first to arrive, bringing a Western Reserve Hospital unit, and they were involved in dealing with the mass casualties reaching Paris in September 1914 from the heavy fighting at the Marne.[10] Cushing's unit followed and replaced Crile's team, and this involvement in Paris helped American medical preparedness for war later.

---

[9] Eric I. Rutkow and Ira Rutkow (2004) 'George Crile, Harvey Cushing, and the Ambulance Américaine' *Archives of Surgery* 139: 678–85.

[10] After the battle of the Marne, 70 miles north of Paris, Crile described how 'the wounded came in 60 at a time, with the operating room in continuous performance and not enough beds to go around'; see John F. Fulton, *Harvey Cushing: A Biography* (Springfield: Charles C Thomas, 1946): 395.

Steadily, by the following spring, the now evenly-matched armies were deadlocked in trenches nearer the English Channel. These trenches soon linked up, and on both sides the complex system extended inland and was eventually continuous for 400 miles. Attacks were planned ahead in detail, with a preceding bombardment, and between battles there was intermittent shelling and sniping.

New Infections

A new pattern of wounds was appearing in the European northern battles. To add to bullet wounds, there were penetrating injuries by jagged shrapnel from shells, which took clothing into the wound. The new wounds, which were uncommon in civilian life and in the relatively recent Boer War, could give new virulent infections. These included tetanus and an unusual, rapidly spreading, life-threatening infection of the limbs, with palpable gas beneath the discoloured skin, eventually called 'gas gangrene'.[11]

It was first noticed in the autumn of 1914 shortly after the War started. By November, British bacteriologists had identified the organism as the anaerobic spore-bearing *Clostridium perfringens*, first identified by Welch at Johns Hopkins in 1892, and named *C. welchii* at that time. The organism is innocuous in most situations but thrives in dead tissue, notably muscle. Detective work was complete when the organism was found to be widely present in the well-manured agricultural soils used for the trenches, and it contaminated military clothing, particularly the heavy trench coats. During battles, the severity of all forms of infection was

---

[11] The unfamiliar situation was described in a circular to the British surgeons on 9 November 1914; see Anthony A. Bowlby and S. Rowland (1914) 'A report on gas gangrene' *Journal of the Royal Army Corps* 23: 514–17. For general accounts of WWI military medicine, see Mark Harrison, *The Medical War: British Military Medicine in the First World War* (Oxford: Oxford University Press, 2010) and Ian R. Whitehead, *Doctors in the Great War* (London: Leo Cooper, 1999). By November 1914, anti-tetanus serum was available and proved effective.

increased when casualties lay injured for long periods between the trenches before rescue.

The Allied military surgeons had, as ever, been ready with management designed for the injuries of the last conflict, which for Britain had been the Boer War, a campaign fought over uncultivated dry, rocky land. Then, most wounds were cleansed with antiseptics and closed with stitches. In the new trench warfare, this was largely ineffective, and at first only prompt amputation could be life-saving. The *British Medical Journal* commented later that

> the complication of gas gangrene was one of the great surprises of this war to all the combatant armies, a calamity before which modern surgery, tutored in the simplicity of asepticism, was at first well nigh impotent.[12]

This revived the debate, one as old as warfare itself, on whether to close recent wounds or leave them open to drain, and then close later.

Policy Shift

After the first months of the War, in autumn 1914, the Belgian surgeon Antoine Depage (1862–1925) led the way.[13] This distinguished civilian surgeon served in the Balkan conflict in 1912 and, working in Constantinople, concluded that it was best to assume that most of the wounds he encountered were infected from the start. This led him to recommend that frontline surgeons 'must repress the desire to close wounds'. Nor were ugly scars the result: late closure gave a surprisingly good cosmetic outcome. Depage was now in charge of the large l'Amulance de l'Ocean at La Panne 12km behind the Belgian front, and he went further, realising that leaving these new war wounds open was not enough. The wound should be explored, looking for any foreign material, and all dead tissue, notably muscle, cut out, any tensions

---

[12] Editorial 'Gas Gangrene' *BMJ*, 11 November 1916: 663.

[13] Thomas S. Helling and Emmanuel Daon (1998) 'In Flanders fields: the Great War, Antoine Depage and the resurgence of débridement' *Annals of Surgery* 228: 173–81.

relieved, and the wound left widely open to drain. This excision of dead issue was a revival of another old strategy, namely wound *débridement,* as the French surgeons had called it from the late 1700s.[14]

Major engagements in the north-west did not re-commence until the spring of 1915 with fighting at Neuve Chapelle during March and at Ypres starting April 22. Over the winter, the new strategy had gained acceptance and from spring 1916 onwards, the new aggressive policy of débridement and delayed suture was in place, and spreading gas gangrene infection was no longer a prominent problem.

Aftercare

But the shift in policy meant that there were now many injured soldiers with open wounds, mostly created by the surgeons, which were ugly but no longer life-threatening. There was now the question of how to dress these wounds. Some surgeons thought that the choice of dressing after débridement did not matter, but others did, and felt strongly about it. Because of the early experience in the first months of the war, there was a lack of confidence in the traditional antiseptics, notably carbolic acid, hydrogen peroxide and iodine.

A debate started on how to treat open wounds after débridement, and the issues were soon clouded by polemical debate. First to take a confident stance was Sir Almroth Wright, the high-profile bacteriologist at London's St Mary's Hospital depicted in George Bernard Shaw's play *The Doctor's Dilemma* of 1906. He had fame as a controversialist and promoted his 'natural' way of defending the body, namely 'stimulating the phagocytes'.[15] Wright had involvement in the Boer War and had managed to introduce vaccination of the troops against typhoid fever. In 1914, Wright was given military rank and, sent by the newly-formed Medical Research Committee

---

[14] In the 18th century, the Paris surgeon Pierre-Joseph Desault (1738–1795) was the first known advocate of wide excision of damaged tissue. For a history of débridement see R.S. Saadia and M. Schein (2000) 'Débridement of gunshot wounds: semantics and surgery' *World Journal of Surgery* 24: 1146–9.

[15] Michael Dunnill, *The Plato of Praed Street: the Life and Times of Almroth Wright* (London: Royal Society of Medicine Press, 2000).

to the No. 14 British Military Hospital in Boulogne on the Channel coast, he obtained laboratory support for a study of wound infection. Wright was influenced by the views of Antoine Depage, who worked at La Panne nearby, and quickly accepted the need for surgical débridement and open wound management. Wright soon had a confident proposal to make for the after-treatment of open wounds, and claimed that antiseptics caused harm by holding back healing. His alternative to antiseptic dressings was to irrigate the wound with a strong salt solution, which would encourage outflow of lymph and hence, he thought, bring the natural defences of the body into action in the wound.[16]

Wright already had an influential surgical supporter in Sir Berkeley Moynihan (1865–1936), based at the British hospital at Rouen, not far from Wright, as a full colonel and advisor to the army on surgical care.[17] Moynihan valued this link with a famous scientist, and praised Wright's contribution as 'the best and the most speedy in securing a healthy condition of the wound'.[18] The two men contributed to a detailed memorandum issued in spring of 1915, from the military medical leadership, on treating war wounds. By now, nine months into the war, it seemed that the matter was settled, and the official advice was to use Wright's saline irrigation method in the open wounds left after débridement.[19]

However, there was one distinguished surgical voice still ready to support the use of antiseptics. Sir William Watson Cheyne (1852–1932) had been Lister's assistant, and he rose to become president of the Royal

---

[16] *The Lancet*, April 10 1915, 737–41 and 843–7.
[17] Colonel Sir Berkeley Moynihan, later elevated in 1922 as Lord Moynihan, was professor of surgery in the University of Leeds from 1909 and was unusual in having the national influence usually held by London-based clinicians. He was president of the Royal College of Surgeons of England in 1926.
[18] Berkeley Moynihan (1915) '"Hypertonic" treatment of wounds' *BMJ*, 29 May, 930 and *The Lancet*, 11 September 1915, 629.
[19] This detailed advice was in F.F. Burghard, W.B. Leishman, B. Moynihan and A.E. Wright 'Memorandum on the treatment of the bacterial infections of projectile wounds' *BMJ*, 24 April 1915, 735–8; Moynihan and Wright's forceful prose is obvious throughout.

College of Surgeons in London in 1914–16. Cheyne was not given any active military role, but as Surgeon Rear-Admiral to the Royal Navy he did some research for the Naval Medical Committee, thus providing some credentials. He soon used an important lecture to enter the debate and to defend against the attack on antiseptics.[20]

Cheyne had reservations about the now-accepted British Moynihan–Wright wound management. He said impishly later:

> Unfortunately, of late years a most unaccountable prejudice has arisen against antiseptics. I need hardly remind my readers that there are two different lines of treatment advocated at the present time.... The first [antiseptics] is at present very unpopular; it is old-fashioned, and savours too much of Teutonic methods. The second [Wright's] is much more popular; it is quite the latest thing in wound treatment; it has a very scientific flavour about it.[21]

Cheyne then criticised Wright's method but at the time, no one heeded his concern.

Carrel's Move

In Lyon, as the War's focus had shifted to the north in late 1914, Carrel had less to do, and was restive. However he had friends in Paris, and it is likely that Carrel's close surgical friends Théodore Tuffier and Samuel Pozzi intervened. Tuffier's post was 'Special Inspector for the Minister of War' and, as described earlier, he had worked closely with Carrel in New York. Tuffier was also one of the small number of guests at Carrel's recent wedding in Paris. Some accounts improbably say that Carrel was only

---

[20] Cheyne's Hunterian Oration is in *The Lancet*, 17 February 1915, 419–30, and the news about the now-essential débridement had not reached him. He still supported direct use of antiseptics but only in new wounds seen early, as he did in his 'Sir Almroth Wright's lecture on the treatment of wounds of war' *The Lancet* 9 May 1915 and 31 July 1915.

[21] W.W. Cheyne (1915–16) 'On the treatment of wounds of war' *British Journal of Surgery* 3: 427–50.

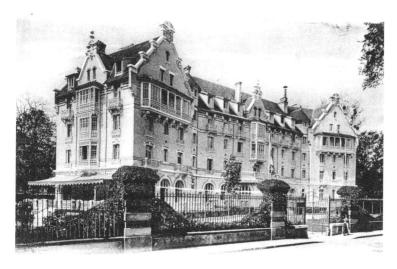

Carrel's hospital, north of Paris, was formerly the Rond Royal grand hotel.

rescued from his lowly post in Lyon by the intervention of James Hazen Hyde, an American businessman resident in France.

The upshot was that in December 1914, Carrel was given the task of surveying the Allies' surgical services. Provided with a driver, Carrel toured the British, French and Belgian front-line medical units.[22] Word of his tour somehow got to the *New York Times*.[23] Carrel then asked his powerful French military contacts to support him with a surgical unit of his own. The local wartime administrator in Paris was told to provide Carrel with a hospital — an 'ambulance' — and for his hospital, Carrel was given the luxury Rond Royal hotel, now renamed Hôpital Complémentaire No. 21 Compiègne, and later sometimes called the 'Mission Carrel'. Compiègne, 50 miles north of Paris, was a town favoured in the past by Napoleon III, and at the time was a country retreat for well-off Parisians. It still had grand apartments, and, converted to a hospital with 52 beds, later rising to 80, it was partly operational by March 1915. Although it was only about 40 miles south from the war

---

[22] Carrel's detailed itinerary is given in Angelo M. May and Alice G. May, *The Two Lions of Lyons* (Kabel Publishing, 1994): 151–4.
[23] 'Carrel On Inspection Tour' *NYT*, 18 December 1914.

frontlines remaining after the battle of the Marne in September 1914, the town was now safe because of the static nature of the conflict and because major actions had moved north-west towards the sea. There were no more major battles close to Paris until the conflict did get close to Compiègne in 1918. It would serve as a base hospital after initial treatment at the distant front lines.[24]

Carrel also enlisted Flexner's support back in New York, and Flexner asked the Rockefeller Foundation, the international part of Rockefeller philanthropy, to assist. The Foundation moved quickly, and gave a $20,000 annual grant towards the costs of medical investigations at Carrel's 'ambulance'. The Foundation was careful to emphasise that they were supporting science rather than the hospital's clinical war work; the Foundation was studiously neutral, and America was not yet at war with Germany. With these funds, Carrel was able to add considerable laboratory back-up for a study of wounds, making it the first-ever military surgical research unit. Carrel showed considerable flair in setting up and administering his hospital and its large staff. On the surgical side, unlike his blood vessel and transplant innovations which he was content to pass on to the surgeons and await their uptake, on this occasion he soon wished the military surgeons to pay immediate attention and follow his lead on wound treatment.[25]

Staffing

Carrel's post was 'Médecin Chef' with the rank of major, but he was paid from his Institute salary. He did not operate himself, and usually had two French-trained military surgeons plus two assistant surgeons to do the

---

[24] The town of Compiègne has lasting military significance because the 1918 armistice ending WWI was signed in the nearby Compiègne Forest. In 1940, when France capitulated to the German invasion, to further humiliate the French, Hitler arranged for the armistice documents to be signed in the same railway carriage.

[25] See Georgette Mottier, *L'ambulance du Dr. Alexis Carrel 1914–1919* (Lausanne: Éditions la Source, 1977), which has many illustrations, and L.G. Walker (2002) 'Carrel's war research hospital at Compiegne: Prototype of a research facility at the front' *Journal of the American College of Surgeons* 195: 870–7.

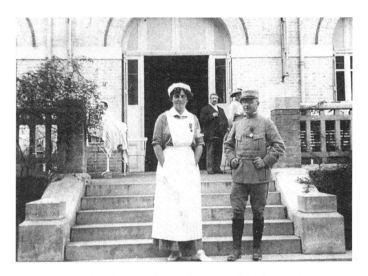

Carrel with his wife, on the steps of the hospital.

work, with two physicians also on the staff.[26] Some nurses came from Emil Kocher's hospital in Switzerland and some via a New York philanthropy set up by Mrs. Post. Carrel's research surgical nurse from the Institute moved to join his hospital. Staffing grew, and when well-established, in addition to his medical staff, Carrel had an administrator, two chemists, a physicist-mathematician, a bacteriologist, and an equipment maker, and he could call on a draftsman and photographer, the French-Italian Francoise-Michel Tonetti (1864–1920), his sculptor friend from New York. Mme Carrel was head nurse, and had a Red Cross ranking of 'infirmière-major de la Croix-Rouge'. To bring in patients from Paris or from the local mainline railway station, they had two ambulances, two cars, one truck and seven civilian volunteer drivers. The former hotel with its chandeliers and painted ceilings retained much of its grandeur, and Carrel's staff may have lived in style. Carrel enjoyed setting up the large organisation and its administration, and the discipline of

---

[26] Dr. Guillot was surgeon-in-chief, with Drs. Dehelly and Woimant as his deputies and Drs. Audiganne and Dumas as surgical assistants. Dehelly would join Carrel in New York in 1917, and was later a surgeon in Le Havre.

military life. He had, as usual, a poor opinion of some of those around him, and his first two bacteriologists, vital in the management of his projects, did not please him, and they were moved out. Of the French surgeons, he reported back to Flexner in New York, 'their purely verbal education makes them take the words for facts. As soon as they have spoken, they believe they have acted'.[27]

At the Institute, the general manager Henry James knew Carrel's weakness for such blunt indiscretion and was concerned. He noted that 'I wish he would not utter his sentiments as freely as he does'.[28] Nevertheless, the Foundation and the Institute were proud of Carrel's high profile; Rockefeller money was again going to a good cause.

Selecting Injuries

Carrel's hospital was one of a network of military medical units, large and small, involved in the war. The workload varied, and there could be an inflow of cases of partly-treated casualties during the short, brutal, inconclusive battles now taking place some distance from Paris, but there were lulls during which there were only sporadic injuries from the skirmishes between battles. The route for the injured was first to a first aid station, then the seriously injured were sent back to casualty clearing stations for more definitive treatment, and the survivors were moved, usually by rail, to base hospitals. The partly-treated survivors reaching Paris were distributed from the railway clearing stations at La Chapelle, and some reached Carrel's hospital, or were picked out by his drivers from the railway trucks passing through Compiègne towards Paris.

At some point, Carrel arranged that he would only look at one type of injury, namely wounds to the legs or arms. These cases usually arrived after débridement carried out at the casualty clearing stations. This case selection gave him adequate numbers for a study of a restricted clinical problem, and only occasionally did he have serious abdominal, chest or

---

[27] W. Sterling Edwards and Peter D. Edwards, *Alexis Carrel: Visionary Surgeon* (Springfield, Illinois: Charles C. Thomas, 1974): 78.

[28] James to Coudert, November 1915, box 2 folder 1, Carrel (Alexis) papers, (1906–1957), FA 231, RUA RAC (note 4).

brain injuries to deal with. This meant that his hospital death rate was low. But leg and arm wounds carried the possibility of amputation, and amputation featured strongly in the public's perception of the effects of war. The public would be interested in Carrel's work.

Diverting one type of injury to a special hospital was not a priority in the triage system and was perhaps a nuisance during busy periods, and was not needed during the lulls between. Carrel complained at one point about 'the bad will of the doctors and hence we received an insufficient number of wounded'. As ever, he was convinced that ways of speeding up wound healing would be found, and he was pleased to hear again from Serge Voronoff, the Russian-born Paris surgeon working nearby, that Voronoff's testicular extract placed on wounds would speed up healing. Carrel wrote to 'mon cher confrère' proposing a joint trial, but nothing came of it. Carrel was less impressed later when Voronoff announced his claims to be able to rejuvenate aging humans using monkey testis grafts, and Carrel then shunned him as a quack.

Crile's Research Meeting

When Carrel arrived, the American surgical presence was already well-established at the Ambulance américaine to the south of Compiègne. On 5 February 1915, while Carrel was still setting up his Paris hospital, George Crile organised what he called 'an impromptu field day' at the Ambulance. It was an international gathering led by a small well-informed group — Crile, Carrel, Wright, Moynihan and Tuffier — and about 100 others attended to listen. The speakers dined at the Ritz in the evening, and Crile published an account of the meeting later.[29] Tuffier and Carrel, who both spoke in French, commented on organisational and wartime research matters, and Crile, by now an early convert to débridement, also described the effects of war on civilians.[30] Wright made his usual case against use of antiseptics and told the group that the British hospitals now used saline lavage for open wound treatment after débridement. Backing

---

[29] George Crile (1915) 'Symposium on military surgery at American Ambulance, Neuilly-sur-Seine, France' *Surgery, Gynecology & Obstetrics* 20: 708–16.

[30] See also George W. Crile (1915) 'Notes on military surgery' *Annals of Surgery* 62: 1–10.

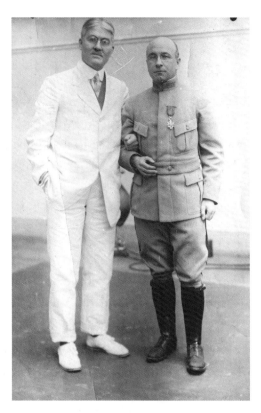

George Crile and his Cleveland Clinic staff were based for a while in Paris and he, like other military surgeons, visited Carrel's hospital. (*Courtesy of the Dittrick Medical History Center, Case Western Reserve University.*)

Wright up, Moynihan said that in wound infections, 'the only thing which is of real value is the salt solution'. Carrel, newly arrived in the north, and with his hospital not yet in action, was listening carefully to this impressive joint advocacy by these British knights.

Cushing Arrives

Shortly after, Crile's group left the Ambulance américaine and, on return home, Crile promptly wrote up his experiences.[31] Harvey Cushing's

---

[31] Crile's report was 'A composite report of the three months' service of the Lakeside Unit at the American Ambulance' *Cleveland Medical Journal* (1915), 14: 421–39.

Harvard unit replaced them in Paris. They had a much quieter time than Crile, but Cushing was to be much busier on his return in 1917 after America entered the war. When Cushing arrived in Paris, he visited Compiègne in April 1915, shortly after Carrel's hospital opened, but before Carrel had developed his new system of wound care which would give him prominence. Cushing had followed Carrel's career closely, and with admiration, from the days of the Frenchman's impressive Johns Hopkins lecture in 1906. Cushing later wrote in his diaries about his tour of the hospital, describing Carrel as 'our little bear in uniform'. He admired the hospital and Carrel's organisation, although, always hard to please, he did think that the dressing changes were badly done by one of Carrel's surgeons. He wrote:

What is known as *Hôpital Complémentaire 21* is in a once fashionable hotel — the Rond Royal — on the very edge of the Forêt de Compiègne — an ideal spot and one which Carrel chose for his purposes on careful survey after he got free from his miserable detail, first in the Lyon hospital and then at the War Office. Here, backed by Rockefeller money and with an admirable staff, a great opportunity lies open for special studies of wound treatment. The lines along which they have started work include the suction treatment of suppurating wounds without dressings; the employment of irrigation with bactericidal fluids which are being worked out by Henry Dakin; methods of increasing resistance to pathogenic organisms by turpentine injections, etc., etc.

There are at present 51 beds with 86 attendants, including slaveys of all kinds — 11 scientific, medical, and administrative officers; 13 experienced Swiss nurses supplied by Theodor Kocher;[32] numerous secretaries, laboratory technicians, linen-room people, scrub women, ambulance men; and 47 soldier orderlies who do everything from boots to waiting on table and keeping up the gardens. It is indeed a research hospital *de luxe* with running water in all the rooms, which are large, most of them having baths, comfortable beds, electricity, and all modern improvements. Over the *dramatis personae* Madame Carrel rules as housekeeper and "general tyrant," according to her husband.

---

[32] Kocher in Geneva had established one of the first nurse training schools not attached to a religious institution.

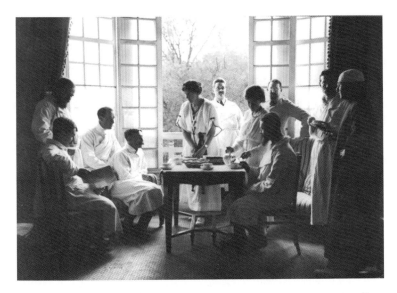

Mme Carrel, head of nursing at Compiègne, serving tea to the medical staff: Carrel is on the far right. (*mesdiscussions.net*)

There are also stables and four chauffeurs whom I had forgotten to mention — one of them a professional racing driver who has figured in international events — another Sarah Bernhardt's leading man on her last tour of the USA — the third an equally celebrated actor from the Odéon — the fourth an underling.[33]

Enter Dakin

Carrel had come a little late to the big debate in the northern sector on wound treatment, but he was to catch up. As Cushing noted, Carrel still had hopes for his suction drainage of closed wounds, but was looking also at the open strategy, having realised that initial débridement was a success. To deal with the resulting open wounds, he was attracted to the Wright–Moynihan perfusion described by its distinguished advocates at Crile's meeting. Even so, Carrel felt that, after all, antiseptics were still important.

---

[33] Fulton, *Cushing* (note 10): 395–7, quoting Cushing's war diaries.

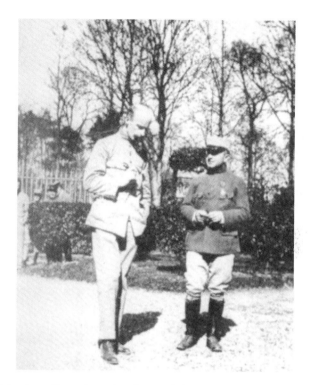

Carrel was joined at Compiègne by the English chemist Henry Dakin where they devised their wound treatment method.

What was needed, he concluded, was a new, potent antiseptic to add to the perfusion of open, débrided wounds.

In March, before his hospital was underway, he gave an interview to the *New York Times* and again said that the number of deaths from infected war wounds was 'small'.[34] He gave a markedly different estimate later.

Carrel had sought expert advice. The antiseptic 'Holy Grail' needed would be a powerful agent which would deal with all bacteria quickly, would not damage the tissues or cellular defences of the body, nor irritate the skin edges. For help with this search for the perfect antiseptic, Carrel contacted the Rockefeller Institute leadership, and their support was

[34] 'Carrel Talks Of His Work' *NYT*, 17 March 1915.

immediately forthcoming. Henry Dakin (1880–1952), an Englishman based in New York, was already keen to assist the British war effort. The two men could hardly have been more different. While Carrel was short, Dakin was tall. Carrel was demonstrative and not averse to publicity, while Dakin was shy and reclusive. Dakin had worked in a private laboratory run by Christian Herter, professor of pharmacology and therapeutics at the College of Physicians and Surgeons in New York, and after Herter's death in 1910, he moved the laboratory to the country, where he led a life of solitary scholarship, without collaborators or pupils, and avoiding academic meetings. Dakin's output of high quality research chemistry was to continue during the War, and he was honoured by election to the Royal Society of London in 1917.[35]

Dakin moved from America and started work in Paris on new antiseptics. He was based temporarily in Tuffier's laboratory in the Hôpital Beaujohn, then moved to Carrel's hospital in March 1915 when it was ready. Dakin tested many likely solutions for use at the Hospital and eventually settled on a modification of sodium hypochlorite (NaOCl), commonly known as bleach, which had, and has, much use in France as 'eau de Javel', and is still the basis of some domestic disinfectants. It was an old remedy. The French surgeon Jaques Lisfranc (1790–1847) used a hypochlorite, as did Ignaz Semelweiss in his famous 1880s studies, and hypochlorite was to be used in other World War I antiseptics, notably the rival Eusol (Edinburgh University Solution of Lime). However, used alone, hypochlorite damages tissues, and Dakin neutralised the damaging alkalinity by adding boric acid. It had the desired action on a range of bacteria and usually did not affect skin. Making up the final Dakin's Solution was quite complex, and being unstable, it had to be made up every few days from fresh. Nor did it last long in the tissues, but it gave off a reassuring whiff of chlorine. With the preparation of this new fluid, Carrel's wound perfusion plan was complete.[36]

---

[35] For Dakin, see *Obituary Notices of Fellows of the Royal Society* 8 (1952): 128–48. It is said that another eponym — the Dakin–West reaction, which gives transformation of amino-acids — deserves to be better-known.

[36] From 1982, hypochlorite became available again in 'Disinfin' or simply as Dakin's Solution; it is used for general disinfection, dental root canal work and emergency treatment of infected water.

Dakin described his antiseptic briefly in the Paris journal *Presse médicale* on 2 August 1915.[37] He humbly pointed out that it was hardly new, but the news reached the *New York Times* shortly afterwards. The New York paper's headline on 6 August 1915 was 'Drs. Carrel And Dakin Find New Antiseptic: Infection Impossible'. The story also appeared in the *Washington Post* that day with less drama and reached the London *Times* on 8 August, and thence to the *The Lancet* on 14 August, causing Dakin concern. He later commented on the 'absurd and extravagant statements made in the lay press'. The newspaper accounts said 200 or so

DRS. CARREL AND DAKIN FIND NEW ANTISEPTIC

Remedy Tested in French Hospital Said to Make Infection Impossible.

PARIS, Aug. 5.—Dr. Alexis Carrel of the Rockefeller Institute of Medical Research, and Dr. Henry D. Dakin of the Lister Institute have discovered, after exhaustive experiments at the Compiègne Military Hospital, what they say is the ideal antiseptic.

The most powerful antiseptic known to science is hypochlorite of lime, but its use is injurious to the tissues, owing to its acidity, and it does not keep.

Drs. Dakin and Carrel have found these two defects are remedied, respectively, by the addition of carbonate of lime and boric acid.

Dakin's contribution to Carrel's method was praised in the *New York Times*.

---

[37] A full description came later — M. Alexis Carrel avec la collaboration de MM. Dakin, Daufresne, Dehelly, et Dumas (1915) 'Traitement abortif de l'infection des plais' *Bulletin de l'Académie de Médecine* 74: 361–8, communicated also to *Presse Médicale*, 11 October 1915, 397–8.

compounds had been tested, and Carrel doubtless saw himself, not for the first time, like Pasteur or Paul Ehrlich, who a few years earlier in 1910 had famously tested 606 chemicals before salversan emerged as the first effective antimicrobial chemical. This announcement in the London press caused others to protest, for other reasons. The Dean of the Medical Faculty at Edinburgh wrote to *The Times* claiming that Edinburgh's 'Eusol', which was also a modified hypochlorite solution, had been devised and announced first. It certainly had been first, in a British journal, by 12 days.[38]

Perfusion System

Carrel worked on how to deliver the new antiseptic to the open wound. Since it was inactivated after two hours in the tissues, it had to be re-applied regularly to the wound. By autumn 1915, Carrel had the new strategy in place, and it would be known as the celebrated 'Carrel–Dakin' treatment, using almost continuous irrigation of the wound. It would soon be forgotten that surgical débridement was the essential first step and Carrel's treatment was a second phase to clear the open wound of infection or prevent infection developing in clean wounds — 'traitement abortif', as he called it. For irrigation he used his octopus-like tubes inserted into all recesses of the wound. The limb was then immobilised in a hammock, and the overflow was soaked up by cotton wool or sphagnum moss or caught in trays under the bed. He aimed to keep a pool of antiseptic in the wound crater, and the cases selected for his treatment were suitable only if they had open wounds on the upper surface of legs or arms.

---

[38] Eusol was described in J.L. Smith et al. (1915) 'Experimental observations on the antiseptic action of hypochlorous acid' *BMJ*, 24 July 1915, 129–36, just prior to Dakin's *Presse médicale* paper. It contained (and still contains) calcium hypochlorite and boric acid, and emerged after research support from the British Medical Research Committee. Edinburgh's grumble also reached the *New York Times* on 7 August 1915 — headlined 'Like Carrel's Antiseptic'. Eusol remained popular among plastic surgeons for skin preparation, but after one hundred years of use, in 2008 Britain's NICE (National Institute for Health and Care Excellence) declared that it could be hazardous.

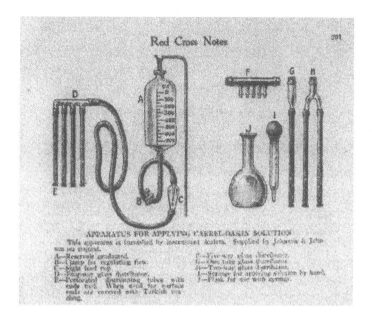

The Carrel-Dakin method was marketed by the Johnson and Johnson Company during World War I. (*Courtesy of the Johnson & Johnson Archives.*)

The progress of the wound was studied daily when the dressing was taken down. A daily bacterial count was made from cultures taken from the interior of the wound, and the figure was charted. He ignored the type of bacteria detected: only the numbers were recorded. When the bacterial count fell below an average of two organisms per high power microscope field, the wound was declared safe to close by stitches or acetate strips, though occasionally skin grafting was required.

Carrel had a disciplined, well-staffed research hospital where he could treat patients with his expensive, labour-intensive method which required weeks of treatment. Carrel's protocol had a rigid complexity which suited the military setting and his personality, and it gained scientific credibility from the many measurements made. The method was witnessed in action later by an advisory group of visiting British surgeons, and they described

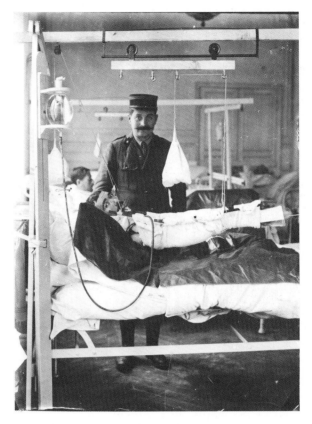

Dakin's fluid from a container (upper left) irrigated the wound via the multiple tubes and the fluid drained on sheeting below.

the fastidious, aseptic, no-touch, five-nurse routine during the dressing round:

> There is a dressing trolley. One nurse goes ahead, loosens safety pins in the dressing, surgeon removes dressing, second nurse holds the slides for surgeon to do [bacteriology] smears, third adjusted combs of the perfusion system, fourth applies Vaseline to edge of wound, a fifth hands fresh outer dressing to the sister who hands surgeon fresh dressing and new tubes. It is elaborate but rapid.[39]

---

[39] See the 'Report to the Director-General British Army Medical Services by The Surgical Committee: The War — Carrel-Dakin treatment of wounds' *BMJ*, 3 November 1917,

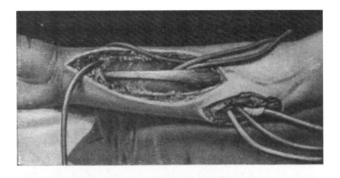

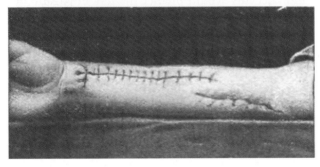

Prompt and wide surgical incision and debridement — removal of damaged tissue then leaving the wound open — was found to be essential early in the War. After this, Carrel added antiseptic irrigation of the open wound, which was closed later.

Carrel urged that the method should never be simplified, and any failures in other's hands were blamed on a failure to follow the *méthode*.

Carrel's method can be seen as a scientific experiment, rather than giving a service.[40] He had selected his patients to be as similar a group as possible, in spite of the diversity of war injuries at the front. He was to make major claims for his method, but one scientific necessity was

---

597–9. The British advisors had one loyal caveat and suggested that Eusol — the 'Edinburgh University Solution of Lime', would be as good a perfusate as Dakin's fluid.
[40] See Perrin Selcer (2008) 'Standardizing wounds: Alexis Carrel and the scientific management of life in the First World War' *British Journal for the History of Science* 41: 73–107.

missing. He had no data on 'controls' — wounds treated by what he called the 'usual' methods of wound care.

Carrel added many observational extras to his treatment. The size of the wound was often studied closely by tracing its outline onto paper, and this area was measured with a planimeter by his physicist Jaubert de Beaujeu, who was followed later by Pierre Lecomte du Noüy. From the progress of these measurements, they derived a formula which mathematically described the events.[41] The formula incorporated various parameters and allegedly would predict the day of closure, if the wound was left to heal in from the edges. It seems that some wounds were left to heal completely in this way.[42] Carrel and du Noüy also claimed that the rate of wound healing depended on age, and that their measurements and the formula showed that 20-year-old soldiers healed twice as fast as 40-year-olds. This was improbable, and common surgical experience shows that healing rates do not change in patients from the late teens until aged over 60.[43]

Publicity for the *Méthode*

By the autumn of 1915, with his *méthode* in use for some months, Carrel was keen to promote it. Carrel took his first steps to tell the French

---

[41] A. Jaubert de Beaujeu (1917) 'Cicatrisation of wounds: V. New mathematical expression of cicatrisation' *JEM* 26, 81–2. It was a time when mathematical analysis was favoured in biology and in Sinclair Lewis's novel *Arrowsmith* (1925), based on the work and attitudes of the Rockefeller Institute, the hero is urged that it is essential to apply mathematics to his bacteriological studies.

[42] The measurements ignored the depth of the wound, as if it were only two-dimensional. For their arcane healing formulae, see the difficult-to-follow articles by P. Lecomte du Noüy *JEM* 24 (1916): 451–3, 461–70, vol. 25, (1917): 721–8 and vol. 29, (1919): 329–50. Du Noüy was acquainted with fellow Paris physicist Louis de Broglie, whose famous equations earned him a Nobel Prize.

[43] See Michael A. Horan and Roderick A. Little, *Injury in the Aging* (Cambridge: Cambridge University Press, 1998). Carrel later often quoted this claim for slower healing in 40-year olds — see his book *Man, the Unknown*, p. 167. An alternative empirical finding, agreed by some at the time, was that the soldiers' bodily vitality related instead to 'trench age' — the length of exposure at the front before injury.

surgeons of his work at the Académie de Médecine on 5 October 1915 and, not being a member, as before, his influential friend Samuel Pozzi presented the paper. On his behalf, Pozzi claimed that Carrel's method gave complete healing in one-tenth of the normal time, that amputations were diminished by 50%, and that 'a great number of lives would have been saved by this means'. Following this, there was a gathering of the Société de Chirurgie, meeting on 5 January 1916, which Pozzi and Tuffier attended. After a bacteriologist gave a presentation on antiseptics, the discussion moved to debate Carrel's claims, and the exchanges became tense. Carrel's caustic private and public comments on France and French surgery were well-known, and his disavowal of French nationality at the time of the Nobel Prize had not been forgotten. Moreover, prior to Carrel's arrival in Paris, the French surgeons had dealt with the huge casualties in the battles near Paris one year before. They knew about war wounds and the new infections. Carrel had come late to the action, nor was he a practising surgeon. The discussion turned to the Carrel–Dakin method, and Pozzi and Tuffier had to defend Carrel against criticism by some of the other surgeons. The distinguished surgeon Edouard Quénu said Carrel's claims were 'exessif', adding that prompt débridement was the crucial factor, and that thereafter the choice of antiseptic was 'secondaire'. Benjamin Broca, professor of clinical surgery in the Faculté de Médecine de Paris, spoke up. Broca declared that he did not like, in the city of Pasteur, being lectured on how to treat infection. Broca commented ' … et nous apporter cela d'Amérique, laissez-moi rire … [and you bring that from America? Pardon me if I laugh]'.[44] Broca added that just before the meeting, an American newspaper had patronised France by saying that Carrel was like 'Vasco de Gama debarking on an unknown land'.[45] Carrel later reported that the atmosphere was of 'culpable levity'. Carrel may again have seen himself as suffering as had Pasteur when

---

[44] The comments of Benjamin Broca are reported in the discussion of the paper by Pierre Delbet (1916) 'Actions de cèrtains antiseptiques sur le pus' *Bulletin et Mèmoires de la Société de Chirurgie de Paris* 42: 92–110. Benjamin Auguste Broca (1859–1924), author of *Chirurgie de guerre et d'après-guerre* Paris 1921 and other surgical texts, was a son of Pierre Paul Broca, the distinguished Paris physician and surgeon.

[45] The American newspaper article quoted by Broca has not been traced.

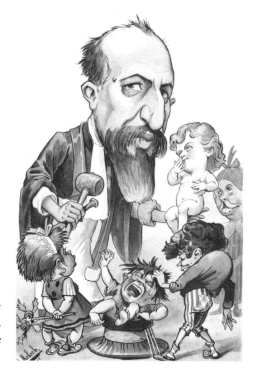

Carrel's critics included the distinguished Paris surgeon Auguste Broca, portrayed in the Paris magazine *Chanteclair* in 1907.

Pasteur, 40 years before, had been ridiculed at the French Academy of Medicine, but fought back.[46]

Carrel's Response

Carrel was exasperated at this criticism. He wrote to Flexner on 18 March 1916, saying that 'there is no chance of our method being extensively used in France on account of the antagonism of the Official Scientific Societies'. In April that year he grumbled in letters to his friend Coudert:

> The irreparable evil that these men do in France shows that science should never officialise itself in the form of Institutes and Académies.

---

[46]This hostile reception of his work is detailed in A. Carrel and G. Dehelly, *The Treatment of Infected Wounds* (New York: P.B. Hoeber, 1919): 11–13.

Académies are the churches which construct dogmas. Unfortunately men of science have adopted the habits of men of religion, by immobilising science in rigid forms. ... They are nearly all against me. I am proud of it. Many will lose their limbs and their life because of the vanity and incompetence of these French surgeons.[47]

But Carrel was not the isolated martyr he made out. He had powerful support from his influential friends Tuffier and Pozzi. Moreover, Tuffier in his official military position had put out a circular in early 1916 to the military surgeons instructing them to use the Carrel–Dakin method.

Carrel now sought wider publicity for his work. He agreed to a visit and an interview by Mrs. Lathrop from the American Fund for French Wounded, which had an office in Paris. She took Carrel's views back to America, and her report appeared in New York's *The Tribune* of 12 July 1916. It contained the news of good results from Compiègne, plus a description of du Noüy's arcane formula for predicting the tempo of wound healing. *The Tribune's* headline was 'Carrel Uses Algebra To Heal — Gangrene Unknown'. Some at the Rockefeller Institute were again restive over Carrel's high profile, and the general manager, Henry James, was again displeased. He rebuked the editor of *The Tribune* for 'sensational half-truths ... . This amusingly sensational story must be an embarrassment to him [Carrel] and his colleagues'. The *Tribune's* editor grovelled and apologised, but the lady president of the Fund was having none of it. She got back to James, pointing out that Carrel had made himself available for the interview and made it clear that the story should be published.[48] James was contrite, and lamely told Carrel that he was concerned that 'the papers were talking about your work in so enthusiastic and free a way'. There was a further Carrel story in the *The New York Times* on 7 October and another on 23 October, which said that at his hospital, healing took 'only one third of the usual time

---

[47] Carrel's letters to Coudert, Compiègne 1916, January to July, boxes 26, 38 and 40, Alexis Carrel Papers, Georgetown University Library, Booth Family Center for Special Collections (GULBFC).

[48] Henry James letters, box 3 file 5, Carrel Papers GULBFC (note 47).

and that amputations were reduced by 50%. In certain cases, healing occurs in one tenth of the time required under ordinary treatment'.[49]

After a demonstration of the method at a Paris Hospital on 15 November, Carrel gave an interview to a reporter from the *New York Sun*.[50] Mme Carrel told a visiting journalist in late 1916 that they took pride in the fact that 'no man had yet died from his wound in our hospital'.[51] Later, the contrarian journalist H.L. Mencken supported Carrel and joined the hyperbole claiming that the Carrel–Dakin method would save tens of thousands of legs and tens of thousands of lives, and that 'at Compiègne the wholesale chopping off of legs and arms has stopped and the death rate has declined enormously'.[52] Carrel's impressive figures, given out freely, are improbable. He had no data for 'usual' healing times, nor for amputation or the death rates in the highly selected wound cases he was treating. Amputation rates for gas gangrene at this time were widely thought to have fallen as a result of early débridement.

Carrel's high profile remained unchecked. His local celebrity led to inclusion in a now-forgotten play *Le père Ubu a l'hopital* by Ambroise Vollard, performed in Paris in 1916, which affectionately described 'le docteur Karrelos'. Mme Carrel featured in stories of bravery near the front when the Hospital was briefly threatened and she appeared, with an illustration of her supervising the perfusion system, in the *Saturday Evening Post* 21 July 1917. The Institute may have hesitated to be involved again in curbing the stories from Compiègne, and they had another reason. About this time, in a rare intervention in the management of his philanthropies, Rockefeller senior told the Foundation to appoint a public relations officer. His view was that the Foundation needed the 'interest, sympathy and moral support of the public and it is therefore its duty to keep the public accurately informed in regard to its activities'. Carrel's work was funded by the Foundation, and Carrel's claims showed that both the Foundation and Institute had made this contribution to the Allied cause and to military surgery in general. The

[49] 'Dr Carrel Prevents Infection In Wounds' *NYT*, 23 October 1916.
[50] *New York Sun*, 3 December 1916.
[51] Lewis R. Freeman (1917) 'Healing wounded soldiers to order' *World's Work*: 430–9.
[52] Mencken's article is in New York's *Evening Mail*, 24 October 1917.

soldier amputee had become an iconic symbol of the war, and the public warmed to the claim that Carrel was able to reduce the amputation rates.

Industrial Interest

In New York Flexner realised that the unpleasant war wounds had an equivalent in peace time, namely the injuries encountered in America's heavy industry. He also knew that the big companies employed their own surgeons and ran their own hospitals. Accordingly, Flexner asked Rockefeller senior for the names of old business contacts in the industry and encouraged surgeons from these companies to visit Compiègne. First to arrive was William O'Neill Sherman (1880–1979), chief surgeon to the Carnegie Steel Corporation in Pittsburgh, and he would be an evangelist for the method thereafter.[53] Following him was Richard Corwin (1853–1929), who was in charge of a hospital for workers of the Colorado Fuel and Iron Co. at Pueblo, Colorado, the 'Pittsburgh of the West'. Corwin visited and said cautiously on return to America that Carrel had halved the recovery time after suffering a wound.[54] Sherman gave even more dramatic figures on his return, saying that at least 150,000 lives and 75,000 amputations and thousand of cripples could have been prevented in the war, had Carrel's method been used earlier.[55] Sherman also passed on his findings to Theodore Roosevelt, no longer President, but active in politics. Roosevelt wrote to Carrel saying 'I was literally astounded at the wonderful results'.[56]

---

[53] William O'Neill Sherman (1917) 'The abortive treatment of wound infection' *JAMA* 69:185–96. Sherman was best known for introducing the 'self-tapping' vanadium screws and plates for fracture fixation in 1912 which remained in favour for 50 years.

[54] Dr. James Burry at the Illinois Steel Company also tried the Carrel–Dakin method, but did not continue with its use.

[55] Although these figures were improbable then, a recent book on Carrel went further and claimed that his method saved 'hundreds of thousands, if not millions of lives'; see David M. Friedman, *The Immortalists: Charles Lindbergh, Dr. Alexis Carrel and Their Daring Quest to Live Forever* (New York: HarperCollins, 2007): 8.

[56] Roosevelt to Carrel, 29 November 1916, folder 7 box 15, War Demonstration Hospital, FA 012, RUA RAC (note 4).

The Treatment of Infected Wounds

In late 1916, Carrel brought out a book on their method and its results. Published initially in French and then translated as *The Treatment of Infected Wounds*, it is a short work largely devoted to the details of the method as used from December 1915.[57] It lacks a historical introduction or references to the literature on wound care. It has a number of case histories but only a short section on his overall results, as if intended as only an instructional work on management of wounds after débridement. In his short section on results, Carrel does not give the important figure of the delay between injury and arrival nor the mix of already debrided or non-debrided wounds. The bacterial counts on arrival are not given, nor the type of bacteria, although streptococcal infections are usually more difficult to eradicate. The number of non-infected cases treated to prevent infection emerging is not given. The overall figures he gives are that 90% of the wounds treated could be closed within one to three weeks. He says this time to closure was one-third of the 'usual methods', and these usual methods meant 'suppuration for several months'.

One odd feature of management was that if a fracture was present, it was regarded as part of the wound and was not treated by immobilisation. Only later was a plaster of Paris applied; the ever-flowing Carrel–Dakin fluid would have softened the plaster.

The Debate Continues

At this stage in the War in 1916, the Allied wound management policy was in considerable private and public disarray. The only progress had been in agreeing that débridement was essential, and this was accepted when success was self-evident. The rival post-débridement Wright–Moynihan and Carrel–Dakin methods both claimed better results and claimed to be based on science. But good data was absent and instead

---

[57] Mme Carrel and one of the nurses wrote a version for nurses, with a Foreword by the surgeon William Keen, who published his own book, the *Treatment of War Wounds* later in 1917.

uncritical assertion and anecdote abounded, and wound treatment remained personal and anarchic.

Wright's saline perfusion method was still supported by the British military medical staff, with influential support from Moynihan. Among the French, Carrel had supporters, notably his old friend Tuffier, but it seemed that other surgeons with the French forces seemed to manage with other simpler traditional methods after débridement.[58] The prominent Lyonnais French surgeon René Leriche, who Carrel taught as a student, was sceptical about his mentor's claims. Leriche worked in the same hospital in Paris as Carrel's supporter Tuffier, and Leriche wrote a wartime text on the management of fractures, including compound fractures. In his management, he did not advocate any complex after-treatment of wounds, and the Carrel–Dakin method was nowhere mentioned in his book.[59] It is unlikely that Leriche was regularly amputating and that his wards were full of infection.

Conferences

This unsatisfactory situation persisted in spite of a mechanism available that should have enabled agreement on best practice in Allied military surgery. The Interallied Surgical Conferences had started at the British hospital at Rouen shortly after the War commenced, and Moynihan is credited with this initiative.[60] The enlarged meetings were handed over, by agreement, to Tuffier, who enthusiastically hosted them thereafter in Paris, providing much support, including secretaries and translators. Depage regularly attended from Belgium, Raffaele Georg Bastianelli came

---

[58] Tuffier notes the resistance to Carrel's strategy in his 'French surgery in 1915' *British Journal of Surgery* 4 (1916): 420–32.

[59] See the translated version, René Leriche, *Treatment of Fractures* (London: University of London Press, 1918).

[60] Berkeley Moynihan (1925) 'The Interallied Surgical Conference' *JAMA* 85: 844. Tuffier was widely respected, and in addition to his many French honours, he was also awarded the U.S. Distinguished Service Medal and was made Knight Commander of the British Empire in 1920.

from Italy and Vojislav Subotić represented Serbia. Between these events Tuffier had informal monthly meetings at his house. But reaching joint policies for wound treatment was difficult. The root of the problem was a lack of clinical data from the frontline medical services. During the major battles, disorder was inevitable, and speedy surgical improvisation was essential. The injured were then moved from stage to stage in the medical evacuation, with only scanty clinical notes accompanying them. Good figures on the outcomes of the 'usual' methods of treatment were not available.

Controversy Continues

Wright's saline irrigation method, though it had won official British approval, had an increasing numbers of critics in Britain. Moynihan, now back in Leeds, but still an advisor to the Army, now dropped his support for Wright, and at a Harveian Society meeting in February 1916 spoke highly of the Carrel–Dakin system and said Wright's method was generally 'not applicable'.[61] Even Zachary Cope, a surgeon at Wright's own St Mary's Hospital, dismissed Wright's method in favour of using antiseptics.[62] Wright in response wrote a new memorandum on wound management which was turned down in May 1916 by the military medical leadership. After his long silence, Watson Cheyne returned in 1916 to his support of antiseptics, perhaps pleased and encouraged by Carrel's high-profile use and support. Cheyne, with new confidence, criticised the Wright–Moynihan method and rode to the rescue of antiseptics. Writing in the *British Journal of Surgery*, and patronisingly using the word 'brine' for Wright's hypertonic salt solution, he made a

[61] Berkeley Moynihan 'The treatment of gunshot wounds' *BMJ*, 4 March 1916, 333–7. Dakin, like Moynihan, was a Leeds graduate and the distinguished Leeds chemist Prof. J.B. Cohen had assisted in preparing Dakin's antiseptics.

[62] V. Zachary Cope 'Fashions in wound treatment' *St Mary's Hospital Gazette*, April 1916, 42–7. Cope in turn was rebuked by Alexander Fleming (of penicillin fame later), who worked loyally under Wright at St Mary's Hospital; see *St Mary's Hospital Gazette*, May 1916, 61–3, which includes a further response by Cope.

lofty attack on Wright's data and his integrity.[63] He thought Wright's failure to publish any data meant that his technique had failed — 'otherwise he would get clinical results which he would show us'. Cheyne ended his article by cheekily suggesting that bacteriologists like Wright should stop thwarting the surgeons. The scientists, he said, should withdraw from France and go back to the lab and get on with what they were trained to do, namely to devise vaccines to assist the surgeons in dealing with the bacteria found in surgical infections. With the scientists gone, he added, 'the surgeons at the front might take advantage of the absence of the bacteriologists to try to see what could be done by more purely surgical methods'.

Wright was invited by the editor to reply to this remarkable attack, and Wright sent in a rambling 16,000 word polemic which strayed far from the issues, and which the editor turned down. The article was then accepted by *The Lancet*, a journal with a tradition of radical journalism, and it was published on 16 September 1916. Wright's long detailed defence of his method started by suggesting that Cheyne was now deranged:

> When an erroneous belief takes firm hold of a man, two bodies of thought will evolve side by side in his mind: one correlated with his obsession, and the other with the data of actual experience; and these will before very long come into open conflict.
>
> But things do not end there. For when truth and untruth lie very unquietly together in a mind, and untruth cannot be thrown out, Nature always steps in and deals with the patient.

The editor of the *The Lancet* felt it necessary to add an editorial deploring the dispute between such senior figures, adding that Wright's tone was unfortunate and that the editor 'should have preferred to see certain crude expressions omitted'. Cheyne made a dignified short response two weeks later, prudently declining to reply in detail.

---

[63] Cheyne 'Treatment of wounds' (note 21).

Wright's Decline

Wright now started to criticise the entire medical management of the war, and lobbied the editor of *The Times* to call for changes. The career soldiers, thus far tolerant of the presence of civilian scientists like Wright, now sought to assert their authority. On 15 January 1917, Sir Alfred Keogh, head of the British military services, took a firm line and said he was prepared to resign if Wright continued to have an influence. Instead it was Wright who was marginalised. Sir Anthony Bowlby, the Surgeon-General to the Army Medical Services, later recalled that

> Wright was a self-seeker, quite ignorant of surgery, the self-styled inventor of the Saline Treatment of Wounds which was now 'as dead as Queen Anne' and the obstructer of all other forms of treatment.[64]

The surgeons — Moynihan, Cheyne, Keogh, Bowlby and Cope — had marginalised Wright, the confident scientist.

This meant that Carrel's system was now unopposed, and Carrel was, after all, a surgeon and 'one of us'. Carrel's own method was the only clearly defined 'system' on offer to use after surgical débridement. Depage, who had first emphasised the need for open wound management and débridement, now advocated using the Carrel–Dakin system as the best after-treatment. Tuffier's circular sent to all the French hospitals earlier now had more authority. At an Interallied Surgical Conference held in March 1917, after almost three years of war, the Allied representatives came out in favour of the Carrel method, helped by the generally favourable report from an Advisory Committee to the Director General of the British Army Medical Services submitted after they visited some surgical units using Carrel's system.[65]

---

[64] Quoted in Whitehead (note 11): 207, and Harrison, *Medical War* (note 11): 97. Bowlby by this time had written the Introduction to Carrel's book on wound treatment, saying that 'it has also renewed faith in antiseptic methods, in spite of the attacks on their utility which characterised the early stages of the war'.
[65] 'Report to the Director-General' (note 39).

Dissent by Others

How far this official advice was taken up is not clear. By 1917, the frontline surgeons were probably less convinced than the leadership that any one method was better than others. Moreover, for military surgeons, coping with Carrel's labour-intensive complexity was not always possible. Even if it could be set up after surgical attention, when the injured were moved from place to place the apparatus would hinder the transfer. Though Dakin's solution was cheap, it had to be made up fresh, and the chemical preparation was tricky and required training. Added to this, the extra staff, tubing, drains and cotton wool padding made the method costly. Moreover, concerns about gas gangrene had disappeared from the surgical reports from the war, poor though the statistics were. If débridement was carried out well, simple after-care seemed to suffice, and a variety of other easily-used antiseptics were looked at.[66] The complex Carrel–Dakin technique was unworkable during major battles. In July 1917, at the time of the battle of Passchendaele, conditions in the Harvard Unit were described by O.H. Robertson, who was trying to introduce blood transfusion at the time. When an offensive started:

> By noon, the wounded began to arrive, then more and more, till there was a solid string of ambulances extending down the road as far as you could see. We were simply deluged. We couldn't operate on more than a fraction of the cases. ... The resuscitation ward was a veritable chamber of horrors, ... blood everywhere ... We had to leave the corpses on the floor as we needed the beds for new wounded. ... I could try transfusion on an occasional one but the majority had to take their chance.[67]

One unexpected critic of the Carrel–Dakin system was Dakin himself. He had departed from Compiègne late in 1915, moving to advise the

---

[66] Antiseptics which found favour late in WWI, as well as Eusol, were hexamethylenetetramine (Hexamine), various flavines and bismuth iodoform-paraffin paste (BIPP), introduced by James Rutherford Morison, professor of surgery at the University of Durham, which is still favoured in ear, nose and throat surgery.

[67] L.G. Stansbury and J.R. Hess (2005) 'Putting pieces together' *Transfusion Medicine Review* 19: 81–4.

British Government on the treatment of the injured in the aftermath of the Dardanelles disaster. In an interesting wide-ranging article in 1917, Dakin reviewed all the innovations from chemists which had assisted the war effort, including the appearance of new antiseptics.[68] While he was proud of his own introduction of the modified hypochlorite in what pointedly called the Dakin–Carrel–Dehelly–Depage technique, he hinted that the results were not as good as Carrel claimed. He compared their method with that of Wright:

> There has been a great deal of discussion as to the rival merits of the two systems, but to some observers at least it would appear that the differences between the so-called "physiological" and "antiseptic" methods of treating wounds are not nearly as great as at one time appeared.[69]

He added disloyally that at Compiègne there were a 'limited number of patients treated. Skin irritation was more of a problem than was thought', adding with characteristic English understatement that

> opinions have varied as to the value of the method, and while it received wide endorsement from many competent observers, it is to be regretted that war conditions made it impossible to secure statistical data of any value.[70]

Enter America

America was drawn nearer to the War when the liner *Lusitania* was sunk in May 1915, and after further German submarine attacks on U.S. merchant ships, on 6 April 1917 America finally entered the European War. The U.S. Army was now expanded rapidly, and Crile and Cushing's

---

[68] H.D. Dakin 'Biochemistry and war problems' *BMJ* June 23, 1917, 833–7. His list of innovations included methods of purification of water, discovery of vitamins, synthesis of dyes and drugs, preparation of antitoxic sera and chemicals which gave protection against poisonous gases. The article helped deflect attention on the chemist's assistance in providing poison gases.
[69] Dakin memorandum, Faculty/Alexis Carrel, folder 1 box 1, FA231, RUA RAC (note 4).
[70] Dakin 'Notes', 3 January, Flexner APS Papers, microfilm reel 27 RUA RAC (note 4).

experience in Paris had already been of crucial value to Surgeon General Gorgas in his preparations. Both these surgeons were ready, once again, to return to Europe, this time with larger trained military medical teams, and they reached and settled in Europe before the infantry men arrived. The Rockefeller Institute now saw a chance for another patriotic initiative. The Institute had benefitted from Carrel's high-profile work in Paris, and Flexner now suggested that Carrel be brought back to teach his method at home, at a 'War Demonstration Hospital', set up and funded by Rockefeller money. Flexner used the impressive figures on success with wound treatment which regularly came from Carrel and had no difficulty convincing the Foundation, yet again, to back the plan.

From late autumn 1916, all was quiet at Compiègne, since any regular military action in the War was far away. Carrel had only received 'old wounds' from 1 September, and he was restive. Flexner's offer to Washington to fund training of military surgeons in Carrel's method was accepted by the U.S. Army and, after he was given leave by the French authorities, Carrel returned to New York in January 1917. He was to be in New York for a full year, teaching the Carrel–Dakin method to military surgeons. He then moved back to France for what turned out to be a final, short, unproductive spell of surgery and research at the end of the War.

CHAPTER NINE

The Demonstration Hospital

C arrel arrived back in New York in February 1917 to start to set up the War Demonstration Hospital, planning to teach his methods from the summer onwards. Flexner arranged for John D. Rockefeller senior and his wife to attend a staff meeting at the Institute at which Carrel presented an account of his work in France, illustrated by 'coloured lantern slides'.[1] Carrel was also entertained at a private dinner at the Rockefeller family home.

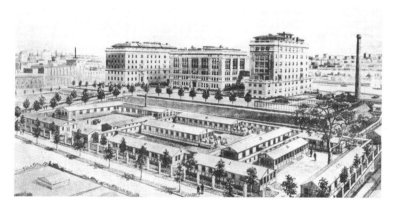

The War Demonstration Hospital constructed in the grounds of the Rockefeller Institute gave tuition in Carrel's methods to military surgeons. (*Courtesy of the Rockefeller University Archives.*)

---

[1] These large glass coloured slides showing the injuries treated in France are well preserved in the Rockefeller University Archives.

The War Demonstration Hospital would be a further Rockefeller-funded contribution to military medicine and the war effort, and it was in action until 1919. It was Carrel's second hospital project in two years. Details of its construction on the Institute grounds were announced in the *New York Times* in March 1917, as well as the news that it was funded by $200,000 from the Foundation, rather than from Institute funds.[2] The project showed that Rockefeller funds were going to a cause popular with the American citizens, and Rockefeller senior and junior were later pleased with its work.

But before looking at this episode in Carrel's life, the earlier war work at the Institute in his absence can be reviewed. Some of the Institute staff moved into military administrative posts or took up projects linked to the War; many had military rank.[3]

Wartime Work

Carrel's assistant Albert Ebeling continued with Carrel's tissue culture studies in a small way. The immortal 'old strain' cells still flourished, though they were often tended by others, since Ebeling changed to work part-time to allow enrollment at medical school. He was also plagued with bouts of puzzling illness, with abdominal symptoms and weight loss, from which he always recovered. In spite of these distractions, he helped Phoebus Levene, the Institute's distinguished biochemist, with his studies on diabetes, by removal of the dog pancreas, but the crucial discovery of insulin came shortly after from Canada in 1920. For Donald Van Slyke (1883–1971), exploring new ideas in clinical chemistry, Ebeling put in a helpful vein loop graft onto the portal vein of dogs which, passing under the skin, enabled regular sampling of portal vein blood. In Carrel's laboratory, some experiments on wound healing were continued by Alice Hartmann, and her dog experiments mimicked Carrel's new method of

---

[2] 'Dr. Carrel Coming for War Work Here' *NYT*, 29 March 1917.
[3] An interesting review of the Hospital's contribution, probably written by Flexner, is in 'War work of the Rockefeller Institute for Medical Research, New York' *The Military Surgeon* 47, (1920): 491–512. Carrel's surgical work figured prominently.

treatment of wounds in France. Carrel and Hartmann published together on the human and animal experiments.[4]

For the other Institute staff, war work involved their traditional experience and skills in investigating and dealing with infectious disease, and this included an unsuccessful hunt for antisera to use in gas gangrene, or in dysentery or streptococcal or staphylococcal infections. But there was partial success in developing antisera to treat the various forms of pneumonia. In Meltzer's laboratory, at the request of the U.S. Chemical Warfare Service, there was work on the effects of mustard gas poisoning and a search for possible antidotes. Rous had patiently continued studying methods of cold storage of blood and successfully established that red cells were usefully preserved in his citrate-dextrose solution. His method would be used when blood banking emerged in the last months of the war.

Murphy's Bold Concept

At this time, one Institute project, unrelated to the war, is of interest. James B. Murphy, as described earlier, had shown the major role of the lymphocyte in the response to tuberculosis, and that this cell was responsible for graft rejection. He then showed that suppressing lymphocyte activity with radiation or benzol would allow tumour homografts to survive longer. He now raised an idea that was to beguile others regularly later, namely that human tumours might be regarded as surviving homografts which had escaped control of the patient's own lymphocytes. If so, it followed that if the activity of the patient's lymphocytes could be increased, these human tumours might be 'rejected'. Practical as ever, he knew of ways to obtain the desired elevation of human or animal lymphocyte counts. In this experimental animal tumour work, he worked with William D. Witherbee (1875–1965), who

---

[4]These wartime activities are noted in Scientific Reports of the Laboratories presented to the Corporation and to the Board of Scientific Directors, vol. 4, 1915–16, box 2 folder 2, pp. 32, 52 and 155, FA 145, Rockefeller University Archives, Rockefeller Archives Centre (RUA RAC). In spite of her contributions, Hartmann's status is unknown, and she is not on any staff list.

was on the staff of the Institute from 1916–1920. He was later a pioneer radiotherapist at the local New York Presbyterian Hospital.[5]

Using Lymphocyte Rebound

The two researchers knew that giving significant radiation to patients or animals caused the lymphocyte count to fall, but a week or so later there was a rebound in the number in the blood, and this count could reach four times the normal level. Murphy considered that this increased lymphoid activity might give a heightened immune reaction, and he had some success with this lymphocyte rebound in controlling tumours in animal models.[6]

If human cancers were homografts, perhaps this lymphocyte rebound could benefit human cancer patients. Flexner seemed interested. The Institute had just received an extra gift of $200,000 earmarked for cancer research, now called the Rutherford Fund, and Flexner applied these funds to support study of Murphy's idea. This joint cancer work featured prominently in the wartime Institute reports in 1915–16.[7] They chose to study cases of breast cancer where the local cancer was advanced and complete surgical removal had not been possible. Three weeks postoperatively, using their powerful Institute radiation source, Murphy and Witherbee gave 'whole body' doses of X-rays to the patients, shielding the area of residual tumour to prevent any local effect of the radiation. After a fall in lymphocyte count, the expected later increase was obtained in most of the nine cases. It was the first attempt at human 'immunotherapy', as the strategy was called later.

---

[5] Witherbee's early textbook (with John Remer) is *X-Ray Dosage in Treatment and Radiography* (New York: Macmillan, 1922). Witherbee credits the inventive Murphy with suggesting that diseases of the tonsil, as a lymphoid organ, could be treated with radiation; see W.D. Witherbee (1921) 'X-ray treatment of tonsils and adenoids' *The American Journal of Roentgenology* 8: 25–30.
[6] James B. Murphy and Ernest Sturm (1919) 'The lymphocytes in natural and induced resistance to transplanted cancer' *JEM,* 29, 25–30.
[7] *Scientific Reports* (1915–16), box 2 folder 2, pp. 10, 95, 126 and 279, FA 145, RUA RAC (note 4).

Murphy initially reported that in this small group of patients some showed a reduction in the remaining cancer, and in others there was no progression. Later, cancer spread did occur, but seemed slower in these patients. But the final results were never published in full and were doubtless disappointing. Exactly the same hypothesis and claims for early success in stimulating the immune response featured in the extensive but unsuccessful human cancer immunotherapy efforts of the 1970s. Murphy also found chemicals which mimicked radiation's stimulating effect on lymphocytes, notably Scharlach (the dye Sudan 3), but did not use it clinically. Almost the entire January 1919 issue of *The Journal of Experimental Medicine* is devoted to Murphy's lymphocyte studies, including eight articles dealing with methods of stimulation of lymphocyte count.

But he took this approach no further. One reason was that Murphy was called up for military service and went to the Surgeon General's Office in Washington, where he helped organise the U.S. military pathology services. Murphy then had a stomach problem which required surgery, and post-operative complications, including clinical depression, followed: he was largely an invalid from February 1918 to September 1920.[8]

The War Demonstration Hospital

The Hospital was built on the grounds of the Rockefeller Institute and on completion it was named Auxiliary Hospital No. 1 (Rockefeller Institute) New York City. An imaginative modular construction was used, based on the design of the British Red Cross Hospital near Boulogne, and for the needs of war, it could be quickly assembled from small units. It could also be dismantled at speed and moved elsewhere.[9] With major involvement by America in the European war, the plan was for 25 similar 1,000 bed

---

[8] Flexner to Carrel, 11 July 1930, box 3 folder 50, Malinin Collection of the Papers of Alexis Carrel and Charles Lindbergh, FA 208, RUA RAC (note 4).

[9] The designer made a Carrel-like grumble about 'the lack of understanding and sympathy which pervade every [military] department in Washington': War Demonstration Hospital, Class Records 1917–18, box 2 folder 16(11), FA 012, RUA RAC (note 4).

WAR HOSPITAL WARD OPEN.

Patients Will Be Under Personal Supervision of Dr. Carrel.

The War Demonstration Hospital of the Rockefeller Institute for Medical Research, at Sixty-fourth Street and Avenue A, New York City, has now opened its second ward. Patients will be admitted who have chronic and obstinate infections that have resisted treatment and those who have compound fractures, chronic osteomyelitis, and varicose leg ulcers.

The purposes of the hospital are to treat patients suffering from infected lesions and wounds by methods which have lately been developed in European army hospitals, especially those developed by Drs. Carrel and Dakin in the Military Hospital at Compiegne, France, and to demonstrate these methods in a practical way to American surgeons. Dr. Alexis Carrel has personal supervision of the work of this hospital. Dr. Adrian V. S. Lambert, Professor of Surgery at the College of Physicians and Surgeons, is aiding Dr. Carrel. The hospital will make no charge for treatment or care. It will admit only male patients over 16 years of age.

Publicity for the Demonstration Hospital in the *New York Times* 8 September 1917.

hospitals to go to Europe eventually. The Rockefeller Institute and Foundation handled the public relations and put out regular press releases on the project, assisted by Carrel:

The present war filled the army hospitals with patients, whose wounds were more than 90% infected and many of whom are suffering from advanced stages of gangrenous or other suppuration. The improvement of procedures for the sterilisation of wounds has been one of the chief surgical achievements of the war. One of the most important of these procedures is the technique of chemical sterilisation of wounds. This technique, as employed at the Compiègne hospital, has reduced the period of disability for infected cases to between one half and one third of the average, and has decreased in a large measure, the number of amputations and deaths from infection. Dr. Alexis Carrel has been granted leave of absence by the French government in order that he may be present to supervise the treatment and conduct demonstrations in person.[10]

The Hospital was officially opened on 12 August 1917 with a ceremony attended by Surgeon General William C. Gorgas and representatives of the Allied government medical departments.[11] Adrian Lambert (1872–1952), father of the baby rescued in 1908 by Carrel's transfusion, and now professor of surgery at the College of Physicians and Surgeons of Columbia University in New York, was appointed joint 'attending surgeon' with Carrel, and a surgical assistant, Dr. George A. Stewart from Baltimore, was in day-to-day charge. The other two assistants were surgeons seconded by the French military, one of whom, Captain Georges Dehelly, was co-author with Carrel of the book on the Carrel–Dakin method. The other was Georges Loewy, who trained under Tuffier in Paris. When fully functional later, they did about 35 surgical operations each month, mostly wound closure, skin grafts and occasional amputations. This was not a great clinical burden for the four surgeons and gave plenty of time, as at Compiègne, for clinical observations and teaching. Paluel Flagg, one of the doctors giving the anaesthetics at the Hospital, became a friend of Carrel's and, interested in resuscitation, kept up an attachment at the Institute after the War.

Carrel, as always, enjoyed the administrative detail and military discipline. Normally he had little interest in teaching, but now he used his huge collection of coloured glass slides and a film on surgical management in the war when teaching the visiting military surgeons. Other Rockefeller Institute experts gave lectures. Tuition was given in 'clinical chemistry', the new field being opened up by Van Slyke, and Peyton Rous described how red cell preservation for three weeks in the cold was possible using his citrate-glucose solution. The trainees were also told of the usefulness of 'hemagenous fluid' — blood plasma — for

---

[10] 'Carrel Will Teach New Treatment Here' *NYT*, 22 July 1917.
[11] 'Army Doctors See Dr. Carrel At Work' *NYT*, 13 August 1917.

transfusion as a blood substitute.[12] John Auer in his lectures described how magnesium could be used to treat the spasms of tetanus although, with antitoxin available, this was largely a thing of the past. He and Meltzer also demonstrated resuscitation using their tracheal tubes, and the visitors were impressed to see that when dogs were paralysed with curare they could be brought back to life in this way. It was an impressive series of novel, practical contributions to military medicine from the Institute staff.

In early October, Carrel gave a lecture illustrated with his slides at the New York Academy of Medicine, and it drew in a large audience. The *New York Times* reported that:

> Long before Doctor Carrel's appearance on the platform, the main hall was crowded and the audience had overflowed into and filled the room at the left of the platform. Many found it impossible to get in and went away.

Carrel told the audience that 'practically every war wound death could have been avoided if the case had been taken in and treated soon enough'.[13]

Civilian Patients

The difficulty at the outset for the Hospital was getting patients. Although war was declared, and American troops were crossing the Atlantic and Crile and Cushing had arrived with their advance 500-bed medical units, the build-up in France was slow. American infantry did not enter the trenches until October 1917, and even then, saw no action for many months. With no American military casualties as yet, the Hospital instead encouraged referral by local doctors of civilian cases of 'infected wounds of the soft parts and chronic ulcers (other than tuberculosis or syphilis)'. No fees were charged, and these patients started to appear at the Hospital

---

[12] See L.G. Walker (2002) 'Carrel's war research hospital at Compiegne: Prototype of a research facility at the front' *Journal of the American College of Surgeons* 195, 870–7.
[13] 'Dr. Carrel Explains Cures' *NYT*, 5 October 1917.

in the autumn of 1917. This was a significant change in emphasis. The original Carrel–Dakin strategy was designed to deal with recent war wounds of the limbs, but Carrel was now treating chronic infections. He had some experience of such cases at Compiègne and was confident that his method was applicable.

As always, he liked having visitors, and among the celebrities he welcomed in 1918 was Winston Churchill. Occasionally there were important patients, and one was Abraham Flexner, Simon's brother, author of the famous report on medical education. After a fracture of his lower leg left him with some skin loss, Carrel took over the treatment of the ulcer on 10 February and Flexner was hospitalised for some weeks before moving to Baltimore for skin grafting by Halsted.

Critics Appear

Shortly after the Hospital opened to patients, the Clinical Congress of Surgeons of North America met in October 1917 in Chicago, and Surgeon General Gorgas chaired a 'War Session'. Surgeons with experience of the European war spoke, notably George Crile, back on leave after six months at the front, and now with serious exposure to the realities of war surgery. A celebrated guest speaker was Sir Berkeley Moynihan, the English surgeon, then on an extensive American tour, which included briefing the U.S. cabinet on military surgery. The Carrel–Dakin method was on the program and Carrel was to be a guest speaker, and show a film. Halsted heard rumours that Carrel's treatment might be criticised and wrote ahead warning Carrel saying that the reception of his lecture would be affected by 'side issues'. This doubtless was unhappiness about the publicity surrounding his methods, including the dramatic claims at his public lecture at the New York Academy of Medicine. Halsted asked Carrel to come to the meeting but 'remain behind scenes and prompt your friends'.[14] Carrel decided not to attend the meeting at short notice, offending his hosts, and making the excuse that he was worn out.

---

[14] Halsted to Carrel, 15 October 1917, box 39 folder 36, Alexis Carrel Papers, Georgetown University Library, Booth Family Center for Special Collections.

At the meeting William Sherman, the industrial surgeon who had visited Compiègne, spoke and was enthusiastic, as before, about the Carrel–Dakin method. Sherman also offered a smaller course on the Carrel system for military officers in Pittsburgh. But others were less supportive, and Crile's view now was that the Carrel technique worked well only if applied in an unhurried way, and that it was unsuitable for use during busy military action. Moynihan then spoke at length. As described earlier, he had been a prominent supporter of Almroth Wright's rival saline perfusion method, but now with Wright and his method discredited, Moynihan seemed disenchanted with any kind of perfusion. He took a new stance, or rather the old view taken by Carrel's French surgical critics. Moynihan said he was now convinced that débridement was the crucial element in wound care, and that thereafter the various added treatments had little influence on outcome. The first stage in wound care was that the surgeon must 'operate ruthlessly, taking away all dead and contaminated tissue'. After that, said Moynihan, almost flippantly, 'you may do such other things as you care to try. One method is as good as another, and no method is the equal of any'. He added gratuitously that the Carrel method 'has achieved its greatest successes in the cases in which it need never have been used'.[15]

Carrel was understandably annoyed at Moynihan's stance, and complained later to Flexner that Moynihan's nihilism had led American military surgeons into error, which 'caused the death of many men'.[16]

Next month there was further disparagement of the Carrel–Dakin method; others seemed determined to rain on Carrel's parade. The first incident was a hostile, anonymous review in the *Journal of the American Medical Association* of the Carrel and Dehelly book *The Treatment of*

---

[15] The proceedings are given in 'Clinical Congress of Surgeons of North America — War Session' *JAMA* 69, (1917): 1538–41. Moynihan had a less hostile version in his *American Addresses* (Philadelphia: W. B. Saunders, 1917): 44–72.

[16] Carrel to Flexner, 9 Aug 1918, Alexis Carrel Papers, Administrative Correspondence 1917–1922, box 2 folder 2, FA 231, RUA RAC (note 4). Moynihan may have been unpopular with surgical insiders — notably for claiming in 1918 that he had been transfusing blood since 1910.

Infected Wounds which mainly criticised Dakin's chemistry.[17] This provoked a sharp response in the journal from Dakin. His name had not been included as an author of the book, Dakin pointed out, and moreover 'he had no previous knowledge of the content of the book'. He then rebuked the reviewer and listed the reviewer's mistakes, notably regarding the chemistry of the Dakin fluid.

Meanwhile the Carrel–Dakin method was assailed from another direction, but in the same journal.

Enter Bevan

One week after the hostile book review in the *Journal*, and just 10 days after the first War Demonstration Hospital course started, the *Journal of the American Medical Association* on 17 November 1917 carried a lengthy public complaint about the Carrel–Dakin method from Arthur Dean Bevan (1861–1943), professor of surgery at Rush Medical College in Chicago. Bevan was a talented surgeon and an influential, opinionated figure in American surgery. Prominent in medical politics, and president of the American Medical Association that year, he was also the long-serving chairman of their Education Committee from 1914–28. The published letter was a long personal one to William Welch, the Rockefeller Institute's president, but Bevan, wishing his concerns to be more widely known, sent a copy of his letter, for publication, to the widely-read *Journal*.

Bevan made a number of points, but the main thrust was that, having studied Carrel's system and spoken to those involved in its use in Europe, he now wished to discourage the take-up of the Carrel method by the American military. He felt the results were not as good as was thought. Bevan noted that Carrel gave few results in his book, nor were there proper comparisons with other methods. He went on:

> The method will have a short popularity among that small corps of enthusiasts of the type that is easily carried away by new startling

---

[17] Book Review, *JAMA* 69, (1917): 1645. But it emerged for the first time that Dakin's solution was hypertonic — an essential part of Almroth Wright's rival strategy.

methods. … The exaggerated claims which have gotten into our medical journals and even into the lay press should be disparaged by those who are in a position to control the situation.[18]

This was a serious public rebuke from a senior figure to both Carrel and the Institute, criticising the data and the publicity surrounding it. But it was perhaps not entirely a surprise. Bevan had a reputation for blunt speaking, and was 'disposed to run amuck', as the senior surgeon William Kean put it. Bevan had earlier annoyed the Rockefeller Institute by attacking Meltzer's pioneering introduction of intra-tracheal anaesthesia. Bevan described Meltzer's method as having 'little place in practical surgery' but also said it was dangerous.[19]

One aspect of this apparently unpatriotic criticism can be traced to some attitudes of Bevan's and the libertarian American Medical Association. They traditionally opposed any standardisation of surgical treatment and

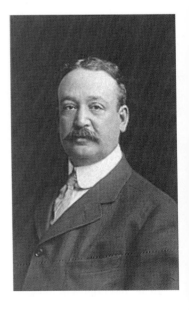

Prof. Arthur D. Bevan, the influential Chicago surgeon, was critical of Carrel's claims. (*www.findagrave.com*)

---

[18] Arthur Dean Bevan (1917) 'The Carrel–Dakin treatment' *JAMA* 69, 1727–8.
[19] A.D. Bevan (1915) 'The choice and technic of the anesthetic' *JAMA*, 65, 1418.

in addition, at this time, were opposed to civilian surgeons moving to join the military effort. For these enlisted surgeons to treat cases by any protocol such as the Carrel–Dakin method was doubly offensive. Added to this, using the lay press for announcements about serious medical and scientific matters was always deplored by the profession, and he rebuked Carrel and the Institute for doing so.

Bevan's letter caused immediate concern at the Institute. They moved quickly to limit the damage, and although Carrel drafted a vigorous response, the Institute lawyer Starr Murphy advised against sending it. Instead Murphy organised supportive letters to the *Journal* from friends of the Institute. Welch replied first and said that Carrel's wound closures were 'amazingly rapid' and said correctly that others in Europe, like Depage, now used the method. He denied that there were any pressure on the military to adopt it as the only method of treatment. But he admitted difficulties in using the method in practice. He made another concession when he added that

> of course, much has appeared in the newspapers which is exaggerated and deplorable, and this is calculated to create a prejudice against Carrel; but I do not think he is responsible for this.[20]

Next week's issue of the *Journal* carried the supportive letters requested from Joseph C. Bloodgood (1867–1935), the Baltimore surgeon trained under Halsted, and the senior public health administrator Arthur T. McCormack of Kentucky. Bloodgood praised Carrel's book and wrote that it had 'scientific precision', adding mistakenly that Carrel's study did include control cases not treated by his method.[21] McCormack's letter was more accurate when he wrote that Carrel's book was simply 'a *précis* or manual … to refresh the memory of those who have participated in the course of study of the treatment'. He wondered, like the *Journal* readers, why Bevan was attempting

---

[20] William H. Welch (1917) 'The Carrel–Dakin treatment' *JAMA* 69, 1994.
[21] J.C. Bloodgood (1917) 'The Carrel–Dakin treatment' *JAMA* 69, 2061–2.

to throw confusion into the Medical Department of our Army. ... in a position of great responsibility, conferred upon him by the profession, he [Bevan] has no right to give publicity to a personal letter which lends the weight of his authority to a destructive criticism.[22]

The Institute seemed pleased with their tactics, and their attorney Starr Murphy noted: 'Evidently Doctor Bevan did not know what he was doing when he pulled the chain of the shower bath. I am glad he is getting a ducking.'[23]

Teaching the Technique

There the Bevan affair rested. The Hospital had opened for teaching on 5 November 1917, and the first 15 medical officers started their 12-day stay, soon called the 'Carrel Course'. Later, up to 28 could be taught on each course, and they came from the 50 or so new army base hospitals throughout the country; it was intended that the method would be taken back and taught locally at the base.[24] In all, by the end of the war, 1,016 medical officers and enlisted men received instruction, as did some Red Cross nurses. In addition to mastering the perfusion technique, instruction was also necessary in the complex preparation of fresh Dakin solution. Assessments were made of the visitors at the end of the course, and the rather fussy military criteria were — 'earnestness, mental alertness, adaptability and potentiality' — criteria which have hints of Carrel's own disciplined approach to using his method.[25]

[22] Arthur T. McCormack (1917) 'A reply by Dr A.T. McCormack' *JAMA* 69, 2062–3.
[23] Vincent to Murphy, 9 Jan 1918, Dr. A. Carrel, box 44 folder 433, RU RG 526–1, RUA RAC (note 4).
[24] For a Canadian surgeon's visit to the Demonstration Hospital, see Herbert W. Baker (1918) 'The treatment of infected wounds with dichloramine-T with special reference to its advantages over the Carrel–Dakin method' *Canadian Medical Association Journal* 8, 805–23.
[25] War Demonstration Hospital, box 1 Class Records 1917–18, FA 012, RUA RAC (note 4).

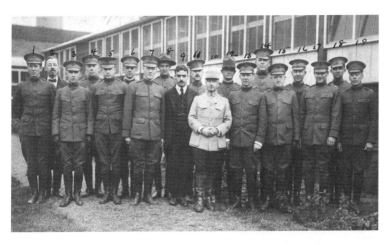

Carrel with a group of enlisted military surgeons attending his teaching course. On his right, in civilian clothes, is Dr. Georges Loewy the French surgeon, and on Loewy's right is Major George Stewart, the surgeon in charge. (*Courtesy of the National Library Medicine/Rockefeller Archives.*)

The enthusiasm of those taught varied. Some trainees felt that by mastering the technique and its mystique they were entering into a privileged brotherhood. But for others, it is likely that the uncertain verdict at the Clinical Congress and the gossip following Bevan's *JAMA* criticism undermined the claims made in the course. On their return to their base hospitals, many did not get senior support. Major Stewart at the Hospital was an evangelist for the method, and when he heard from his ex-pupils that there was local resistance to its use, Stewart told them to be firm and to 'stick to the principles'. When there were failures, he was convinced that the detailed method had not been properly used.[26]

Cases Arrive

Not until 31 August 1918, nine months after the Hospital started work, did convalescent military American casualties arrive back by sea in the U.S., and they were triaged at the New York docks. The threat of gas gangrene in

[26] Perrin Selcer (2008) 'Standardizing wounds: Alexis Carrel and the scientific management of life in the First World War' *British Journal for the History of Science* 41, 73–107.

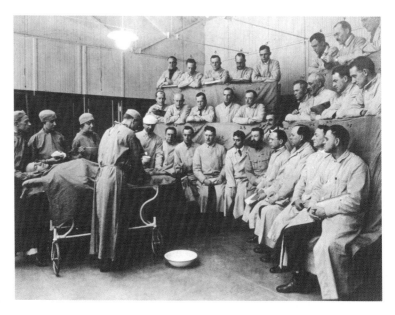

Carrel in the surgical theatre of the War Demonstration Hospital watching Major Stewart change a leg dressing, with a nurse ready to take a bacteriology swab. (*Courtesy of the National Library Medicine/Rockefeller Archives.*)

the mud of the Western Front was long gone. Those sent to the Demonstration Hospital were cases of chronic wound infection, otherwise recovered, and included chronic bone infection — osteomyelitis — as a complication of compound fractures. These cases usually showed a chronic discharging track out to the skin.

In treating chronic cases, no further débridement was usually necessary. The perfusion with Dakin's solution was now directed at open ulcerated surfaces or used down the track to areas of osteomyelitis within bones. Carrel now claimed a new success. He said that normally only in 1% of cases of osteomyelitis could treatment be effective and the sinus be closed. With his perfusion via the sinus he reported that 60% of cases were sterilised, and this included success in civilian cases of several years duration. In the remaining 40% usually only a dry sinus remained. He also claimed, more dramatically, that he could clear tuberculosis from bones by his perfusion methods.

Extending the Technique

Carrel's new confidence meant he now felt justified to go further, and he envisaged the universal application of his method to any focal infection. In war wounds he proposed that it be applied to infection in the chest, abdomen and brain. Shortly after the Hospital opened, a new opportunity arose to apply it to a common life-threatening localised infection.

In late 1917, New York had a serious pneumonia epidemic and many cases reached the Rockefeller Hospital, known for its special interest in the infection. A serious complication of pneumonia is empyema, a collection of pus in the chest cavity between the lung and the ribs. With an established empyema, it was, and is, necessary to obtain proper drainage of the pus. It was usual to attempt drainage with a needle first then, if necessary, proceed to surgical removal of a portion of rib over the collection and insert a drain. In spite of this, the death rate was still high. The new venture was to apply Carrel's method in these cases, and the Rockefeller Hospital sent these cases over to Carrel at his hospital to treat them with his new approach.

To add to the surgical drainage, Carrel now used perfusion of the cavity with Dakin's fluid via the drain. He and Stewart at the Demonstration Hospital were enthusiastic about the first results in the Hospital's post-pneumonia cases. In Paris, Tuffier loyally took up the method and somehow the news of the new treatment for empyema reached the *New York Times*.[27] At the Demonstration Hospital, they recommended to the surgeons on the courses that when they returned to their base hospitals they use the method when treating any cases of empyema occurring after pneumonia.[28]

Influenza

There was soon a sharp increase in cases of empyema at the base hospitals, not from the usual type of pneumonia, but as a consequence

---

[27] 'A New Pleurisy Treatment: Carrel Tubes Inserted' *NYT*, 7 October 1917. Tuffier wrote of his early experience with Carrel's pleural perfusion technique in 'Traitement des suppurations de la plèure' *Bulletin de l'Académie de médecine* (1917), 76: 11 and 16.
[28] 'Empyema in base hospitals', *Review of War Surgery and Medicine* 1, (1918): 1–40.

A NEW PLEURISY TREATMENT

Carrel Tubes Introduced and Inflamed Surfaces Sterilized.

The Paris correspondent of The Medical Record sends this brief account of a new method of treating pleurisy:

" Professor Tuffier, at a recent meeting of the Academy of Medicine, reported a series of cases of purulent pleurisy and extravasations of blood into the pleura which had become purulent. After having exposed the technique of his procedure, which consists in evacuating the pleural cavity, introducing the Carrel irrigating tubes and sterilizing the inflamed surfaces until all infection is shown to be absent by the microscope, then closing the pleural opening to heal. Dr. Tuffier gives the result in twelve cases thus treated, ten of which were purulent. All were cured, but the remarkable feature of the cure was that the lungs recovered all of their functional activity, which infrequently follows the other forms of treatment."

Carrel had strong support for his perfusion treatment method from Théodore Tuffier, his distinguished surgical friend in Paris. (*New York Times* 7 October 1917.)

of influenza. The influenza pandemic, which was to spread world-wide and have a huge death toll, possibly arose in U.S. military training camps in early 1918 and was spread thereafter by the military. Infections like measles, mumps, scarlet fever, meningitis and pneumonia were to be expected in the young recruits gathered in the overcrowded barracks, but influenza was a new and unexpected killer. The first serious outbreak was at Fort Riley, Kansas, in mid-March, and soon all the training camps in America were affected, with the virus spreading via the troop movements to Europe. The severity and spread were alarming and eventually 30,000 were to die in the U.S. army alone. There were two waves during 1918, and the epidemic was a major killer in civilian life before it burnt out mid-1919. U.S. Army morale fell, and there was a sense of hopelessness with this defeat in spite of the successes against infectious disease earlier. The old adage that more troops died of disease than in combat was now resurrected. A major factor in causing death from influenza was secondary bacterial pneumonia, and this in turn caused empyema.[29]

Although there was no treatment for influenza, there were choices in the management of the empyema which could follow. In March 1918, the Surgeon General's office, in response to the new challenge, set up an Empyema Commission to study the problem. This led to a conference on the problem held at the Base Hospital, Camp Hancock, Augusta. Captain Evarts Ambrose Graham (1883–1957), later a distinguished chest surgeon in St. Louis, was in charge of the study and sent out questionnaires on the 'new scourge' of empyema.[30]

His survey showed that physical examination was relied on for the diagnosis, with aspiration following, and the newly available X-ray examination was used only when in doubt about localisation. Rib removal and drainage followed if necessary. The Carrel–Dakin perfusion had been tried in the majority of camps, but the Report said that no obviously beneficial results were obtained thus far, except in diminishing the odour of the discharge. From the reports from the base camps he drew up a consensus document, as an 'Empyema Report', which was submitted to the Surgeon General in April 1918.[31]

Setbacks

But with further experience, complications were encountered. Dakin's solution slowed the natural resolution of the infection, notably by delaying the contraction of the empyema cavity. More dangerously, it emerged that perfusion with Dakin's solution could unplug the tiny

---

[29] For a full account, see Carol R. Byerly, *Fever of War: The Influenza Epidemic in the U.S. Army During World War I* (New York: New York University Press, 2005).

[30] Peter D. Olch (1989) 'Evarts A. Graham in World War I: the Empyema Commission and Service in the American Expeditionary Forces' *Journal of the History of Medicine and Allied Sciences* 44, 430–6.

[31] Publication was seriously delayed and the Report's findings were included by Evarts A. Graham in his book *Some Fundamental Considerations in the Treatment of Empyema Thoracis* (St Louis: C.V. Mosby, 1925).

tracks from the lung into the pleural cavity which led to the empyema in the first place. During perfusion, Dakin's fluid could pass back along these tracks into the air passages and the irritant perfusion solution was then coughed up. One military surgeon blamed this strategy for some deaths:

> We believe the injection of any solution into the pleural cavity is fraught with some danger. In these cases the fluid proved erosive and the patient drowned ...[32]

Meanwhile, the New York civilian post-pneumonia cases treated in this way were also not doing well, and Stewart had to report 12 deaths out of 46 empyema cases treated with this method; even Flexner was concerned at the events.[33] The influenza epidemic was over by 1919, and the Carrel–Dakin strategy for empyema was dropped thereafter by the military and the method was never successfully revived in civilian practice.

But Carrel also advocated his method for infection in the abdomen. Peritonitis can result from injuries, or follow abdominal inflammation or a leak from bowel. Again, it seemed an attractive idea to flush out infection from the abdomen, but when the Carrel–Dakin method was applied to sepsis in the abdomen, problems arose which were similar to those encountered with chest perfusion. The irrigation with the solution dislodged the thin mobile sheet of the greater omentum which can wrap round the septic area, and it also broke down the protection given by adherent loops of bowel.

Use of the Carrel–Dakin method in abdominal sepsis may have already claimed one early and prominent casualty in late 1917. Halsted at Baltimore had been following the news of the Carrel–Dakin method of wound treatment in France and New York, and he was interested in its extension to these other situations. In late 1917, Halsted operated on his Hopkins friend and colleague, the distinguished anatomist Franklin P. Mall (1862–1917). The surgery for gall-stones did not go well, and bile leakage and infection followed. Drains were in place and Halsted, taking

---

[32] War Demonstration Hospital, box 16 folders 15, 16, FA 012, RUA RAC (note 4).
[33] War Demonstration Hospital, box 16 folder 11, FA 012, RUA RAC (note 4).

advice, used the Carrel method, irrigating the abdomen via these drainage tubes. But the internal bile leak worsened and Mall died, aged 55.[34] Halsted later publicly warned against using Dakin's solution to perfuse the abdomen in this way.[35]

Dakin's New Antiseptic

Dakin had returned to America after his Dardanelles involvement, and continued to work on antiseptics. He soon announced a new antiseptic which could be used instead of what he still called 'the older Dakin-Carrel-Dehelly-Depage method'. The new chemical was chloramin(e)-T, soon replaced by dichloramin(e)-T, which was applied in a spray after mixing with chlorinated eucalyptol and liquid petrolatum. It was tested in use at the Pennsylvania Hospital's industrial accidents clinic.[36] The new antiseptic was said to cut down the hospital stay by one third, and others started to use this simple treatment at the military base hospitals.[37] By 1918, and the end of the War, an increasing range of methods of wound management was in use.

Reports

Clinical data were carefully reported from the Demonstration Hospital. The first results were for the year December 1917 to December 1918,

---

[34] Details of the surgical events leading to Mall's death are given in Gerald Imber, *Genius on the Edge: The Bizarre Double Life of William Stewart Halsted* (New York: Kaplan, 2011): 322–5.

[35] W.S. Halsted (1919) 'The omission of drainage in common duct surgery' *JAMA* 73, 1896–7.

[36] H.D. Dakin, Walter Estell Lee, Joshua E. Sweet, Byron M. Hendrix and Robert G. LeConte (1917) 'A Report of the use of dichloramin-T in the treatment of infected wounds' *JAMA*, 69, 27–30 and *Annals of Surgery* 67, (1918): 14–24. Lee had worked at the American Hospital in Paris and then returned to the Pennsylvania Hospital.

[37] Carrel accepted Chloramin-T as a useful antiseptic for maintenance of sterility; see *JEM*, 24 (1916): 429–50. He used it on suitable human wounds at Compiègne from June 1916, and it was used in animal experiments on wound healing at the Institute by the mysterious Alice Hartmann (see note 4).

though this involved a mixture of civilian and the early military cases from August 1918 onwards. The total number treated and discharged in the year was 253, of which 168 were classed as 'Recovered', 59 were 'Improved', and 4 as 'Unimproved'. Twenty-two had died in the Hospital, mostly the empyema cases in which the Carrel–Dakin method was tried.[38] The Hospital had bad luck with dealing with three civilian cases of gas gangrene in patients involved in road traffic accidents, since two needed an amputation of a leg.[39]

Return to France

Carrel returned to Paris at the end of February 1918, leaving the running of the Demonstration Hospital in others' hands. But it was to prove to be only a short spell of work for him in France until the end of the War in November. On his return, there was military action close to Compiègne, and the German front line advanced from the north, where it had been for almost three years, gaining about 20 miles and bringing the conflict closer. Carrel's hospital was bombed from the air, and although there were no serious injuries, the staff and patients were evacuated south on 21 March. Carrel obtained a new base hospital at Noisiel, to the east of Paris and much further south. He had laboratories there and also at St. Cloud. He did not return to his earlier wound treatment work, and instead moved into other areas.

The War's military surgical priorities were changing. In particular there was a new interest in 'shock'. The typology of shock at the time included immediate 'neurogenic' shock, 'wound' shock, and 'surgical' shock. Added to this was shell shock — a psychiatric state. It was taught that the nervous system was involved in all types, and George Crile in particular considered that over-stimulation of the nervous system was responsible for all kinds of shock.[40] But with blood pressure measurements now more commonly used, it was accepted, after urging by Bradford

---

[38] War Demonstration Hospital, box 3 folder 3(2), FA 012, RUA RAC (note 4).
[39] War Demonstration Hospital, box 16 folder 11, FA 012, RUA RAC (note 4).
[40] Peter C. English, *Shock, Physiological Surgery, and George Washington Crile* (Westport, Conn: Greenwood Press, 1980), chapter 10. Crile's memoirs claim he had been the pioneer of blood transfusion in WWI.

Cannon, the Harvard physiologist, that blood or fluid loss was often responsible for the shock seen after serious injury. This led to treatment by replacement of fluid, and at first, simple saline or blood substitutes like Bayliss' 6% gum, Hogan's gelatin or horse serum were used. But blood seemed best and by the end of 1917 steps were taken to set up the first blood banks. Fluid replacement proved to be successful, and by the spring of 1917, the casualty clearing stations started to set aside space for resuscitation of the seriously injured.[41]

New Projects

Carrel was well-placed to be involved in these new areas of interest. He was a pioneer of blood transfusion through his remarkable operation on the New York infant. At the Institute, he had watched at first hand the emergence of the simple blood storage method devised by Rous and Turner which would now make blood banking possible.[42] With the new interest in treating abdominal injuries, he thought that a more dilute Dakin's solution would safely deal with abdominal infection.

In his new laboratories, he had facilities for animal experiments and studies of shock commenced. He reported to Flexner that blood pressure might indeed be useful in assessing shock and that du Noüy, his physicist, was looking at ways of measuring blood loss. The French surgeon Dehelly had returned with him from New York, and he started work on the use of plasma in resuscitation. Carrel must have been close to offering whole blood transfusion, but he took no steps towards this. It was others who first thought to obtain blood during lulls in the war and store it ready for the next wave of casualties. A Canadian army doctor, Oswald H. Robertson, who had recently worked with Rous at the Rockefeller Institute on blood storage in this way, in November 1917 set up the first 'blood bank'. He took donations at the front from lightly

[41] Kim Pelis (2001) 'Taking credit: the Canadian Army Medical Corps and the British conversion to blood transfusion in WWI' *Journal of the History of Medicine* 56, 238–77.
[42] P. Rous and J.R. Turner (1916) 'The preservation of living red blood cells *in vitro*' *JEM* 23, 219–48 and *JAMA*, 70, 219.

injured or convalescent 'universal' group O soldiers during quiet times and stored it for future use.[43]

For his plans to study shock in the injured, Carrel needed to be near the front line. Although he had a base and laboratories at Noisiel, to deal with casualties early he needed to reach the action, and he was now further away. Once again he turned to Flexner and the Rockefeller Foundation and obtained generous funding for a mobile field hospital with 100 beds. It was the third hospital project for Carrel in the three years. Although Dr. Woimant, who had served at Compiègne, was appointed as surgeon-in-charge, little is known of this project or further appointments. The field hospital's first location was placed near the German lines at Soissons to the north, and it may have been involved in dealing with the 168,000 Allied casualties during the four-day Battle of Soissons starting on 18 July. No studies of shock or perfusion of abdominal or brain injuries were reported.[44]

Because of this, Carrel had a low profile at this time, and the newspapers carried no news of him. Another reason was that the attack on Carrel and the Institute by Bevan in the previous autumn may have made the Institute cautious about publicity, yet again. Related to this, in August 1918, Carrel's Rockefeller Institute secretary was dismissed. Flexner wrote to Carrel saying 'have you been informed we let Mrs. Doane go? … She was leaking stories to the newspapers'. Mrs. Doane was married to the editor of the New York *Sunday Mirror*.[45]

The Last Battles

The U.S. Army saw their first action, on a small scale, at the end of May 1918, but later there were mass casualties at the Battle of Hamel to the

---

[43] O.H. Robertson (1918) 'Transfusion with preserved red cells' *BMJ*, 18 June, 691–5. See also Lynn G. Stansbury and John R. Hess (2009) 'Blood transfusion in World War I: the roles of Lawrence Bruce Robertson and Oswald Hope Robertson' *Transfusion Medicine Reviews* 23, 232–6.

[44] Walker 'War research' (note 12).

[45] Flexner to Carrel, 7 August 1918, Simon Flexner APS Papers, Microfilm roll 21, FA 746, RUA RAC (note 4).

north of Paris on 4 July. Further serious action followed in the successful drive launched by the Allies in August 1918, and in this 'Grand Offensive', three major battles over 100 days decided the war in the Allies favour. It is likely that methods other than the Carrel–Dakin routine were used by the American medical corps during these major engagements. Simpler methods of wound care were desirable and traditional methods probably sufficed.

But a newly-arrived American surgeon soon successfully urged the adoption of a radically different method of wound care. Winnett Orr (1877–1956), an enlisted military surgeon from Lincoln Nebraska, made a puzzling observation. For American convalescent soldiers with open wounds or compound fractures starting on their long journey back home by land and sea, he and others often applied only a simple dressing, then encased the limb, with its open wound, in a plaster of Paris. On the journey, the plaster often remained unchanged for long periods, but when the sodden, odorous cast was eventually removed, the messy open wound beneath was easily cleaned up. Moreover, maggots in the wound added to the success and the tissues were surprisingly healthy and healing was proceeding well. This empirical advance lacked scientific credentials but offered a simple workable routine, and it found favour.[46]

An armistice was declared on 11 November 1918, and the war was over. Carrel was discharged from the French Army on 1 January 1919 and returned to New York. The Demonstration Hospital remained open for a while, and after the last course of instruction in March 1919, the Hospital discharged its last patient and closed on 1 April 1919. The fixtures and fittings were given to the Association for Improving the Condition of the Poor.

Carrel's awards for his wartime work were Belgium's Leopoldsorde (1916), Serbia's Royal Order of Saint-Sava (1917), Sweden's Grand Commander of the Polar Star (1918), Britain's Knight Commander of St Michael and St George (1918) and the U.S. Distinguished Service

---

[46] Orr's method was used after WWI in the surgery of osteomyelitis; see his review H. Winnett Orr (1928) 'Listerism properly and improperly applied' *American Journal of Surgery* 4, 465–85.

Medal (1921). From France, he was already an Officier de la Légion d'honneur from 1915 and was raised to Commandeur level in 1917.

The End of the Method

Carrel moved away from surgical studies after the war, and the Carrel–Dakin treatment was almost forgotten in peacetime. Significantly, in the official U.S. history of the war, the volume on 'Surgery' does not mention the technique.[47] In post-war civilian American surgical practice, wounds were simpler and débridment seldom needed: rigid treatment by protocol was in any case anathema to the profession, as it devalued clinical judgement and discouraged individualised treatment. The growth of laboratory science and the influence of non-clinicians in patient care was also seen by the medical profession as a growing threat. Medicine in the 1920s generally retrenched into holistic attitudes with disease management reverting to being an art rather than a science, using empirical skills gained from bedside experience. Wound management could return to being a matter of individual clinical judgement.

Wartime surgery, like warfare itself, needs discipline and group action based on agreed protocols. Carrel responded to this opportunity by offering a standardised practice, an approach which suited his personality and attitudes. His system for wound after-care had all the characteristics of a Carrel project. It had scientific credentials, it was intuitively attractive, it caught the public's attention and it had complexity and mystique. Displays of his method were available for distinguished visitors, and he made confident public statements about his achievements.

A few enthusiasts, like the industrial surgeon W. O'Neill Sherman, continued to treat their company's occasionally severe industrial limb injuries with the full Carrel–Dakin method. Dakin's solution has had a longer public life, and is commercially available simply as Dakin's

---

[47] *Medical Department of the United States Army in the World War, Volume 11: Surgery* (Washington: National Museum of Health and Medicine, 1927). But Carrel had been praised earlier in an enthusiastic review by the Surgeon General Merritte W. Ireland (1921) 'The achievement of the Army Medical Department in the World War' *JAMA* 76, 763–9.

Solution™.[48] There have also been occasional short-lived returns to enthusiasm for perfusion treatment of wounds, seen as a useful alternative to antibiotic use.[49]

By early 1919, Carrel had settled back at the Institute and was ready to resume where he had left off in 1914. But he reasonably wished to have a bigger unit. Flexner soon took an opportunity to use Carrel's name again when dealing with the Rockefellers, and was once again successful in obtaining more Rockefeller money.

---

[48] See Jeffrey M. Levine (2013) 'Dakin's Solution: Past, present and future' *Advances in Skin & Wound Care* 26, 410–14. Dakin's Solution is marketed in various strengths by Century Pharmaceuticals Inc.

[49] The V.A.C.VeraFlow™ system gives controlled delivery of solutions when treating chronic wounds, and Dakin's solution is one of the recommend agents. NPWT (Negative pressure wound therapy) is offered in addition in the more complex V.A.C.Ulta™ System.

CHAPTER TEN

Early 1920s Research

'Sorry to disturb your vacation,' Simon Flexner wrote hesitantly on 16 July 1919 to John D. Rockefeller senior, then out of town at his Maine retreat. Flexner's letter was apologetic for a good reason — he was looking for more money. The War had been a trying time for the Institute management since serious inflation had led to a fall in the buying power of their investment income. Added to this, one of Rockefeller's bonds in the Institute's endowment had defaulted. With the staff returning from war work to their usual Institute posts, the scientific directors had met and, looking to the future, agreed that Flexner approach the Rockefellers, father and son, in the hope of reviving their financial position. Flexner was not confident that further money would be produced soon, or at all, since Rockefeller junior had warned Flexner privately of 'cries on every side of rising expenses'. Junior added darkly, using the language of business, that granting some of these financial pleas 'would not increase output'.

In Flexner's summer letter to Rockefeller in support of his case, he played the Carrel card. Flexner was aware that although Carrel's war work did not please everyone, the Rockefellers had noticed it favourably. The family had entertained Carrel in New York and Carrel also gave a talk to the lady helpers at Abby Rockefeller's Red Cross Auxiliary group. Flexner now had Carrel back in New York, rather unexpectedly, and ready to resume his Institute work. Prior to the war, Carrel's Division of Surgery was quite small, but in France, he had set up and ran a well-staffed, well-equipped surgical hospital, and, to follow, then set up the War Demonstration Hospital in New York. Carrel's scientific and administrative skills were clear. Flexner now asked him what he required, and Carrel, not surprisingly, first suggested that he be given a surgical research hospital; more realistically, he then settled for a substantial research unit in the Institute. Flexner hinted in his letter to the Rockefellers that Carrel had a new grand project, and for this, more money was needed:

> The Scientific Directors feel Dr. Carrel should be given better facilities. His work besides advancing surgery to a huge degree has shed lustre on the Institute, as you know. His plans of work … will be even more important than his discoveries in the relation to the treatment of war wounds.[1]

This new plan was not described. But Carrel was not intending to go back to the transplantation studies at which he excelled and which had been left tantalisingly close to major developments on the eve of the War. Nor was he going back to his pioneering heart or blood vessel surgery: instead, he wished to expand his tissue culture work.

New Funds

The starting point for this new direction came when Rockefeller senior, with advice from his son, agreed to add a further $2 million to the Institute's endowment, lifting the Institute's annual income to nearly $250,000. Flexner and the scientific directors were understandably relieved and delighted at the news, and recorded their 'exaltation inspired by the news of Mr Rockefeller's last generous gift and the alluring outlook it opened up'.

With his new money, Flexner prioritised Carrel's needs, and a generous top slice went towards 'rehabilitation and development of the Division of Experimental Surgery'. Others in the Institute gained some

---

[1] Minutes of the Board of Scientific Directors, October 1917–June 1920, Entries from June 1919, FA 856, Rockefeller University Archives, Rockefeller Archives Centre (RUA RAC).

extra support, and it seems that Flexner took this opportunity to intervene and make the changes in the research direction of some members. These were not always for the better.[2]

Carrel's Expanded Division

A reconstruction of the entire fifth floor, costing $184,000, gave Carrel four large laboratories and operating rooms, and he had an increased annual budget of $12,089 for staff and supplies. Carrel was now paid $16,000, and he obtained salaries for three more scientists to add to his existing assistant staff member, Albert Ebeling, who had been with him from 1911. In spite of Carrel's regular complaints about his French compatriots, both his new posts went to staff who had been with him at Compiègne or the War Demonstration Hospital. To expand his division's chemical research, he brought in Maurice Daufresne, who had worked in France on developing Dakin's solution and its successor chloramine-T.[3] When Daufresne left in 1925, he was replaced by Lillian E. Baker (born 1890), who had obtained her PhD degree from Columbia University nearby, as an early appointment of a woman scientist in America. She was to work closely with Carrel until his retirement, hoping, without success, to develop a fluid that would sustain cells without the need to add the chicken embryo extract.

Carrel's other appointment in February 1920 was of the physicist Lecomte du Noüy (1883–1947) who had been with him in France and who had introduced the mathematical analysis to the war wound healing work.[4] Carrel had said correctly before the war that the 'principles of

---

[2]The senior staff, i.e. the 'members' of the Institute, now were Loeb, Levene, Meltzer, Carrel and Noguchi. Rufus Cole was in charge of the Rockefeller Hospital and Theobald Smith headed the Animal Pathology Division.

[3]Daufresne died during the Allied bombardment of Le Havre in 1944.

[4]Du Noüy's wife declined to move from Paris to America, and their divorce followed. He remarried in 1923 into the Harriman dynasty and his second wife Mary's helpful account is Mary Lecomte du Noüy, *The Road to "Human Destiny": A Life of Pierre Lecomte du Noüy* (New York: Longmans, Green and Co., 1955). He had career

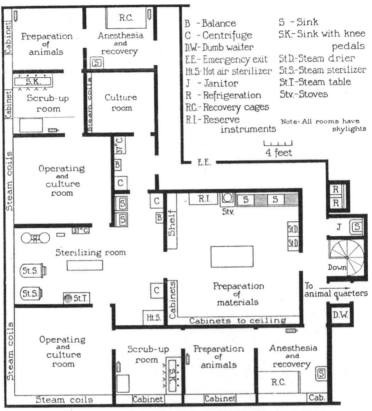

Fig. 2. Operating rooms in the laboratory of Dr. Alexis Carrel at The Rockefeller Institute, New York.

After the War, Carrel obtained extensive new facilities at the Institute in 1920, including this operating suite and experimental area. (From Raymond C. Parker *Methods of Tissue Culture 1938*.)

immunity' should be applied in an attempt to understand organ grafting, and du Noüy's new project in the new unit had a hint of that strategy. He applied his training in physics to antigen–antibody reactions, but not, with hindsight, in a profitable direction. He measured the surface tension of serum taken from animals before and after immunisation by a protein,

---

difficulties later at the Pasteur Institute and there was some criticism from fellow physicists of his research.

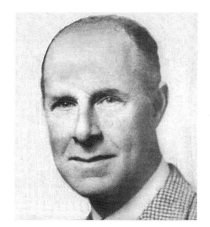

Pierre Lecomte du Noüy in Carrel's laboratory was first to apply the methods of physics to biology. (*Wikipedia*)

and surprisingly showed a prompt and major change in surface tension. But little came out of the work, other than an exploration of the surface tension of biological fluids, and a new measuring device of his own design. His work was mostly well regarded, and his call for the introduction of the methods of physics into biological research was a perceptive one, ultimately vindicated, and his viewpoint was noticed. He was later asked by the newly formed U.S. National Research Council to chair an expert international Committee on Molecular Physics in Relation to Biology, and this reported in 1929 and had influence.[5]

Technical assistance for the four scientists in Carrel's expanded unit was increased, and he now had three technicians, two 'skilled helpers', and three 'helpers', giving a staff of 12, as well as their own 'supervising nurse' in the enlarged animal facilities.[6] He also gained a personal secretary, and Miss Crutcher was to work with him, and be devoted to

---

[5] *Molecular Physics in Relation to Biology* (National Research Council of the National Academy of Sciences: Washington, DC, 1929). Joining du Noüy on his international Committee were Donnan (of the Donann Equilibrium) and Michaelis of the Michaelis–Menten Equation).

[6] The lower grade staff had 2–3 summer weeks holidays: their hours were 9 a.m. to 5.30 p.m. daily and they worked on Saturday mornings. See the plan of Carrel's operating suite in Raymond Parker's book *Methods of Tissue Culture* (New York: Hoeber, 1938).

him as the 'Chief', until his retirement in 1939, and beyond. She soon coped with reading and writing French documents and eventually dealt with much of his routine correspondence, including the steady flow of letters from the public. During his long absence in summer, she increasingly acted for him.

In Carrel's expanded laboratories, Albert Ebeling now extended Carrel's tissue culture work, which he had kept going during the War. Ebeling, now qualified as a doctor, was upgraded to the assistant grade and at the Institute, his MD degree allowed him to wear a white coat rather than the scientists' brown version. Ebeling and the technicians did all of the rather monotonous tissue culture work, and eventually even Ebeling may not have been involved in tending the cultures from day to day. Though made an associate from 1922, Ebeling was never promoted beyond this level, nor was encouraged to leave, although Flexner's usual policy was that junior staff should either show promise or move on. Carrel and Ebeling were not particularly close, and had one major disagreement later, but it seems that Ebeling was too valuable for Carrel to lose. Ebeling's health problems, mainly puzzling abdominal symptoms, continued and in one of Simon Flexner's long friendly summer letters to Carrel, Flexner had a clear view on the diagnosis and the best management. After Ebeling had been absent for an extended period, Flexner confided that:

> I am inclined to believe that he [Ebeling] was kept from falling into what might have been a long period, if not a permanent one, of invalidism and hypochondria, by being got back to work. I shall not be surprised if it takes two or three years to get him completely on his feet again. In the meantime, it is important to put him to work and not to humor him.[7]

Carrel's Laboratory

Daily life in the new laboratories had its frustrations. Strikes had delayed constructing the new extension, supplies were difficult to obtain and slow to arrive. The city of New York was expanding northwards, and drilling

---

[7] Flexner to Carrel, 11 July 1930, box 3 folder 50, Malinin Collection of the Papers of Alexis Carrel and Charles Lindbergh, FA 208, RUA RAC (note 1).

and blasting nearby for new buildings created fumes and dust that affected the tissue culture experiments. Two of the technical staff were feuding, and one had to go. The secretary Miss Crutcher was overloaded with work but was allowed to send typing out for completion.

In his laboratories, Carrel favoured rigid procedures and protocols. He was a respected disciplinarian in his unit, but was supportive of his technical staff. He could be testy at times and might turn away even old friends who arrived to visit him. Carl Beck in Chicago, Carrel's mentor earlier, made repeated attempts over many years to arrange to see him, and René Leriche, visiting from France, was annoyed when turned away twice, before being admitted at the third attempt.

Carrel ran his laboratory in a quirky way. Everything was cleared away into cupboards at night. The labs had no windows and there were water sprays to cut down dust. Asepsis in his dark-walled operating theatre suite on the floor above was unusually strict, and the tissue culture lab staff wore dark gowns and burka-like masks. A visitor noted 'an atmosphere of mystery and complication. The grey walls, black gowns,

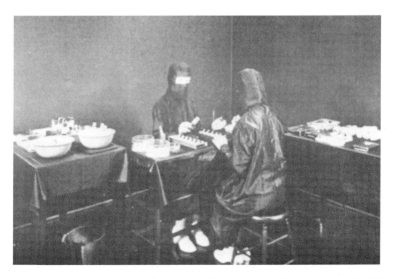

Carrel insisted on rigorous asepsis for tissue culture work, including unusually elaborate gowns for the staff. (*Courtesy of the Rockefeller University Archives.*)

masks and hoods; ... [the] enclosed microscopes and huge witches' cauldrons'.[8]

By now, scientists in other laboratories, notably Warren and Margaret Lewis at Baltimore, Christian Champy and Constantin Levatidi in Paris, Albert Fischer in Copenhagen and Giusseppi Levi in Italy had taken up tissue culture, as had Thomas Strangeways at Cambridge. Their view was that some of Carrel's fastidious extras were not required:

> Carrel caused the method [tissue culture] to be wrapped up from the beginning in a considerable cocoon of mumbo-jumbo. ... Thus tissue culture, though a delicate and exacting technique and one in which rigorous asepsis is absolutely essential, gained a spurious and unfortunate reputation for difficulty and almost for mysticism.[9]

Carrel's Choices

Flexner had agreed that Carrel should expand his tissue culture work. With this done, Flexner looked back and gave this odd assessment of Carrel's career:

> For many years Dr. Carrel and his associates devoted themselves to the study of problems and the perfection of the techniques of vascular suture, wound healing, etc., in the search for the factors governing the preservation and regeneration of tissues and organisms. Since his return to the Institute in 1919 Dr. Carrel has transferred his studies from the entire living animal to living cells, separated from the body ...[10]

Flexner was rather tortuously suggesting that before the War, Carrel had developed blood vessel and transplant surgery not primarily for

---

[8] P.R. White, *The Cultivation of Animal and Plant Cells* (New York: Ronald Press, 1954): vi.
[9] E.N. Willmer, *Cells and Tissues in Culture* (London: Academic Press, 1965): 4. For criticism at the time that 'the necessity for elaborate aseptic precautions has been over-emphasised', see H.M. Carleton (1923) 'Tissue Culture' *British Journal of Experimental Biology* 1: 131–51.
[10] Scientific Reports of the Laboratories Presented to the Corporation and to the Board of Scientific Directors, FA 145, October 1922, vol. 10, p. 331, RUA RAC (note 1).

human surgical use, but to explore fundamental mechanisms. Flexner further suggests that the reductionist move away from study of the whole animal and into tissue culture was a logical progression from this earlier work. Flexner then added the reassurance that surgical relevance had not been entirely forgotten. Carrel's tissue culture studies, he said, had already 'opened up a wide and fruitful field in which accurate surgical technique becomes the handmaiden of precise cellular physiology'. If Flexner was serious, this was an unusual aspiration.

Carrel also reflected on his shift away from his innovative practical surgery, but he was also prepared to defend it, in a way similar to Flexner. Writing to a doctor who requested news of his surgical research, Carrel explained that at the Institute

> surgery [here] is not to be studied from its direct application but from its foundation and it is essential to pursue it in accordance with its relation to physiology, chemistry and physics. This is what we are endeavouring to do. For this reason, there is no actual surgical work being done here at present.[11]

These glimpses into Flexner's and Carrel's thinking may explain some of the puzzling events of the 1920s. It seems that there was a hope that a shift into studies of cellular biology would assist in the advancement of clinical surgery. But, in retrospect, this policy was seriously mistaken, and nothing of surgical interest came from Carrel's cellular studies in the next 20 years.

Loeb's Lead

A major influence on Flexner and Institute policy at the time came from the biologist Jacques Loeb (1859–1924).[12] From his arrival at the Institute in 1910 onwards, and during the War, he had urged that the animal body

---

[11] Carrel to Mistachi, 20 June 1923, box 86 folder 10, Alexis Carrel Papers, Georgetown University Library, Booth Family Center for Special Collections.

[12] Jacques Loeb founded the *Journal of General Physiology* in 1918 with Winthrop J.V. Osterhout, also at the Rockefeller Institute, as joint editor.

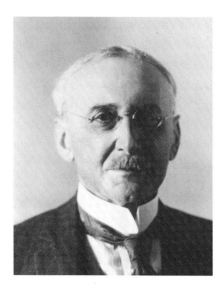

Jacques Loeb's advocacy of reductionist studies in biology had a dominant influence at the Rockefeller Institute until the mid-1920s. (*Courtesy of the National Library of Medicine.*)

could be explained in engineering terms, discarding the vitalist's old view that a 'life-force' directed the living matter of the cell. Loeb called for a retreat from studying the responses of the entire animal, suggesting instead that the integrated mechanism of the whole animal should first be separated into its components. After understanding these elements, the insights would be put together, and enlightenment would follow: the whole was not greater than the parts. At the Institute, Loeb's teaching was well enough known for Loeb to be a central character in Sinclair Lewis's *Arrowsmith* of 1925, the earliest novel based on day-to-day life in scientific research.[13]

---

[13] Sinclair Lewis was briefed on details of life at the Institute by Paul de Kruif, a former Institute staff member, and author later of the best-seller *Microbe Hunters* (1926). In his autobiography, de Kruif mentions his contact with Carrel, but Carrel is not immediately identifiable in the novel; he could be part of the character of blunt-talking Terry Wicket.

Carrel knew that his cell culture work fitted Loeb's strongly held, influential reductionist views and Carrel was content to follow. Tissue culture apparently held out hopes for a fundamental understanding of the cell in health and disease, including reaching the important goal of understanding the cause of malignant change. Even beyond this, perhaps re-engineering the cell was a possibility. Loeb wrote that 'the idea hovering before me is that man can act as creator, even in living nature, forming it eventually to his will'. Carrel doubtless warmed to these challenges which would be regularly issued by Loeb at the Institute lunch table and hoped that the solutions would eventually trickle through to surgical practice. Also probably affecting Carrel's plans was Meltzer's earlier criticism that surgery was not a fundamental enough topic for a scientist. Carrel may have now wished to add to his creditable position in the world of basic biology and drop all the surgical studies for which he was so well suited. In putting surgical studies behind him, he made a mistake.

Carrel's Forgotten Grafts

Before the War, Carrel had used a successful animal kidney transplant model and he had firmly established that the slowly developing graft loss after some days (termed 'rejection' later) was the inevitable fate of homografts. Carrel heard of ways of dealing with graft rejection from his Institute colleague Murphy, namely using radiation or benzol. As described earlier, Flexner had enthused about this work before the War, saying 'it is needless to say that these results have fundamental bearing on the problem of transplantation'.[14]

Before the War, Carrel was apparently poised to make organ transplantation possible. He had a clear path ahead and a practical road

---

[14]The properties of benzol were well known in New York at the time; see Alwin M. Pappenheimer (1919) 'The effects of intravenous injections of dichloroethylsulphide in rabbits' *Proceedings of the Society for Experimental Biology and Medicine* 16: 92–3. The War had produced yet another effective immunosuppressant, since the soldiers surviving from the German use of poisonous mustard gas showed marked reduction in white cell count and difficulty resisting infection. It was 'an effect comparable to that of benzol', as one perceptive New York study of the poison noted.

map. Carrel could easily have tried the effect of benzol or radiation on kidney grafting in dogs, using the Institute's powerful radiation source used by Murphy for his wartime human 'immunopotentiation' studies.[15] Benzol (and also toluene and nitrogen mustard) were available and their actions, dosage and usage known. It was not unrealistic to consider human kidney transplantation. Carrel and the Institute were not isolated from the challenge of human chronic renal failure, then a major cause of death, and the Rockefeller Hospital even had a special clinic set up in 1924, run by Van Slyke, in which, using his new blood chemistry tests, he carefully followed patients with serious chronic kidney disease, eventually publishing a classic work on his studies.[16] In addition, Karl Landsteiner, who discovered the blood groups, joined the Institute in 1923, and had ideas about tissue 'groups'. Nor had the public forgotten about transplantation. Requests for organ grafts still came in regularly to Carrel's office. He even received a playful letter from Baltimore's Sir William Osler, now in Oxford, saying:

> Dear Sir,
>
> My kidneys are worn out, my heart is used up and my liver has struck work. How much will it cost to have ones put in at yr Institute?[17]

But Carrel made no moves to continue his transplant work, poignantly abandoning the technical side of surgery. In retrospect, it is clear that if he had studied the action of benzol on his organ grafts in animals, with a bit of luck in getting the right dosage and timing, he was within a few weeks of successfully prolonged organ grafts.[18]

---

[15] Thomas Schlich, *The Origins of Organ Transplantation: Surgery and Laboratory Science 1880–1930* (Rochester: University of Rochester Press, 2010): 223, puzzled at the 1920s failure to proceed with transplantation studies, wrongly invokes the dangers of radiation use.
[16] Van Slyke's Rockefeller Hospital study of kidney disease brought in the first tests of renal function; see his team's huge publication 'Observations on the courses of different types of Bright's disease' *Medicine* 9 (1930): 257–386.
[17] The letter was sent under Osler's *nom de plume* Egerton Yorik Davis; see Harvey Cushing, *The Life of Sir William Osler* (Oxford: Oxford University Press, 1925) vol. 2, 239–41.
[18] There is danger in making this irresistible retrospective judgement, as emphasised by

Nor did the surgeons take up his lead in organ grafting, and the topic was not revived until the emergence of transplantation studies in the 1950s.[19] A later historian said of Carrel's insights that 'the great surgeons dropped the ball', but they seemed uninterested in even receiving this helpful pass.[20] Surgical progress in the 1920s and 1930s slowed, and Sir Berkeley Moynihan was not alone in believing that 'the craft of surgery has in these days almost reached the end of its progress ... '[21] Looking for possible reasons for this apparently inexplicable hesitation, one obvious factor is that the European surgical research departments were weakened by the War. Added to this, the highly successful pre-war German science and technology was widely regarded with suspicion. It was equated with Prussian rigidity and narrow specialism; the Germans were seen as scientific giants but moral pygmies whose soul-less scientific success had contributed to their military aggression. Internal medicine in the 1920s showed a hesitation similar to the slow-down in surgery, and medical practice increasingly returned to neo-Hippocratic thinking, with treatment based on holistic ideas.[22]

Murphy Diverted

Carrel was not alone in moving away from successful pre-war accomplishments at the Institute. James B. Murphy, who had opened up the perceptive strategies for immunosuppression and immunopotentiation,

---

David Hackett's *Historian's Fallacies: Toward a Logic of Historical Thought* (New York: Harper Torchbooks, 1970). But the other error — Whig history — would try to deny that any gap existed in the evolution of organ transplantation.

[19] Radiation was used, without effect, in the 1950s revival of dog kidney transplantation studies. Radiation is a very effective immunosuppressant in most species, including man, and this misleading species variation concealed for a while that low doses of radiation would give survival of human kidney transplants.

[20] Julius H. Comroe, Jr. (1979) 'Who was Alexis who?' *Cardiovascular Diseases* 6: 251–70.

[21] Berkeley Moynihan, *The Advance of Medicine: the Romanes Lecture* (Oxford: Oxford University Press, 1932): 24.

[22] David Cantor (ed.), *Reinventing Hippocrates* (London: Ashgate, 2002), describes the inter-war revival in holistic medicine, as do Christopher Lawrence and George Weisz, *Greater than the Parts: Holism in Biomedicine 1920–1950* (Oxford: Oxford University Press, 1998).

did not return to work until September 1920, delayed by war service and illness. But Murphy also changed direction, moving away, or being moved away, from these now-famous studies on the lymphocyte.

Flexner may have had a role in this shift as part of his realignment of Institute projects after the war. Flexner sounded pleased when he announced that

> Murphy has gradually modified his studies in cancer to determine the effects of conditions other than those affecting lymphocytes ... [He] will publish his monograph on the lymphocyte and move on and leave the extension to others.[23]

No one did. Murphy finished his monograph slowly. It would become famous, but only four decades later. Instead, Murphy now took up worthy studies of accelerators and inhibitors of coal tar skin cancer induction. A Rockefeller colleague noted poignantly at the time that 'Dr. Murphy is insistent on the validity of his long series of experiments in establishing a significant role for the lymphocyte in tumour resistance [i.e. rejection]'. This hints that Murphy was reluctant to shift from the lymphocyte work, and that there was pressure on him from Flexner to change projects.[24]

Rous Changes Course

These moves by Carrel and Murphy away from organ transplantation are a historical puzzle, and the historian watches in perplexity as they failed to enter what seems in retrospect to be an open door. In the many changes of project by the Institute staff at this time, Peyton Rous' change of direction is stranger still. After the War, he moved, or was moved, out of his celebrated studies on his virus-induced, lymphocyte-controlled sarcoma,

---

[23] *Scientific Reports* (1926–27), vol. 11 1922–23 p. 252, FA 145, RUA RAC (note 1).
[24] Theophil M. Prudden's unpublished history of the Rockefeller Institute in 1924 sympathised with Murphy and noted that his lymphocyte work was left 'with legs dangling in the air'.

which later gained him a much-delayed Nobel Prize.[25] Rous now gave up this work and took up a surgical challenge, investigating the formation of bile and the origin of gallstones.[26] Rous went to work with enthusiasm on this project and from 1920 until 1925 published 19 papers on bile secretion, importantly showing that the gall bladder concentrated bile coming from the liver. Rous would return to cancer work in 1934 when he took up the study of the cancer-inducing Shope virus, and he gained his belated Nobel Prize for the virus work in 1966.

All Change

These were puzzling career 'musical chairs' shifts at the Institute. Murphy moved into cancer induction, Rous moved out of cancer induction and into surgical studies, and Carrel shunned any surgery to expand his cell culture work. But these talented men had no significant success in their new research fields in the 1920s. All three scientists eventually gained posthumous fame in the 1960s, but for their pre-World War I contributions. For the Institute generally, the 1920s and early 1930s were an undistinguished period, and the historians of the Institute are largely silent when dealing with this post-war period. In particular, accounts of Carrel's life all move quickly from his World War I Carrel–Dakin wound infection work to the more dramatic events of his career in the 1930s.[27] Flexner's role in these changes of project

---

[25] Eva Becsei-Kilborn (2010) 'Scientific discovery and scientific reputation: the reception of Peyton Rous' discovery of the chicken sarcoma virus' *Journal of the History of Biology* 43: 111–57.

[26] Flexner may have had a part in this odd choice of one new project by Rous. In Flexner's early work at Philadelphia, before moving to New York, he had made the important discovery that reflux of bile could cause pancreatitis: see S. Flexner (1900) 'Experimental pancreatitis' *Johns Hopkins Hospital Medical Reports* 9: 743–71, and he spoke to the Association of American Physicians on the same topic in Washington in May 1905: see their *Transactions* 20 (1905): 537–41.

[27] Flexner's policies as director after WWI are largely ignored in the otherwise helpful material on him in *Obituary Notices of Fellows Royal Society* 6 (1947): 408–26. Among the successes of this period, Phoebus Levene identified the sugars ribose and deoxyribose as components of DNA, but he did not think DNA carried genetic information.

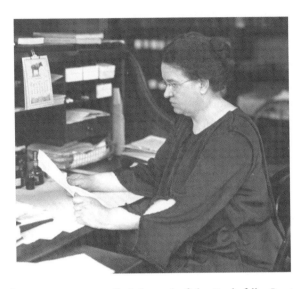

Florence Sabin's appointment signalled the end of the Rockefeller Institute's successful interest in the lymphocyte and tuberculosis. (*Courtesy of the National Library Medicine/ Smith College.*)

may have been significant. Though he generally left his scientists free to work on their own projects, from time to time he did suggest new directions for staff, and he had the power to do so.[28] In the early 1920s, with the new funds available, it seems he did intervene in this way, and his judgment must be questioned.

To add to this, one puzzling appointment at the Institute at this time was favoured by Flexner. In 1924, Flexner recruited the anatomist Florence R. Sabin (1871–1953) to be head of the Institute's new Department of Cellular Studies.[29] She, like Murphy, also worked on tuberculosis, and she saw no merit in Murphy's correct identification of

---

[28] Darwin H. Stapleton (ed.), *Creating a Tradition of Biomedical Research: Contributions to the History of The Rockefeller University* (New York: The Rockefeller University Press, 2004): 21–33.

[29] Florence Sabin was the first woman to be appointed to a senior post at the Institute. She was also the first woman to graduate from Johns Hopkins University and first female full professor in America.

the lymphocyte as the body's defence against that disease. Her own explanation was non-immunological and instead involved the monocyte cell. Even her approach was outdated; it relied entirely on reasoning from traditional microscopy of tuberculous tissues, ignoring the Institute's 'New Cytology' that studied the capabilities of living cells.[30] A Rockefeller insider wrote of Sabin's rigid views at the time:

> It is usually fatuous to draw sweeping conclusions from [microscopic] examination of such devitalized [formalin fixed] tissues. … when investigations like those of Murphy begin to throw new light on the problem, these high priests of morphology use these energies of their minions in the attempt to prove he was wrong.[31]

Surgical World

With Carrel's stimulating surgical influence gone, organ transplantation was off the clinical agenda in the 1920s, and some in the surgical world even resumed using homograft skin or gland slices grafted from one human to another. At this time, Emil Kocher's son loyally continued with his father's belief in thyroid homografting and claimed that half of their clinic's thyroid deficiency patients treated by homografts were cured or improved.[32] Other surgeons uncritically returned to attempts with human skin homografting, notably for burns, and convinced themselves that the grafts survived, unaware of the observational traps so clearly identified and warned against by Lexer, Ullmann and Carrel.[33]

In this disorderly decade, there was also a growth of transplant quackery. The French surgeon Serge Voronoff (1866–1951) now claimed success when using monkey testicle grafts to deal with the ills and

---

[30] See Carrel's paper on 'The New Cytology' *Science* 20, March 1931, 297–303. It carried a rebuke to those who shunned the new 'cellular biology' and used classical microscopy only.
[31] Paul de Kruif, *Our Medicine Men* (New York: The Century Co., 1922): 213–4.
[32] Albert Kocher (1923) 'The treatment of hypothyroidism by thyroid transplantation' *BMJ*, 29 September, 561–2.
[33] This self-deception when claiming success with gland and skin homografting is analysed in David Hamilton, *The Monkey Gland Affair* (London: Chatto & Windus, 1986).

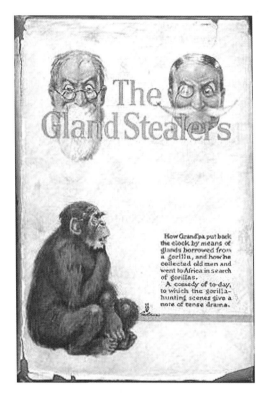

The 1920s confusion about graft rejection encouraged human grafting with monkey tissue. This met satire in Bertram Gayton's 1922 novel.

decreasing potency of senior human males. He made a high-public-profile visit to New York in July 1920, claiming in the *New York Times* to have worked with Carrel. Carrel promptly and wisely denied the link, but the newspaper grumbled that America was now lagging behind Europe in gland grafting. Adding to this anarchic world of transplantation came the claims of Theodore Koppányi, a refugee from Vienna.[34] He found work in Chicago's Hull Physiological Laboratory, Carrel's former location, now

---

[34] Koppányi moved to Syracuse University and then to Cornell Medical College in 1930 as a pharmacologist. In his popular work *Conquest of Life* (New York: D. Appleton and Company, 1930) he predicted routine eye and ovary transplants. His book was one of the Scientific Book Club's 'Book-of-the-Month' picks that year.

headed by Anton J. Carlson, and Koppányi carried out whole eye homografting in rats, simply inserting and fixing the detached donor eye in the empty socket. After a popular account of his improbable claims appeared in *Scientific American*, the press lionised him as the 'juvenile phenomenon of the scientific world — a *wunderkind* still only 23 years old'. Doubts about his work were reinforced when news came from Vienna detailing earlier allegations of scientific misconduct against the Austrian.[35]

Carrel must have thought the world of organ transplant studies had gone mad in the 1920s, but he made no comment on this bad science. But others did so, and Waro Nakahara, working in Murphy's unit at the Rockefeller Institute, attacked transplant quackery in the widely read *The American Mercury* magazine. Perhaps prompted or assisted by Carrel, Nakahara reaffirmed Carrel's view that homografts always rejected. But no one was listening.[36]

The 'Old Strain' Cell Line

Carrel's 'immortal' chicken heart cells had survived the War, even though the tiny disc of cells, growing in hanging drops of culture fluid on cover slips, required subculture every second day. Ebeling was responsible for sustaining the cells during Carrel's wartime absence, but Ebeling was often absent through illness or his medical studies and the tricky work of sub-culturing the tiny growths was left in the hands of the technicians.

Public interest in the immortal cells revived when an illustrated article appeared in *Cosmopolitan* magazine on 20 September 1920, entitled 'Must we grow old?' In 1922, Ebeling encouraged further journalistic interest when he gave a vivid description of the cells' vitality in the *Journal of Experimental Medicine*, saying that the expanding disc of cells doubled in size every 48 hours and had to be trimmed regularly. Without this restraint, he added, if all the culture tissue had been kept, 'today their

---

[35] See Joseph Imre (1924) 'Transplanting the eye' *JAMA* 83: 1097, and the rebuttal from Carlson and Koppányi is in *JAMA*, 11 October (1924): 1185–6.
[36] Waro Nakahara (1925) 'Tissue transplantation: real and bogus' *American Mercury* 17: 456–7. Edited by H.L. Mencken, this magazine had a reputation for good science and exposing fraud.

mass would be very much larger than the sun'.[37] The New York newspapers believed his calculations, and since Ebeling gave the origin of the cell line as 17 Jan 1914, the press thereafter celebrated this January birthday. Journalists also described how a group of young female laboratory assistants tended and guarded the frail cell line, adding to the mystique surrounding Carrel's laboratory. Often omitted was the less exciting detail that the cells were no longer the beating heart cells of the original growth, but were ordinary connective tissue fibroblasts.

Senescence

If cells are immortal, as Carrel's cultures suggested, then it followed that aging must be due to other, non-cellular influences, notably something in the body fluids. Carrel was quick to support this new paradigm that a blood deficiency limited human life span, but he was open-minded on what non-cellular factor was involved. He backed up the blood-deficiency theory with claims that in his cultures, cells grew better in young plasma than in older plasma.

This 'humoral' view of aging now became central to gerontology — the study of aging — starting with Raymond Pearl's important text of 1922, *The Biology of Death*, which was entirely based on the consequences that followed the existence of Carrel's immortal cells. Carrel's work also gave comfort to the gland-grafters like Serge Voronoff and the idea that decline in circulating hormones was important in explaining senescence. Their mantra was — 'you are only as old as your glands'.[38]

Carrel regularly sub-cultured his cells into fresh media to lengthen their life, and this appealed to others who thought that disease, decay and old age were not caused by a deficiency but that the body tissues were being poisoned by a build up of toxins of some kind. The London surgeon Sir Arbuthnot Lane, who, as noted earlier, had visited Carrel, still took this view and believed that accumulation of life-shortening poisons could come from the colon; he took appropriate surgical steps. Carrel had earlier taken

---

[37] Albert H. Ebeling (1922) 'A ten year old strain of fibroblasts' *JEM* 35: 755–9. Flexner suggested privately to Ebeling that his calculations may have been faulty.
[38] For an account of Voronoff's gland-grafting, see Hamilton, *Monkey Gland* (note 33).

out much of an old dog's blood, removed the serum and replaced only the cells, and claimed that the dog's decline was reversed. Flexner for once was sceptical.[39]

Some Concerns

The long-lived 'old strain' cell culture was not given away to others to study. Plenty of the exuberant culture was discarded, yet his colleagues and critics did not apparently ask for, or receive, a gift of the cells. To have a robust standard cell line, always available in the laboratory, would be a hugely attractive asset. The private and unwritten explanation was that Carrel had been lucky in some way or it was a product of Carrel's skills and resources, particularly the obsessional attention to detail in avoiding infection and in the tricky, labour-intensive transfer of tissue from one hanging drop to another by his staff. Nor did anyone else create a similarly robust 'eternal' cell line of their own by following his lead.[40]

Culture Projects

With his expanded staff, Carrel could carry out a large number of cultures, attempting to grow every variety of normal or abnormal cell, in all conditions of culture. Bold hypotheses were tested, but there was also much deliberate random experimentation in the hope of serendipitous discovery. In his simple test system, all influences, chemical or physical, in high enough dose or concentration, would enhance or inhibit growth of his cells. The problem was knowing the significance of any such findings. This work occupied him for most of the 1920s. He was still ambitious and was characteristically productive, authoring many substantial publications each year, plus many short reports, two-thirds of

---

[39] Claims for rejuvenation by transfusing young blood still appear regularly in fringe scientific work; earlier, Alexander Bogdanov (1873–1928) was the most celebrated advocate of this strategy.

[40] J.A. Witkowski (1979) 'Alexis Carrel and the mysticism of tissue culture' *Medical History* 23: 279–96.

which were in French journals. But his achievements in the 1920s were only modest, and are largely forgotten, and there were a number of claims which could not be confirmed. His successes included improving tissue culture techniques and working towards improving the artificial solutions used in culture work, hoping to obtain culture of cells without the necessity of the added mysterious chicken embryo 'soup'. He made cine-microscopy films of living cells, and he imaginatively made the first attempts to grow viruses in his cultured cells. Less convincingly, he claimed to have created malignant cells in culture, and also to have understood the nature of the malignant cell. He felt he could turn one cell type into another, hinting at stem cell technology to come. In tackling the entrancing challenge of how cells communicate with each other, he probably did identify the presence of what are now known as cytokines.[41]

His Projects in Detail

On the technical side, he improved on the traditional hanging drop culture method first with a larger chamber based on the 'Gabritschewski box', but

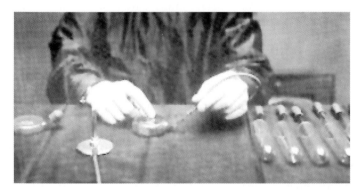

Carrel's improved tissue culture flask avoided entry of infection, but detailed microscopy was not possible. (*Courtesy of the Rockefeller University Archives.*)

---

[41] Malinin's biography has only eight pages on Carrel's contributions in the 1920s and Edwards' book has only two; Corner's history of the Institute is silent on Carrel's work in this decade.

in 1923 he successfully introduced new flat-bottomed culture flasks, his series of D-flasks, made of sterilisable Pyrex glass. Their greater volume of fluid allowed for a longer period of incubation without changing the medium, but they did not allow higher power microscopy. They had a side port that could be flamed during change of contents, reducing the chance of infection, and the new flasks gave better quantification of growth. Even so, the tissue culturists of the 1920s were still working awkwardly with clumps of outgrowing cells, and relying on measurement of clump size was risky, since it depended on not only new growth but also outward migration. It was still not until 1937 that the enzyme trypsin was found to liberate the cells and give the now-familiar dispersed culture of separate cells spreading in a monolayer. Curiously, Carrel had studied trypsin in his World War I wound healing experiments in France, poignantly missing the great benefit of its use in tissue culture. Always interested in photography from his contact with the Lumière brothers in Lyon, Carrel heard in 1913 that Levatidi at the Pasteur Institute in Paris had managed to make films of cells in culture, using time-lapse photography. Carrel visited the Paris laboratory and on return used a talented local New York photographer, Alesandro Fabbri, to make similar films. On Fabbri's death in 1923, Heinz (or Heim) Rosenberger, the Institute's instrument maker, a former German aerial photographer in World War I, continued the work, and Carrel produced his own cine films of cells and their movements. These became well known, and there were regular requests to borrow them to use for teaching or study. They were on display at the important Congressional hearing on the Ransdell Bill in 1930, which established the National Institutes of Health. However, again Carrel had some bad luck, since his pioneering films failed to show that cell membranes could form little vesicles to capture outside matter and take it into the cell. The tissue culture group at Johns Hopkins first noticed this phenomenon of pinocytosis in 1929.[42]

---

[42] The sustained interest in tissue culture at Baltimore is described in A. McGehee Harvey (1975) 'Johns Hopkins — the birthplace of tissue culture: the story of Ross G. Harrison, Warren H. Lewis and George O. Gey' *The Johns Hopkins Medical Journal* 136: 142–9.

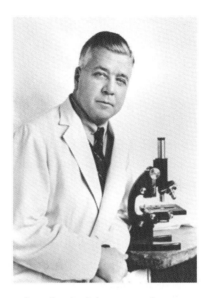

Tom Rivers, the 'father of virology', did some early joint work with Carrel at the Institute. (*Courtesy of the Rockefeller University Archives.*)

The role of viruses in human disease was increasingly of importance to the Institute, and Flexner had a continuing interest in poliomyelitis and its prevention. The study of viruses could only prosper when they could be grown outside the body, as was routinely possible with most bacteria. Only when large quantities of the virus were grown could a vaccine be made, but obtaining success in cultivating viruses was proving to be elusive. Carrel imaginatively added viruses to his tissue cultures in the hope that the cells would assist viral growth, and he obtained short-term growth of some viruses, notably that of horse vesicular stomatitis and the Rous sarcoma virus.[43] He was on the right track. Tom (Thomas) Rivers (1888–1962) arrived at the Rockefeller Hospital in 1922 and imaginatively used Carrel's tissue culture methods to grow vaccinia virus, taking another important step on the long road to later success, particularly with the polio virus. Rivers was editor in 1923 of the multi-author book *Filterable Viruses*, and it became the standard work on this

---

[43] Alexis Carrel (1926) 'Some conditions of the reproduction *in vitro* of the Rous virus' *JEM* 43: 647–68 and A. Carrel, P.K. Olitsky and P.H. Long (1928) 'Multiplication du virus de la stomatite vésiculaire du cheval dans des cultures de tissus' *CRSB* 98: 827–8.

new field. Carrel contributed a chapter on tissue culture of viruses which still reads well, almost prophetically, since he suggested that cultured cells might provide 'industrial production' of virus.[44]

Other Studies and the Trephones

Carrel was mistakenly convinced for a while that he could 'type' monocytes into groups, like red cells, and that culture of these cells in serum from another individual would change the 'type' of the monocyte into that of the serum donor.[45] He was probably wrong again in his bold claims to have cultivated lymphocytes long-term and to be able to turn fibroblasts into monocytes.[46]

However, among this group of these forgotten projects, he had one remarkable success, still hardly noticed. He rightly felt that the tissue cells must communicate locally with each other, not only in normal life, but particularly during tissue repair. He set about trying to identify and isolate these necessary signalling agents from the fluids of his cultures. It seems he did detect what he was looking for. In 1923, he announced that he had identified 'leukocyte secretions', growth-promoting substances made by white blood cells in culture, which when added to other cultures, stimulated cell division. Encouraged, he called these extracts 'trephones'. He wrote:

> Leucocytes may be regarded as unicellular glands, which set free their
> secretion in the circulation. … Lymphocytes remain throughout life as
> a store of embryonic growth promoting substances or trephones, which

---

[44] See Alexis Carrel 'Tissue cultures in the study of viruses' in Thomas M. Rivers (ed.) *Filterable Viruses* (London: Baillière Tindall & Cox, 1928) 97–112. Rivers, a prickly and pugnacious colleague, later unfairly grumbled about the quality of Carrel's chapter, which he said he had requested 'only because of Carrel's celebrity' — see Tom M. Rivers, *Reflections on a Life in Medicine and Science* (Cambridge: MIT Press, 1967) and their paper 'La fabrication du vaccin in vitro' *CRSB* 96 (1927): 848–50.

[45] Scientific Reports of the Laboratories Presented to the Corporation and to the Board of Scientific Directors, FA 145, RU RG 439, vol. 16 p. 6, RUA RAC (note 1).

[46] Alexis Carrel (1925) 'The mechanism of the formation of sarcoma' *JAMA* 84: 157. See also Carrel in *Annals Surgery* 82: 1–13; he quickly dropped these claims to have produced malignant cells.

may cause a resumption of cell activity when it is needed.[47]

It is possible that Carrel had revealed the group of substances now called cytokines, which were regularly detected from the 1950s. Now much studied, they are intercellular cell-signalling proteins, which include interleukins, chemokines, lymphokines and interferons.[48]

Into Cancer

Carrel ceased work on the trephones in 1924 and moved into cancer studies instead. His first view was that cancer was caused by a virus and that cancer cells in turn emitted the cancer-causing virus.[49] He claimed to have created cancer cells when he reported that the Rous virus would induce malignancy in his tissue culture cells; he was instead observing the diagnostic cytopathic effect of a virus.[50] His explanation of malignancy later changed to proposing that the cancer cell had a greater ability to use the tissue constituents around them and hence multiply in an uncontrolled way. This concept had little impact.[51] However, his work had some celebrity at the time, and in 1931 he was awarded the Sofie A. Nordhoff-Jung Cancer Prize for his 1920s work, nominated by a distinguished panel of German scientists.[52] Previous winners included the chemist Otto

---

[47] Alexis Carrel (1923) 'Leucocyte secretions' *Proceedings of the National Academy of Sciences* 9: 54–8 and *JEM* 36: 645–59. Fischer from Copenhagen worked for one year with Carrel from 1921–22. Fischer set up his own lab, wrote a text, *Tissue Culture* (1925), and made a growth-stimulating extract from calf embryos, marketed by Messrs Lundbeck of Copenhagen as 'Epicutan'. Other users were less impressed with it.

[48] Commendably, Stephen S. Hall in his *Commotion in the Blood* (New York: Henry Holt, 1997): 129, names Carrel as the 'patron saint of cytokines'.

[49] Alexis Carrel (1925) 'Mechanism of the formation and growth of malignant tumours' *Annals of Surgery* 82: 1–13.

[50] Alexis Carrel (1925) 'Essential characteristics of a malignant cell' *JAMA* 84: 157–8.

[51] Alexis Carrel (1929) 'The nutritional properties of malignant cells' *Proceedings of the American Philosophical Society* 68: 129–32.

[52] 'Dr. Carrel Honoured For Cancer Studies' *NYT*, 20 and 29 March 1931. Sofie Nordhoff-Jung, widow of the Washington German-born associate professor of gynaecology at Georgetown University, funded the Prize.

Warburg (1883–1970), Nobel Prize winner in 1931, and Katsusaburo Yamagiwa (1863–1930), originator of the 'chronic irritation' explanation of cancer. The award and $1,000 were presented at a ceremony in Washington, with French and German diplomats in attendance. Ironically, by this time, Carrel had moved away from tissue culture studies.

Carrel's work in the later 1920s will be described later. But first, his life outside the laboratory at this time can be looked at.

CHAPTER ELEVEN

Life in the 1920s

Carrel and Mme Carrel had returned to New York after the War. Before the War, she had lived in the city only for a short time in 1914 before they left for France, and she now had the prospect of living far from France. At first, all seemed well, and Mme Carrel worked productively with him as a volunteer, bringing in skills from her work in Tuffier's surgical laboratory in Paris. She briefly took up Carrel's old interest in corneal homografting, with one initial success, but, perhaps surprisingly, this work was not carried through. Mme Carrel's name is included in the reports of some of the other projects and publications, including an update on the dogs surviving from his pre-WWI cardiac surgery, which showed no long-term deterioration. She also published with du Noüy in 1921 on the last of the healing studies carried out in Compiégne.

Mme Carrel had some bouts of ill health. Carrel described one of her problems as 'pleurisy', which he said followed the bombing at his Paris hospital, but in a family letter in 1920 he was also concerned about her 'mental and emotional equilibrium'. These may have been the alarming, short-lived 'turns', noticed by visitors later, but she seemed vigorously well otherwise and was to have a long life. She and her husband took little part in the social life in New York, declining most invitations although, probably because of his military interest, they did go to a 'brillant dîner chez Miss Cornelius Vanderbilt avec le Général Pershing et tout le haut monde de New York'.[1]

---

[1] Alain Drouard, *Alexis Carrel (1873–1944): De la mémoire à l'histoire* (Paris: Éditions L'Harmattan, 1995): 112.

Living in New York, they did not use his apartment, but stayed first at the Blackstone Hotel, paying $220 a month, then at the fashionable Garden City Hotel in Long Island outside the city. They made moves to purchase a home and nearly took one in Long Island with 12 rooms and 20 acres of land. They returned to France in summer, as before, visiting her mother, now in her 80s, in Anjou in Brittany and meeting up with his family in Lyon. When in Lyon, Carrel would consult with his brother and adjust his investment in securities and land.[2] Mme Carrel also had an apartment in central Paris in the Place de la Tour-Maubourgh.

The Island

However, each autumn, Mme Carrel was increasingly reluctant to return to New York, and it was soon clear that New York life did not suit her. By 1922, she decided to remain in France throughout the year. With this decision, in 1923, never short of money, Carrel bought an island on the northern coast of Brittany, reasonably close to his wife's mother's chateau home to the south. The island of Saint-Gildas, for which he paid

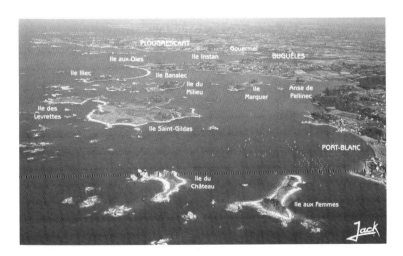

In 1923, Carrel purchased the French island of Saint-Gildas, one of a group close to the Brittany shore.

---

[2] Drouard, *Carrel* (note 1): 42.

$16,000, is one in a complex archipelago close to the shore, exposed to the Atlantic's 40-foot tides and storms. To reach the mainland nearby they used a rowing boat, and they kept a car in the nearby coastal village of Port Blanc. The island had a two-story house, a walled garden, an ancient 9th century chapel and an orchard, and the rest of the island was a small farm. The farmer and his wife acted as caretakers for the Carrels, and Mme Carrel now divided her time between the island, her elderly mother's house, and Paris. In summer, when he returned from New York, the island also became Carrel's base. It was an arrangement which suited them both; they shared many interests and were supportive of each other, particularly during the difficult times later. Mme Carrel's son, now a teenager, was at an international school near Paris. He married in 1929, at age 21, and moved to Argentina to work on his father-in-law's ranch.

New York Life

In New York, Carrel reverted to a bachelor life, and at first rented a small apartment close to the Institute, later moving uptown in the 1930s to a penthouse at 56 East 89th Street which had a terrace and a view of Central Park to the west. Carrel bought another car in February 1922 for $2,043 but was an erratic driver and used it little, though garaging it in New York required $32 per month. For his annual summer spell in France, there were many liners on the transatlantic route available and a return journey cost about $450. During his summer absence, his clothes went into cold storage to defeat the problem of moths which appeared in the New York summer heat, and while abroad, he cancelled the apartment's services and the delivery of milk and cream.

Newspaper pictures taken of Carrel departing for Europe show him smartly dressed with a flower in his buttonhole. In winter in New York he used large gauntlets and wore a jacket with a fashionable wallaby fur collar. Carrel used his membership at New York's The Century Association (annual dues of $80) for dinner about twice a week, usually having pork chops or minute steak (well done), plus baked apple or peaches and cream. The club's artistic and academic membership included scientists

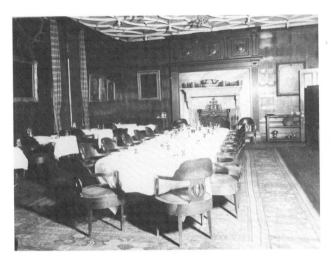

Carrel was a member of The Century Association club and might dine at their communal table. (*Courtesy of the Century Association.*)

from the Rockefeller Institute, and senior staff from the Rockefeller Foundation and Columbia University. Henry James the philosopher, John Dewey the educationalist and Dwight Morrow, diplomat and politician, were members, as was the geneticist and Nobel Prize winner Thomas Hunt Morgan before he moved to the West Coast. Another Prize-winner, Robert A. Millikan, was a country member, as was Harvey Cushing. Carrel belonged to the Riding Academy operating from Central Park West and used the Fencing Club until the mid-1920s. A lawyer friend had arranged for Carrel to join the fashionable Piping Rock Country Club, and encouraged him to do more horse riding at the club, adding the suggestion that Carrel play golf, though he 'expected it to be resisted'. Carrel entertained guests at The Century Association or at a local French restaurant. He had no obvious involvement in the city's art or music world, although he talked much about culture in his later writings. Carrel deplored risqué novels and avoided the cinema, confessing that he occasionally 'shamefully' saw a movie. One painter he admired was W. Langdon Kihn (1898–1957), who specialised in naturalist images of North American Indians. Carrel did not smoke, and although he might have a pre-dinner cocktail when at his club, he deplored the heavy drinking he witnessed on his transatlantic voyages. Now living alone in

New York, he joined a group of male friends who met together regularly, but otherwise he avoided social life as much as possible. He was always charming to women and wrote to one:

> The reason I left before the speeches [at the American Institute dinner] was that after listening to your illuminating conversation, I felt I did not need to hear the addresses.

In his religious life, he attended mass irregularly in New York but contributed money to local Catholic churches. He subscribed to the *Catholic Digest* and *Our Sunday Visitor*, the widely selling popular Christian magazines of the time, but his own religious views were not orthodox, as was clear in his writings later. When living on his island, since his wife was a devout Catholic, they attended mass together on the mainland.

The Paranormal

Carrel was attracted to mysticism and would soon consider that 'mysticism plus science' could give a description of the whole person. His colleagues often described him as a 'mystic', but there is no description of him regularly practising withdrawal or contemplation. Carrel took physiognomy seriously, and studied strangers and visitors intently at a first meeting, believing that mental capacity and personality were revealed in the face via the nerves from the brain. Carrel was a believer, as was his wife, in clairvoyance (the ability to perceive remote events) and in telepathy (transmission of thought), and in other related psychic powers.[3] Belief in such 'parapsychology' was widespread at this time, and was a fashionable pursuit; it was the golden age of the séances, which 'asked incredulity to dinner'. Serious-minded societies were growing up, particularly in Europe, to study the occult, and this attachment to psychic phenomena was prominent in France at the time. The philosopher Henri Bergson had

---

[3] James D. Newton, *Uncommon Friends: Life With Thomas Edison, Henry Ford, Harvey Firestone, Alexis Carrel and Charles Lindbergh* (New York: Harvest Books, 1989): 134 has an account of Mme Carrel's alleged powers, as has Anne Morrow Lindbergh in her diaries *The Flower and the Nettle* (New York: Harcourt Brace Jovanovich, 1976).

given his support, as did Charles Richet, the 1912 Nobel Prize-winning immunologist. The British Society for Psychical Research had distinguished adherents, notably Arthur Conan Doyle, and the London physicists Sir Oliver Lodge and Sir William Crookes. Carrel was therefore in good company, and he claimed when attending Paris séances with his wife that he studied the proceedings with the necessary scientific detachment. He failed to impress one acquaintance, Max Thorek, the Chicago surgeon, who was critical of Carrel's beliefs, and Thorek recalled that

> I had an impression that when I talked with Alexis Carrel that in spite of his professed deep devotion to mysticism, he was one of the wraith-chasers. Was his mystic philosophy more than a feeble defence of miracles, of clairvoyance, of psychic power? He tried to prove to me that he had good reason to believe in the miracles of Lourdes. A triangular bedsore had resisted all treatment. One day at the holy shrine had reduced the sore to half its size.[4]

Mme Carrel's interest in the paranormal led her to study a villager in France near their island who claimed to be able to see through screens.[5] Carrel took an interest and reported from his laboratory that he found people who could see light waves above and below normal frequencies, commenting however that these subjects 'were prone to serious nervous disorders'.[6] Believing that his wife had these gifts, when she worked in his laboratory he had tried to test and confirm her powers. He described in his reports to Flexner that she could detect light waves passing through opaque screens, and that he was searching for the wavelength of the radiation which came from her fingers.[7] Mme Carrel supported her husband's belief

---

[4] Max Thorek, *A Surgeon's World* (New York: Somerset Books, 1943): 398. See also Carrel to Flexner, 3 September 1909, Carrel (Alexis) papers, (1906–1957), box 2 folder 1, FA 231, Rockefeller University Archives, Rockefeller Archives Centre (RUA RAC).

[5] Carrel to Flexner, 4 August 1921, Flexner APS Papers, roll 21, FA 746, RUA RAC (note 4).

[6] This does not appear in any of his reports: but see Carrel to Clifford, 23 February 1928, box 39 folder 85, RUA RAC (note 4).

[7] Carrel to Gigou, 29 April 1917, box 39 folder 58, Alexis Carrel Papers, Georgetown University Library, Booth Family Center for Special Collections (GULBFC). There was a plan at this time, never fulfilled, to describe her powers in Charles Richet's journal *Revue de Metapsychique*.

that unexplained healing could occur, and she told of an experience when accompanying the sick from our home in Brittany to Lourdes, when she saw a baby's sight restored while she held it in her arms.

Pursuing this interest, in 1926 Carrel attended New York's Selwyn Theatre to see the performances by Rahman Bey, a celebrated Egyptian 'fakir'. With the support of the local Institute of Psychic Research, Bey demonstrated thought-reading and hypnotism, and also apparently entered into a comatose, cataleptic state during which he claimed his breathing and heartbeat ceased. Carrel was sceptical about Bey's act, but was to retain an interest in any account of Indian holy men's powers and their ability to enter trance-like states. About this time, Carrel became a supporter of J. B. Rhine, the Duke University parapsychologist.

Carrel Encountered

Carrel continued to have many visitors to his laboratories and had an impressive guest book on show. Any visitor would notice his two-colour eyes, and his monk-like shaven head. He had 'thin firm lips, tightly shut, almost stern, if it were not for an ever-lurking smile that illuminates his countenance' and 'an impression of youth, strength and power'. He leaned forward while standing and walked quickly. Friends compared him to a 'jaunty Maurice Chevalier figure who could on occasions be pleased with himself' or said he was 'like one of those little Italian abbés one meets in Rome'. Others noted 'réserve distante, and a 'peu d'égoïsme'.[8] A young staff member thought that Carrel had 'carefully preserved his French accent, which made him sound to me even more learned than he was ... I secretly practice a French accent'.[9] His intense, restless manner was a feature, suggesting 'inner force controlled by a hair-trigger'. At a first meeting with him, visitors were interrogated closely, then dazzled by his wide-ranging discourse and erudition. A journalist noted: 'Carrel delivers himself of his ideas. He does not arrange them. ... They press him, they

---

[8] These impressions are taken from many sources, including GULBFC, (note 7) box 38 folders 33 and 41, box 37 folder 8 and J.-J. Gillon 'Les aspects essentiels de l'oeuvre scientifique d'Alexis Carrel' *Le Concours Médical* vol. 73, 11 and 17 October 1951, 525–28.

[9] Paul de Kruif, *The Sweeping Wind* (New York: Harcourt, Brace and World, 1962): 17.

harass him.' Friends, though fond of him, could still find him impossible at times:

> I do not argue [with him], because Dr. Carrel makes all argument impossible. He does not say mildly or sympathetically "I think you don't understand, or I think you are mistaken." It is always "No, you are quite wrong about that." ... And there is nothing more to say.[10]

Those who understood his intense manner explained, with regret, that

> He used such sweeping statements to emphasise his points that only those who knew him well were able to draw the kernels of fact from the husk of fantasy. ... He could act with an abandon which laid him open to the thrusts of the enemies he tactlessly and fearlessly created.[11]

He might say that 'all surgeons are butchers'; 'the clinical ignorance of physicians today, is as great in France as in the United States'; the 'Scandinavians are a highly civilised people, what a shame they have lost the will to live'; and 'Nobody in New York is in sufficient condition to do best intellectual effort'. There were also Delphic and enigmatic views and aphorisms: 'Every institution which lasts has to be unbending, autocratic and intolerant.' One of his friends, who took a charitable view of his utterances, yet admired his insights, had an amusing assessment, saying that if 'Carrel is right 20% of the time, it is enough'.[12] Less supportive verdicts were that he was 'naïve' and 'a misanthrope' and 'childish'. The gossips in New York spread the tale of a doctor's encounter with Carrel on an Atlantic crossing:

> Dr. Carrel said his prayers dutifully every morning in the chapel at 6 a.m. and one night when he couldn't sleep, he and W. encountered one another. ... Carrel then put the question, 'Who do you think were

---

[10] Ann Morrow Lindbergh, *War Within and Without: Diaries and Letters of Anne Morrow Lindbergh 1939–1944* (New York: Harcourt Brace Jovanovich, 1980): 637.

[11] Lindbergh's 'Introduction' to Carrel's *Voyage to Lourdes* (New York: Harper & Brothers, 1950) has an assessment of Carrel which was accepted as fair by other friends of Carrel.

[12] Joyce Milton, *A Biography of Charles and Anne Morrow Lindbergh* (New York: Harper Collins, 1993): 266.

the three greatest men in the history of the world?' The doctor thought the question rather juvenile. ... So W. turned the tables, which was evidently what Dr. Carrel expected, and said 'who do you think were the three greatest men in history?' Without hesitation, or apology, Dr. Carrel replied, "Julius Caesar, Napoleon, and Mussolini."[13]

Carrel's views were delivered without humour, which would have softened the impression of dogmatism, and there was also a lack of insight. He could say without self-awareness that when 'a man becomes blinded by the idea that he is 'a big man' he is liable to make all sorts of utterances'.[14] When a British scientist's work and deeds appeared in the press, Carrel tut-tutted to Flexner, without any sense of irony, that 'It is most unfortunate that such methods are used by a scientist. ... the confidence of the public should not be played upon'.[15] This lack of insight also meant that his 'blunt indiscretion lost him allies' and that he had 'a special knack of insulting the wrong people at the wrong time'. These failings did not cause him regular problems since, within the Institute, he was well-established, independent and unassailable.

Probably the most important observation was that his many utterances often had ambiguity: massive certainties could soon be followed by opposing stances. His asides on scientific method and his aphorisms often contradict each other. Friends noted with concern that his 'shifting and opposing moods [meant] many would misinterpret the kind of person he really was'.[16] Others agreed and said that he was 'endowed with this incessant ambivalence ... he was constantly changing his views' and in particular that 'politics was a field in which he flew around with a dangerous innocence'.[17]

---

[13] 'Alexis Carrel: an Anecdote', Carrel (Alexis) papers (1906–1957), box 1 folder 13, FA 231, RUA RAC (note 4).

[14] For these sentiments see Carrel's *Man, the Unknown* (New York: Harper & Brothers, 1935): 46–7.

[15] Carrel to Flexner, 24 July 1925, Flexner Papers, American Philosophical Society microfilm, FA 746, roll 21, RUA RAC (note 4).

[16] Gros to Durkin, Alexis Carrel Papers, box 37 folder 8, GULBFC (note 7).

[17] See Gillon, *Les aspects* (note 8).

These are important insights. His many dramatic remarks and jibes were not necessarily his settled view, but were instead the whim of the moment, and he might soon contradict himself. This analysis explains much, and when he began to comment and write on the broader issues of the day in the 1930s, notably on European politics, this variety of confident but contradictory written and spoken opinions have left behind a wide range of material to choose from. It allowed both friendly and hostile commentators and biographers to produce evidence to support their contrasting verdicts. A French colleague noted these possible choices and perceptively warned future biographers about the 'terrible responsibility of those who would accurately and fairly interpret Carrel's thoughts'.[18]

The 'Philosophers'

On a transatlantic voyage in 1908, Carrel met a man who was to be a close, life-long friend. Frederic Coudert Jr. (1898–1972), a New York lawyer from a French émigré family, now headed the family firm founded in 1853. Dealing with French and Spanish immigrants at first, in 1879 they opened a Paris branch, as the first U.S. law firm to have an overseas office. Coudert was fluent in many European languages and following America's increasing involvement in international affairs, by the 1920s his firm had gained important international legal work from the U.S. Government. After World War I, the French embassy in New York employed Coudert as an advisor, and his other clients also included exiled Russian czarist supporters in various parts of the world. He was a Republican politician later. Coudert and Carrel enjoyed each other's company and shared many views and attitudes; Coudert acted as Carrel's lawyer and named his son Alexis Carrel Coudert.

Coudert had many contacts, notably at nearby Columbia University, and entertained regularly at his home. Carrel and another guest, Father Cornelius Clifford (1859–1938), a New Jersey priest and Columbia lecturer, started to join the Coudert family meals from about 1912.

---

[18] Gros to Durkin, box 98 folder 50, GULBFC (note 7).

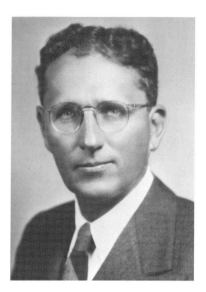

Frederic Coudert's friendship with Carrel led to the formation of an evening discussion group, dubbed 'The Philosophers'. (*Courtesy of the U.S. House of Representatives Archives.*)

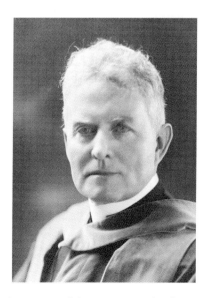

Father Clifford, a parish priest and lecturer at Columbia University, was a regular attendee at Coudert's evening meetings. (*Courtesy of the Century Association.*)

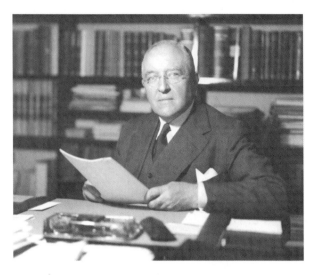

Boris Bakhmeteff, professor of engineering at Columbia University. (*Courtesy of Columbia University Library.*)

Clifford, when studying earlier in Britain at Campion Hall, Oxford, fell under the influence of George Tyrrell, the Catholic moderniser, who sought to reconcile science and religion, but, as a result, the Jesuits expelled him.[19] On his return to America he was given only a small parish in New Jersey. But Clifford had friends at Columbia University and they appointed him as a part-time lecturer in mediaeval theology. He was a member at The Century Association and enjoyed jousting with Carrel on theological matters, including reform of the Catholic Church. Clifford's many letters to Carrel, who he called 'Magister Humanissime', were full of self-deprecating put-downs and Latin and Greek tags.[20] The three men, Coudert, Clifford and Carrel, were soon close, enjoying each other's

---

[19] Clifford's impact at Oxford is described in William S. Abell, *Laughter and the Love of Friends: Reminiscences of the Distinguished English Priest and Philosopher Martin Cyril D'Arcy* (Westminster, Maryland, 1991): 73–5. There is a portrait of him at Oxford but the annual Cornelius Clifford Dinner has lapsed.

[20] Clifford's only publications are *Introibo: A Series of Detached Readings on the Entrance Versicles of the Ecclesiastical Year* (New York: The Catholic Library Association, 1904, reprinted 2008 and 2012), and *The Burden of Time: Essays in Suggestion* (New York: The Catholic Library Association, 1904, reprinted 2010 and 2012).

company, and the inner group expanded to four later when Boris Alexandrovich Bakhmeteff (1880–1951) joined in regularly. Bakhmeteff, an engineer born in Russia, was appointed by the post-revolution Russian Provisional Government as their ambassador to America in 1917. However, out of sympathy with the political events which followed, and dismissed as ambassador, he never returned to Russia, and Columbia University eventually appointed him as their professor of engineering.

In the 1920s, others were brought in, often also members of The Century Association or with Columbia University links, and it evolved into a group which might meet every two weeks over the winter on Tuesday evenings for dinner and discussion at Coudert's house at East 124th Street and 5th Avenue. At these 'hebdomadel suppers' as Clifford called them, he hoped that 'the origins of life will be discussed thoroughly, but perhaps not wholly solved'.[21] One of the early members, the jurist Benjamin N. Cardozo (1870–1938), who soon moved to Washington and was later appointed to the Supreme Court, christened the group as the 'The Philosophers' and the name stuck; the meetings were to continue until the late 1930s.[22] The numbers and personnel varied over the years, but there were usually about eight attendees. Visitors from Europe might join in as guests.[23]

Those attending fairly regularly had differing backgrounds. One was Nicholas Murray Butler (1862–1947), president of Columbia University,[24]

---

[21] Clifford's many letters to Carrel are in box 40 folio 19, Alexis Carrel Papers, box 42 folder 28, GULBFC (note 7).

[22] Some of the 'Philosophers' are listed in Andrew L. Kaufmann, *Cardozo* (Cambridge: Harvard University Press, 1998) p. 148, Virginia K. Veenswijk: *Coudert Brothers* (New York: Dutton, 1994): 218 and also *The Reminiscences of Frederic René Coudert*, 1949, 1950, Columbia University Oral History Research Office 1972, NXCP87-A43, Mss. Fiche 6: 112–15.

[23] Occasional guests included Henri Bergson, who held the chair of Modern Philosophy at the College de France in Paris; he spent time at Columbia University during WWI and after.

[24] Nicholas Butler, Nobel Peace Prize winner in 1931, also had a Saturday lunch group called the 'Sage and Occasional Thinkers', which Coudert joined regularly. For a hostile contemporary assessment of Butler, see Dorothy D. Bromley 'Nicholas Murray Butler: portrait of a reactionary' *The American Mercury*, March 1935, 268–98.

and joining in occasionally was Alfred Noyes (1880–1958), the lecturer at Princeton and a poet in the 'Romantic' tradition.[25] Columbia's philosopher Frederick Woodbridge (1867–1940)[26] might attend, and he was, with Dewey, one of the 'American Naturalists' who revived interest in Aristotle. Spenser Nichols, John W. Davis the former Democratic Solicitor General, George L. Burr (1857–1938) and Foster Kennedy (1884–1952) the Irish-born Cornell University professor of neurology and ardent eugenicist, came occasionally.[27]

Attitudes and Interests

The group discussion was robust and suited Carrel's assertive discourse. The members were deeply interested in current affairs, early literature and philosophy, and there would be a sympathetic hearing for anti-materialist thought. Those, like Carrel, who believed in the paranormal, would not be ridiculed, and religious scepticism would not be prominent. Cardozo was the only Jew, and many of the others, perhaps all, were Roman Catholics. In politics, the Republican Party was favoured, and they were hostile to Roosevelt's 'New Deal' interventionist policies from 1932 to deal with the Depression. The group's interests were strikingly international. Coudert and Carrel were particularly well informed on the unstable and complex events in France in these interwar years. Bakhmeteff had his insider's authority on Soviet politics and communism, and had insight into the developing European struggle between fascism and communism. If a choice had to be made, fascism was favoured by many at the time, and when Butler attended the gatherings in the mid-1930s, his pro-German sympathies and admiration for Mussolini would be noticed. Carrel also

[25] Alfred Noyes, an anti-war activist who converted to Catholicism in the 1920s, published *The Unknown God!* in 1934.
[26] Frederick Woodbridge, an anti-reductionist who rejected mind–nature dualism, worked at Columbia University from 1902, served as Dean of the Faculty of Philosophy from 1912–29 and founded the *Journal of Philosophy* in 1904.
[27] Foster Kennedy as late as 1942 advocated euthanasia of feeble-minded children; see F. Kennedy (1942) 'The problem of social control of the congenital defective: education, sterilization, euthanasia' *American Journal of Psychiatry* 99: 13–16.

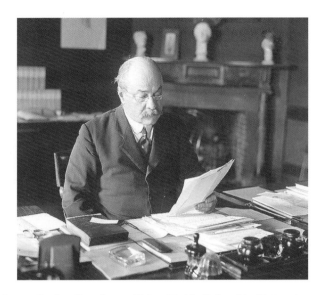

Nicholas Murray Butler, President of New York's Columbia University, attended the 'Philosophers' meetings occasionally and for a while shared Carrel's admiration for Mussolini's Italy. (*Wikipedia*)

admired Mussolini's firm leadership at the time, and Coudert gave him a friendly warning in one of his many personal letters:

> I am afraid that with an iron despotism, even under such a great man as Mussolini, a man of your free thinking and critical mind would be the first to find himself imprisoned, exiled or executed. This is a high price to pay for having the railroads run on time.[28]

The group were split on a major issue. Some, like Carrel, were 'declinists' who believed that the Western nations were in serious decline; others in the group were less sure.

Somehow the activities of 'The Philosophers' were leaked to the newspapers, and in 1923 their gatherings were the theme of a satirical novel *The Talkers* by Robert W. Chambers, a fellow-member of The Century Association.[29] He portrayed a 'Fireside Club' which favoured

---

[28] Coudert to Carrel, 15 August 1934, box 97 folder 10, GULBFC (note 7).
[29] Robert W. Chambers (1865–1933) used science-fiction themes in his historical and romance novels.

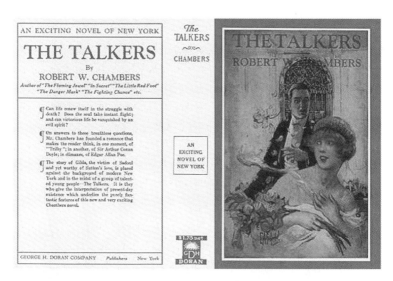

Carrel's group of 'Philosophers' were gently satirised in Robert Chambers' 1923 novel.

'talk not work'. In the novel, Carrel, aka 'Pockman', the miracle-working surgeon, has a central role, since he can revive the dead by grafting the 'nymphalic' gland. The action of the novel includes a visit to Pockman's laboratory, where gifted subjects undergo psychic testing.

Carrel and France

In spite of his World War I clashes with the Paris surgeons and his frequent complaints about France and the French, Carrel never cut himself off from the nation of his birth. He retained his French citizenship and instead had a visa for 'permanent residence' in America. He appointed Frenchmen to his staff at the Institute, and remarkably the majority of his publications in the 1920s were still in French journals. On his Christmas card list at this time, one third were French recipients, including Pasteur Vallery-Radot, soon to be head of the Pasteur Institute.

Carrel's extended three month summer break in Europe was based on his island in France, from where he travelled to visit scientists and hospitals. He and his wife supported some French organisations and attended occasional meetings, and he was beginning to take an interest in the unsettled world of French politics. He had hopes for his nation, taking the view that France had latent greatness which suitable policies could reveal. Carrel, as a Frenchman, had no particular admiration for Germany at this time and refused to take into his lab a 'too nationalistic' young German scientist, who went instead to Tom Rivers' new virus lab.[30] In the mid-1920s he applauded a new 'renewal' effort in French politics, namely the Fédération des Républicains Rénovateurs. He also saw merit in the volatility of French politics and the occasional emergence of new Republics. In 1920, he remarked with pride: 'I suppose France will be, as it always has been, the experimental field of the world for the new forms of democratic government.'[31]

At other times, he could behave towards France with pettiness, as he had done at the time of his Nobel Prize. In 1920, Marie Curie came by invitation to America, to assist American fund-raising for her Marie Curie Radium Fund. Carrel declined to lend his name to the drive, and did not attend the White House event at which President Harding presented one gram of the precious material to Marie Curie. Carrel wrote:

> I regret I cannot help and it is out of the question for the U.S. to help for this. A good many men in industrial France made a great deal of money during the war and it is the duty of these Frenchmen to give to the hospitals and to the poor the radium they need.

He added ungraciously that Curie was 'ugly'.[32]

Academic Activities

Carrel, now in his mid-50s, was content with his position at the Institute and the considerable facilities given to him. Moreover, he had the full confidence and admiration of his director, and had no desire to move. But Carrel had one worldly ambition left and explains his regular publication

---

[30] Saul Benison, *Tom Rivers — Reflections on a Life in Medicine and Science* (Cambridge, Massachusetts Institute of Technology, 1967): 132.
[31] Carrel to Tuffier, Malinin Collection of the Papers of Alexis Carrel and Charles Lindbergh, box 3 folder 25, FA 208, RUA RAC (note 4).
[32] Carrel (Alexis) papers (1906–1916), box 2, folder 2, FA 231, RUA RAC (note 4).

in French journals. He longed to be one of 'les immortels' of the French Academy, the elite group of 40 savants drawn from French intellectual life. He nearly reached this honour later. Lower level awards came in steadily, and his first honorary degree came from the City College of New York in 1913, followed by degrees from Columbia University (1913), Belfast in Northern Ireland (1919), Brown University (1920), and Princeton (1920), and he later would be similarly honoured at the University of California in 1936. At first, he accepted most academic invitations but later increasingly declined to attend all but the more important occasions.

He spoke well and could enthuse an audience. He gave the prestigious Janeway Lecture in 1929 at Mount Sinai Hospital on the nature of the cancer cell, and wound healing was his theme in his McArthur Lecture to the Chicago Institute of Medicine in 1930. But when he spoke earlier at the University of California Charter Day in 1927, usually an occasion for a broad optimistic theme, he surprised his audience with a gloomy assessment of the state of the world, picturing an unhappy mankind in which individuality was gone and 'the weak are aided and often admired'.

He kept up his membership of the main clinical, biological and physiological societies of the day and received their journals, but he seldom attended these organisations' meetings. He wrote well-crafted formal letters to colleagues and friends, which were uniformly polite. But Carrel was a highly critical reviewer of the scientific work of others. Papers for consideration for publication in the Institute's *Journal of Experimental Medicine* came to him via Flexner as editor, and Carrel's reports could be scathing: 'It would have had some slight interest in 1911, but it has none in 1929' ... 'he [Levaditi the pioneer microcinematographer] is working in a filthy lab' ... [Another author] 'has discovered that a toxin is toxic – a waste of money' ... 'Really childish; the drawings mean nothing and even the colours are bad' ... 'The author is perhaps not sufficiently familiar with the extensive literature published outside his country [UK]' ... 'Professor Hueper has conceptions which would have greatly surprised Pasteur ... they have the freshness of innocence'.[33]

---

[33] Malinin Collection of the Papers of Alexis Carrel and Charles Lindbergh, box 4 folder 13, FA 208, RUA RAC (note 4).

These views would not endear him to his scientific colleagues, but at this time he was unassailable. To add to his scientific writings, he obliged friends and colleagues by writing short introductions to their published books. The first author he helped in this way was Paluel Flagg, formerly the anaesthetist at the Demonstration Hospital, whose *The Art of Anaesthesia* of 1919 was a success and sold steadily thereafter. Carrel had links with the talented much-travelled Edmund V. Cowdry (1888–1975) of the Anatomy Department at Washington University in St. Louis, and Carrel did the introduction to Cowdry's important multi-author book *General Cytology* in 1924. Carrel also wrote a chapter for Cowdry's monumental three-volume *Special Cytology* (1928).[34] Carrel wrote the entry on 'Tissue Culture' for the *Encyclopaedia Britannica* in 1926, for which he was paid $45.

Committees and Associations

Carrel took up few posts on outside committees or organisations. He avoided such involvement, since although he was a capable administrator, he had little interest in influencing any outside bodies by his presence. He declined to be president of the new International Society for Experimental Cell Research, although he was the obvious choice, and did not attend its early meetings from 1930.[35] He was, however, a trustee of the ambitious Institute for Advanced Studies, near Princeton University, established in 1930 as a major intellectual centre for independent research and intellectual inquiry. It soon added Albert Einstein to the faculty, but it proved to be only partly successful in its endeavours; no influence on its

---

[34] The chapters in Cowdry's book came largely from the scientists who gathered each summer at Woods Hole Marine Biological Station in Cape Cod. From 1931, he served as chairman of the Division of Medical Sciences of the new National Research Council.
[35] Carrel's professional correspondence is unfailingly polite — a rare unpleasantness occurred in exchanges with the formidable German scientist Rhoda Erdmann, who deplored his lack of support for this new International Society; see Theodore I. Malinin, *Surgery and Life: the Extraordinary Career of Alexis Carrel* (New York: Harcourt Brace Jovanovich, 1979): 57.

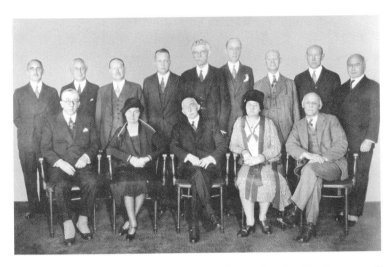

Carrel usually avoided added administration and outside roles, but he was a founder trustee of the Institute for Advanced Studies at Princeton. (*Courtesy of the Institute for Advanced Studies.*)

work by Carrel can be found.[36] His links with the Roman Catholic Church meant that he was later elected to the Pontifical Academy of Sciences in Rome which, in a change of policy for the Church, aimed to reconcile religion and science. He briefly assisted the French cause in America via the Council on Foreign Relations, which towards the end of World War I gathered a small group of scholars together to advise the U.S. president on European policy. His liking for the military life meant that he supported French and American veterans organisations, notably the American Legion, and sent money to them in response to one-off appeals. He attended the occasional Legion social event, even purchasing annual single Patrons Ball tickets, not to attend, but as a contribution to their local funds.[37] Carrel was also on the board of American Fund for French Wounded.

---

[36] Steve Batterson, *Pursuit of Genius: Flexner, Einstein and the Early Faculty at the Institute for Advanced Study* (Wellesley: A.K. Peters, 2006).

[37] The American Legion's politics at the time were conservative and, reluctantly headed at this time by Teddy Roosevelt, they sent an invitation to Mussolini to address their conference in 1930.

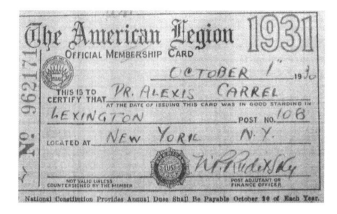

Carrel enjoyed his military service and supported veterans organisations, including the American Legion. (*Courtesy of the Georgetown University Library, Booth Family Center for Special Collections.*)

Eugenics

Much earlier, in 1914, before he left for war service, Carrel had accepted an invitation to advise one of the early U.S. eugenic organisations then growing in prominence and confidence. Previous biological understanding of heredity was that each new generation involved a blending of parental qualities, giving a dilution of earlier qualities. But the new genetics showed that genes, often called 'germ-plasm' at the time, were passed unchanged from one generation to another. Those who sought to improve the human race considered that the 'good' genes of the 'superior classes' could be encouraged by suitable mating (positive eugenics), and the 'bad' genes of those judged 'unfit' in some way could be removed from the population by negative eugenics — using incarceration or sterilisation to prevent breeding. Eugenic thinking, positive and negative, had general support and respectability at the time.

In 1910, a Eugenics Record Office was set up at Cold Spring Harbor, New York, funded by the philanthropy of Mrs. Averell Harriman, and with some Carnegie Institution of Washington and Rockefeller family assistance. William H. Welch added to his many involvements by being the first vice-chairman of the Office, and it soon established a 'Committee to Study and to Report on the Best Practical Means of Cutting Off the

Defective Germ-Plasm in the American Population'. The Committee's secretary was the controversial activist Harry H. Laughlin.[38] Helping the main Committee was a 19-strong Expert Advisory Committee, which included Carrel as representing 'Surgery'. The 'Medicine' expert was Lewellys F. Barker, the Johns Hopkins physician-in-chief who succeeded Osler, and Harvard's Walter Cannon represented 'Physiology'.[39] The committee reported in 1914, and the surgical methods of male and female sterilisation were mentioned. Carrel looked like the person on the Committee who could advise on the details.[40]

After the War, to assess in more detail the practicalities of sterilisation of the 'unfit', a small executive sub-committee with Laughlin again as secretary emerged. But Carrel was not on this new committee. Instead, they brought in the surgical expertise of Dr. Everett Flood, who used castration as a treatment at the State Hospital for Epileptics at Palmer, Massachusetts. Carrel's lack of interest in further involvement does not mean that he was uninterested in eugenics.

One other eugenic organisation watched by Carrel was The Race Betterment Foundation organised from 1911 by John Harvey Kellogg (1852–1943), the Seventh Day Adventist, surgeon and medical director of the huge Battle Creek Sanitarium in Michigan. He held a Race Betterment Conference in 1914 at Battle Creek which 400 attended, and it met again in 1915 at San Francisco. After Kellogg moved his institution to Miami, Carrel attended the Foundation's third conference there in 1928, and the speakers included the increasingly strident eugenicists Charles Davenport, Madison Grant and Harry Laughlin. Carrel gave a purely technical paper on cells in tissue culture, making his familiar claim that all tissues were immortal. Kellogg believed he could remove alleged

---

[38] Later, when American support for simplistic eugenics declined in the mid-1930s, Laughlin's bad science, crude racism and anti-Semitism were deplored; his work reflected badly on the Carnegie Institution, and the Record Office was closed.

[39] Others on the Committee included the psychologist H.H. Goddard, author of the notorious study of the Kallikak 'degenerates'. Theological advice came from Newell Dwight Hillis, the deeply conservative and controversial Brooklyn minister.

[40] *Eugenic Record Office Bulletin* No. 103, February 1914 (New York: Cold Spring Harbor, 1914).

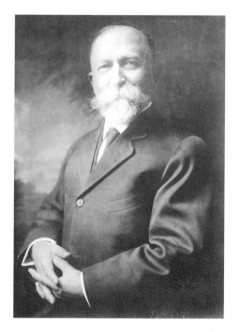

Carrel supported John H. Kellogg's views on 'race betterment' and eugenics and visited his Florida 'Sanitarium'. (*Wikipedia*)

poisons from the body, and the regimen at his health clinic included a focused diet and enemas. The two men corresponded and later Carrel visited Kellogg again in Miami to discuss ideas about ageing and longevity. Nearer home, in 1927 Carrel attended the inaugural meeting in New York of the Aristogenic Association, set up by Laughlin and other eugenicists. They announced that man's future was in his own hands and that lifespans could be increased. 'Strong leaders' were also required, and the Association hoped to study and find the secret of the physical and mental attributes of great leaders, 'on whom the survival of the white race depends'.[41]

Publicity

Carrel was now well established as a celebrity. The French Line company offered him upgrades on their Atlantic liners if he decided to travel with

---

[41] 'Launch Move To Raise Human Standards' *NYT*, 3 February 1928.

them, which he did. Carrel was still offered free tickets for first night openings on Broadway sent to him by the theatres in the hope that he would appear, but he did not. In 1926, he featured on the list of 20 chosen for Frederick Houk Law's *Modern Great Americans* (1926), and he appeared along with Andrew Carnegie and Franklin D. Roosevelt.

Letters from the public came in steadily. The enquiry pattern changed, and since Carrel was now the authority on ageing, enquirers asked how to gain a long life or, if ageing had brought a problem, how to obtain rejuvenation. There were detailed questions about immortality, some from ministers of religion requiring help with their sermons, and from school children who wished to repeat the chicken heart experiment at science fairs. As before, all got a polite response. Some better-known correspondents like Joseph Pilates (1883–1967), who sent impressive pictures of himself and his physical training methods, were invited to visit the Institute to discuss matters with Carrel.

Carrel's newspaper appearances were relatively few during this period in the 1920s. One reason for Carrel's lower profile was that in the 1920s, the Institute yet again had sought to cut down on publicity. The adverse public comments by Bevan in 1919 on the Carrel–Dakin method had meant new caution in the Institute's public relations, and soon there were other reasons for care. Paul de Kruif arrived as a young scientist at the Institute and in 1922 wrote a series of article in *The Century Magazine* poking fun at the medical profession and its allegedly intellectual and scientific shortcomings when compared with full-time researchers. The New York doctors reasonably resented this attack from within the Institute, and Flexner had to dismiss de Kruif.[42] Added to this, in the early 1920s Flexner's star microbe-hunter Hideo Noguchi was again causing concern when he wrongly claimed to have identified the organism responsible for yellow fever, and his much publicised vaccine, which followed, proved to be ineffective.

---

[42] These controversial articles by de Kruif in *The Century Magazine* were collected as *Our Medicine Men* (New York: The Century Co., 1922). Later, de Kruif's *Microbe Hunters* (1926) sold extremely well and Sinclair Lewis' *Arrowsmith,* with de Kruif's briefing, also cast the Institute in a generally good light.

As a result, the Institute again sought a lower and more dignified profile. In 1921, the Institute ruled that all announcements were to go out via the business manager E. B. Smith. The magazine *Popular Science Monthly* grumbled in 1921 that they were not getting press releases from the Institute, notably about the upcoming birthday of the immortal chicken heart cells, but Smith declined to help, saying that 'there had been enough written on the matter'.[43] In any case, post-war scientific journalism had become less credulous and avoided extravagant stories. Carrel's work on trephones was hardly newsworthy, nor did the press warm to his cancer work. However, Carrel still had contacts with the editor of *McClure's* and hosted him at the Institute. He also met his old friend Hitchcock, editor of *Harper's Magazine*, at The Century Association. Carrel soon found a way round Smith's embargo. When *Harper's Magazine* wished to obtain an interview, he agreed to answer questions 'provided it did not appear as an interview'. On another occasion he congratulated another magazine on their article about him which, 'without it appearing to be an interview given at the Rockefeller Institute, I greatly appreciate your handling of our conversation'.[44] Another journalist submitted a short piece to him for his comments and Carrel replied:

I have just received your letter. As you understand, I cannot give any interviews. However, at the same time, my studies and opinions are not being concealed. I have modified the statement in your letter as follows ....

Later he explained rather pompously to another editor, declining to help, that 'Men of science should not attract the curiosity of the public.[45]

Carrel added to his stock of personal portraits taken at private studios in New York and Paris, often at the request of the newspapers or

[43] Smith memos, Carrel (Alexis) papers (1906–1957), FA 231, box 2 folder 2, RUA RAC (note 4).
[44] Malinin Collection of the Papers of Alexis Carrel and Charles Lindbergh, box 4 folder 31, FA 208, RUA RAC (note 4).
[45] Theodore I. Malinin, *Surgery and Life: The Extraordinary Career of Alexis Carrel* (New York: Harcourt Brace Jovanovich, 1979): 172.

magazines, and this explains the large variety which have survived. He also made himself available for photographers and journalists when embarking on or returning from his visits to Europe.

Carrel's non-attributable assistance to the American newspapers was skilful and even helpful to biologists in the tissue culture field. His private briefings to the friendly press headed off the idea that there were any sinister features in the culture techniques. In Britain, the culturists at the Strangeways Laboratory decided they would shun the newspapers, and in 1935, the director advised the staff to 'refuse to see, or to communicate with any newspaper reporters'. The papers interpreted this hostile silence as evidence of dubious practice and that there was something to hide. British journalists then wrote stories alleging that tissue culture was able to create life and even 'test tube babies'.[46]

Fiction

Carrel appeared in another Maurice Renard novel *Les Mains d'Orlac* (*The Hands of Orlac*). First published in 1920, and filmed later, it borrowed heavily from the novel *Mortmain* (1907), described earlier, written by Carrel's New York friend Arthur Train. In Renard's new novel, Carrel was thinly disguised as the famous 'Dr Cerral':

> At that time one name alone dominated surgery, just as that of Foch had dominated military science. His fame spread worldwide. The whole world knew the life-story of this Frenchmen of genius ....

The plot featured a pianist with damaged hands, and the surgeon replaces them with donor hands taken from a guillotined murderer. The deceased donor hands then try to murder again.

Carrel's tissue culture also featured in other fiction, and in the magazine *Amazing Stories* of August 1927, the British scientist Julian Huxley published a short story 'The Tissue-Culture King', which told of the adventures of a Rockefeller-trained biologist-explorer who reaches a

---

[46] See Duncan Wilson (2005) 'The early history of tissue culture in Britain: the interwar years' *Social History of Medicine* 18: 225–43.

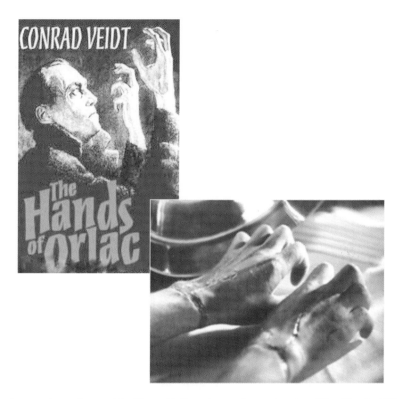

Hand transplants featured in Renard's French novel translated as *The Hands of Orlac*, and film versions followed.

remote tribe in an African jungle. He takes tissue from the king and this is cultured, tended and guarded by a special cadre of young women. Subculture gives copious spare tissue for the king to disburse as a royal blessing.[47]

Withdrawal

Carrel kept up his clinical surgical contacts for a while in the early 1920s, but these steadily faded and Carrel's correspondence with surgeons like Cushing slowly ceased. His Paris friend and supporter Samuel Pozzi had

---

[47] *Amazing Stories* was the first science-fiction magazine and from April 1926 offered 'extravagant fiction today … cold fact tomorrow'.

died in 1918, as did Halsted in 1922. Another surgical link was lost when Théodore Tuffier died in France in 1929.[48] The hostile reception to his Carrel–Dakin treatment at the French medical societies meetings during the war had not pleased him, nor had he much support from the American surgeons. The rather nebulous proposal at the Institute that fundamental cellular biology would bring benefits to clinical surgery had come to nothing. The American surgical societies still visited the Institute in the 1920s, but attendance at these sessions was beginning to fade. A telling incident came in 1931 when the Institute hosted a visit for surgeons attending the American College meeting in New York. Few turned up at the Institute, and the College's secretary wrote afterwards to the Institute with an apology for the poor attendance. Carrel and Rous were unconcerned and joked that 'next time they will doubtless send us an audience even if they have to drug them and transfer them in bulk'.[49] But the surgeons disinterest was understandable: Carrel's surgical contributions on organ grafting and blood vessel surgery were still unexploited and were increasingly forgotten. He had also long since cut himself off from the surgical world.

By the late 1920s, Carrel was also losing interest in his laboratory studies. He was restive, and he and Flexner embarked on a new, very different, grand project.

---

[48] Carrel later contributed a heart-felt tribute to the French surgeon — Alexis Carrel (1932) 'Tuffier' *Revue de Paris* 39: 347–59.

[49] Carrel to Rous, Malinin Collection of the Papers of Alexis Carrel and Charles Lindbergh, box 4 folder 13, FA 208, RUA RAC (note 4).

CHAPTER TWELVE

Confidence Gone

By the end of the 1920s, little new was coming from Carrel's tissue culture work. The expected significant insights into cellular mechanisms had not emerged, and in particular, after many false trails, the hopes of understanding the cancer cell had not resulted. The status of tissue culture at the end of the 1920s was that:

> By some, optimists, it has been regarded as a magic key to the understanding of the life processes, by other pessimists it has been slighted as a valueless craft which has contributed nothing to science.[1]

Harrison's early pioneer work on tissue culture was again considered for a Nobel Prize in 1933, but it was not favoured by the Committee 'in view of the rather limited value'.

Carrel was losing interest in cellular studies. Up until 1928, he was averaging four or five substantial papers a year, plus numerous preliminary communications, but in the year 1929, he published only one brief review and nothing of consequence in the next year.

The rest of the Institute was also rather unproductive at this time. Science in general in the interwar period was under criticism and seen by some as a threat to progress, even moral progress, being uninvolved in matters of the mind and spirit. Public criticism of science was on the increase, and in America, the Scopes trial in 1925 banned the teaching of

---

[1] E.N. Wilmer, *Cells and Tissues in Culture* (New York: Academic Press, 1965) vol. 1, xx. For earlier pessimism, see *The Lancet*, 28 April 1923, 858, which concluded that the technique had been oversold both within and outside of science.

evolution. There was a revival of the antivivisection movement, and in New York in 1927 there was a successful prosecution of Dr. David Shelling, an expert on rickets, at the Jewish Hospital of Brooklyn, resulting from his dietary experiments on dogs. This led to local bills presented to the New York State legislature, and some controls on animal experiments followed. The newspapers' uncritical admiration and coverage of science and scientists had also gone. Carrel's public profile was also declining by the end of the decade, as judged by his press cuttings count.[2]

Institute Policy

Flexner, now in his late 60s, and close to retirement, was aware of the slowdown at the Institute. Jacques Loeb had died in 1927, and his crusade at the Institute to understand the body as a machine seemed to peter out with his death, signalling a rethink.[3] Flexner acknowledged the new holistic mood of interwar medicine, and he noted wryly the return by some physicians of the day to 'more mystical doctrines ... as defined by Hippocrates, and especially by Sydenham'. Carrel was also taking an interest in this revived 'alternative' medicine. In summer, in his home city, he encountered the Groupe lyonnaise d'etude médicales philosophique et biologique and back in New York kept in touch with their activities. The new (or rather very old) 'constitutional' explanation of disease proposed that, for instance, in infectious disease the invading organism was not the main factor but that instead the host response was dominant in the outcome of the contact. Flexner decided to get involved, and with his staff member Leslie T. Webster, they set up large colonies of mice at the Institute and studied the spread of infectious disease within the groups.

---

[2] Carrel's collection of press cuttings in the Alexis Carrel Papers, Georgetown University Library, Booth Family Center for Special Collections (GULBFC) show they had fallen to single figures annually in the early 1920s, then rising to 39 in 1925, and falling again to single figures by 1930.

[3] For a hint of a rethink, see Simon Flexner (1927) 'Jacques Loeb and his period' *Science* 66: 333–7. Jacques Loeb's, *Mechanistic Theory of Life* was republished with a useful Introduction by Donald Fleming (Cambridge: Harvard University Press, 1964).

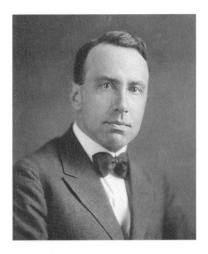

Raymond Fosdick had a major influence on Rockefeller Foundation policies in the interwar period, and his declinist views influenced Carrel's later writings. (*Courtesy of the Library of Congress.*)

Flexner called the approach 'experimental epidemiology'.[4] Flexner went further and suggested the need for an Institute of Hygiene, whose staff were to 'assimilate knowledge and deal with man and his environment notably light, soil, water, dwellings, ventilation, heating and lighting, food and clothing, occupation, eugenics and safety appliances'.

There were also policy changes at the Rockefeller Foundation, taking them into holistic realms when they announced a program to study 'the modern science of man'. Raymond Fosdick, the dominant figure at the Foundation, produced a book in 1929 with the intriguing title *The Old Savage in the New Civilisation*, and he suggested that man was now a victim within the world he had created, and that the race had declined. He wrote: 'The challenge of this situation is obvious ... can we develop some sound and extensive genetics that we hope to breed in the future, superior men?' Fosdick's view was that the Foundation, rather than support laboratory science, should take up the study of human behaviour,

---

[4] See Simon Flexner (1922) 'Experimental epidemiology', *JEM* 36: 9–14 which describes his encounter with the nostalgic mood of a 'neo-Hippocratic' meeting at London's Royal Society of Medicine in 1919.

and its control, which he called 'human engineering'. Fosdick also wished to rejoin the mind with the body, and the Foundation now offered large grants for psychiatric research. They even hoped that psychoanalysts might develop a scientific attitude and contribute verifiable insights into the mind.[5]

Carrel's Choices

At this time of uncertainty, and with cellular studies out of favour, there were other projects for Carrel to explore, or rather re-explore, which appear obvious in retrospect. He could have collaborated with Karl Landsteiner, of blood group fame, who as noted before, had arrived at the Institute in 1922 and was beginning to look beyond his blood groups to explore the ideas of tissue groups. Landsteiner wrote that 'one is led to the idea that every person might have a peculiar biochemical structure'.[6] When the Society of Clinical Surgery visited the Institute in November 1930, Landsteiner gave a presentation, and afterwards Carrel wrote to him saying that the surgeons 'understood fully the importance your researches will have in the selection of the proper donor for the transplantation of skin or organs'.[7] But otherwise Carrel seemed uninterested in reviving the work he had done on 'matching' with Ingebrigtsen in 1912. Carrel's letters from the public requesting grafts had declined, but in his replies he often said that the future of transplantation 'depends on the progress and knowledge of individuality'. Flexner noticed that the Mayo Clinic had taken up Carrel's earlier dog kidney transplantation studies, though they had not added to it, and wrote to Carrel about this, but Carrel did not

---

[5] Fosdick's remarkable, forgotten sentiments are found in the *Rockefeller Foundation Annual Report* 1933: 198–9.

[6] K. Landsteiner and J. van der Scheer (1927) 'On the production of immune sera for tissues' *PSEBM* 25: 140–1, and see also Karl Landsteiner (1928) 'Cell antigens and individual specificity' *Journal of Immunology* 15: 589–99. Landsteiner was handicapped in his search by his reasonable view that these putative human tissue 'groups' would be found on red cells.

[7] Carrel to Landsteiner, 24 November 1930, box 42 folder 'Karl Landsteiner 1923–37', GULBFC (note 2).

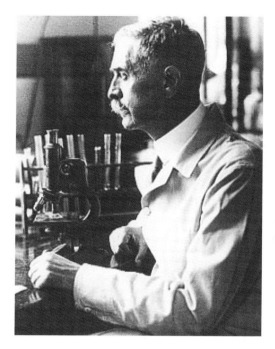

Although Karl Landsteiner joined the Institute in 1923, and worked on tissue matching, Carrel did not resume any similar studies. (*Courtesy of the National Library of Medicine.*)

respond nor seem interested.[8] Carrel might now have understood 'individuality' in a broader sense and accepted the new holistic teaching that everyone had a unique constitution and a varied susceptibility to disease. This might also apply to tissue transplantation and that the power to reject a graft might vary from person to person, and even vary in the same person from time to time. Perhaps the 'rejection deniers' were right.

Doubts about the Cells

Carrel's 'old strain' cell line continued to be well known and influential. Carrel had these 'immortal' cells on show under a microscope as a fixed

---

[8] For an account of the cautious Mayo Clinic work, which repeated Carrel's kidney homografts, but did not take his work any further, see David Hamilton, *A History of Organ Transplantation* (Pittsburgh: Pittsburgh University Press, 2012): 149–52.

exhibit in his laboratory. George Corner, the historian of the Rockefeller Institute, conceded that the culture was a 'consummate piece of scientific enterprise and showmanship'. Other labs reported that they managed to obtain short-term growth of some cells, but no other long-lived cell cultures emerged. If Carrel's long-lived cells were given out to other laboratories, none of them were reported to be in use.

The first concerns about the long-lived chicken-heart-fibroblast cells appeared at this time. Ralph Buchsbaum, then a PhD student at the University of Chicago, concerned at his inability to repeat the experiment and obtain long-lived cells, decided in 1930 to visit Carrel's laboratory to study the famous strain. On arrival, he was disappointed to be told by Ebeling (Carrel being absent) that the cells were too delicate to be shown to visitors. As he made to leave the building, he saw Ebeling and others departing, and the student returned to Carrel's department and pleaded with a technician to let him see the cultures. She said that 'Carrel and

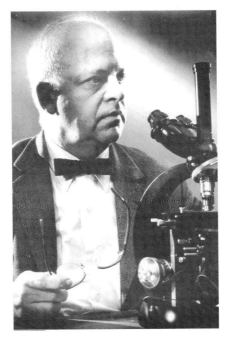

Ralph Buchsbaum, as a young post-graduate student, visited Carrel's laboratory in 1930 and formed private doubts about Carrel's 'immortal cells'. (*Wikipedia*)

Parker would have a fit' if they knew, but nevertheless showed him the cells. They were full of fat globules and were dying in the way familiar to him during his own attempts. The lab assistant then added: 'Carrel would be upset if we lost the strain and we add a few embryo cells now and again. We make new strains for new experiments.' On his return to his department in Chicago, and reporting this news, the student met a mixture of disbelief and amusement.[9]

There was some low level gossip at the time that all was not well in Carrel's laboratory.[10] It was not until 1965 that a new understanding of cellular lifespan emerged when Leonard Hayflick established that normal cells only divide a finite number of times. None are immortal.[11] As a result, as described later, attention returned to Carrel's earlier claims, which seemed improbable.

At the start Carrel had handed over the project to Ebeling and, as was usual with Carrel, unless he was personally involved, he did not look closely at results. Ebeling, in turn, was often absent, and the laboratory work relied on the technicians. They would believe what they were told by Ebeling and Carrel about the immortal cells, and would fear being responsible for the failure of the famous cell line. If so, their method of rescue of the dying cultures may have started even before World War I. Nor did the laboratory run smoothly at all times. In the mid-1920s, Carrel wrote to the general manager that:

> Only two of the technicians are in good health. The other four are more or less ill — Miss Johnston has left for several months, probably for a year. Miss Todd is at home with a surgical infection. Miss Hollander and Miss Griffin are still working, but both are far from well.[12]

---

[9] Quoted in J.A. Witkowski (1980) 'Dr. Carrel's immortal cells' *Medical History* 24: 129–42, at 139.

[10] Witkowski (note 9): 139 notes these rumours.

[11] L. Hayflick (1965) 'The limited in vitro lifetime of human diploid cell strains' *Experimental Cell Research* 37: 614–36.

[12] Carrel to Smith, 1 December 1926, Alexis Carrel Papers, (1906–1957), box 2 folder 3, FA 231 Rockefeller University Archives, Rockefeller Archives Centre (RUA RAC).

The stressed technicians may have known by then how to keep the 'old strain' immortal cells alive by taking short cuts. It is interesting that the visiting Chicago student was told by the technician that they made new cultures for new experiments; the immortal cells were not, after all, routinely used then as an easily-available standard cell line.

Another, more charitable explanation, is that the chicken embryo 'soup' necessary for growth of the famous cells from the start contained fresh chicken connective tissue cells and that these replaced those dying. Carrel never described the preparation of the embryo extract in detail, and his letters in reply to those enquiring about the matter are rather casual about the methodology. Carrel did investigate the soup, and an important finding was that Berkefeld filtration, which removed particles the size of bacteria, or irradiating the extract, annulled its power, as did prolonged freezing, again suggesting that there were cells in the soup. There was also a strong chance of cellular transfer on other occasions. Carrel said in a letter that 'sometimes we use just the juice after mincing in the 'Latapie apparatus' without adding any fluid and without centrifugation'.[13]

This was a strange admission to make — and it is possible it was deliberate. If Carrel now knew that the famous cells died out unless refreshed in this way, he may have been relaxed about the deception. He probably expected that other 'immortal' cell lines would be developed shortly, and that his premature claim would not be noticed, with credit remaining with him for being first. But this did not happen. His laboratory was stuck with their famous exhibit and its birthdays, and a retreat was unthinkable.[14]

---

[13] Carrel to Kopeloff, 29 April 1927, box 44 folder 3, GULBFC (note 2). Carrel told another inquirer that sometimes the chicken embryo was minced with scissors, suspended in a few drops of Tyrode's saline, and centrifuged for 10 minutes at 3,000 revs. In Ebeling's *JEM* (1913) 17: 284 first description of the power of the extract, he saw 'scattered cells grow [sic] in a medium due to extract'.

[14] Carrel has only one cautious supporter in Henry Harris, *The Cells of the Body* (Cold Spring Harbor: Cold Spring Harbor Laboratory Press, 1995): 45, who suggests that Carrel's cells might have been transformed, i.e. were malignant cells, having been contaminated with the Rous sarcoma virus; Leonard Hayflick (personal communication) firmly rejects this explanation.

If fraud was involved, the affair is one of the first cases of scientific misconduct in the world of biology.[15] It would certainly explain why no one could repeat the experiment at the time and why the cells, if gifted, did not survive in other laboratories.[16] When George O. Gey obtained the first genuinely immortal cell line in 1951 — the human cervical cancer 'HeLa cells' — he immediately gifted samples to anyone interested. It grew easily and was widely used from the outset.[17]

But no one openly disputed Carrel's claim at the time, shrinking from making distasteful allegations, thus avoiding bringing discredit to the newly-emerged world of cellular biology. The Rockefeller Institute was a major research organisation and it also published the respected *Journal of Experimental Medicine*. The Institute and the Rockefeller Foundation dispensed considerable external funds to American universities and medical schools. Johns Hopkins University received $68,000 annually and their tissue culture lab received an extra Rockefeller grant. If there were doubts, a professional *omerta* prevailed: Carrel was unassailable.

The press kept up their interest in the cells in the 1920s, and on 10 February 1932, Waldemar Kaempffert, the respected science correspondent of the *New York Times*, enthused about the 'tenderly guarded living flame in the Rockefeller temple of science … it may become as sacred in a scientific sense as a venerated religious relic'. Carrel was so pleased that he asked Kaempffert to send him a signed copy of the article.

Decline in Output

In the doldrums by 1928, after years of largely fruitless effort, there were other difficulties and Carrel could show some frustration. In November 1928 he made an uncharacteristic complaint about the Institute's services,

[15] Carrel's 1912 claim preceded Kammerer's 'midwife' toad fraud, revealed in 1926. Gregor Mendel was first to be accused retrospectively of misconduct, but allegations that he tampered with the 1860s data from his pea-growing experiments are still resisted by his supporters.

[16] Albert H. Ebeling (1942) 'Dr. Carrel's immortal chicken heart' *Scientific American* 166: 22–4 vaguely describes gifts to other laboratories.

[17] Rebecca Skloot, *The Immortal Life of Henrietta Lacks* (New York: Crown Publishing Group, 2010): 48.

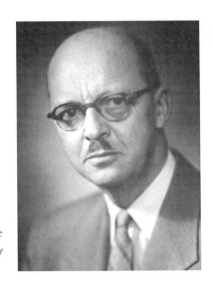

Raymond Parker moved to the Institute in 1930, strengthening Carrel's group. (*Courtesy of Sanofi Pasteur, Canada.*)

notably 'the ridiculous amount of time and energy to get things done ... our inability to obtain a proper and efficient service'.[18] He also had some staff problems. In January 1926, du Noüy, his physicist, went to the Carnegie Institute in Washington to learn methods of X-ray studies of crystals, and the Institute bought the new apparatus for his use on return. This would have given an early start with the use of this crucial investigative method in biological physics. But when du Noüy returned to New York, he promptly took a year off to work at the Pasteur Institute in Paris, and he did not return. Another setback for Carrel was that Ebeling was off work for three months in 1928 suffering, as before, with the vague abdominal symptoms and weight loss from which he had always recovered in the past. But this time John Finney, the Baltimore surgeon, was consulted and a diagnosis of chronic appendicitis made; removal of his appendix followed. Post-operatively, Ebeling had a near-fatal pulmonary embolism and was off work for a year. With Ebeling absent, and du Noüy gone, Flexner urged Carrel to accept a new post and take on an established scientist to support the tissue culture work.

---

[18] Carrel to Smith, 23 and 30 November 1928, box 44 folder 48, Alexis Carrel Papers, GULBFC (note 2).

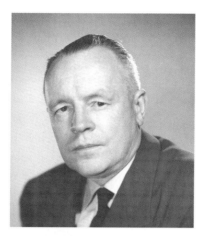

Ralph Wyckoff, the pioneering molecular biologist at the Institute, later was one of Carrel's few supporters. (*Courtesy of the National Institute of Health.*)

Raymond Crandall Parker (1903–1974) was appointed as an assistant in 1930. Parker, experienced already in tissue culture studies at the University of Pennsylvania, had also worked with Carrel's close colleague Fischer in Berlin.[19]

Carrel was now not in favour with the rest of the staff. Ralph W. Wyckoff (1897–1994), a newcomer to the Institute in 1927, was impressed with Carrel but noted the isolation of Carrel and his group, even in the dining room:

> The fact that Carrel's group had its meals always isolated from the rest of the staff was the consequence of the disfavour with which many of the Institute's influential members saw him and his work. The situation revealed, on the one hand, the sentiments of jealousy elicited by his brilliant scientific accomplishments, his Nobel Prize; on the other, it was the result of the unrestrained manner with which he frequently expressed his critical judgments. Soon after my arrival ... a member of

---

[19] Parker had criticised the leadership of the Cancer Research Laboratory at the Pennsylvania Graduate School of Medicine, and was keen to move elsewhere after being accused of 'non-cooperation and selfishness'.

the Institute informed me about this antipathy and let me know that to succeed I would have to give up my friendship with Carrel.[20]

Now rather isolated, Carrel grumbled to friends that 'Simon Flexner is the only person who really understands me', and that the scientists of the Rockefeller Institute 'were not complete humans'. He told a visiting journalist that the Institute 'was not a place for personal research and individual thinking'.[21] He now rarely attended scientific gatherings and had not spoken at a surgical meeting since World War I. Carrel declined to join the lunch parties in honour of visiting surgeons organised in New York by the distinguished surgeon William S. Bainbridge, saying it was impossible to get away during the day.[22] He also routinely declined to join evening social events, pleading pressure of work. He later excused himself when invited to join the Alfred Nobel Centennial celebration dinner for the American holders of the Prize organized by Columbia University. The event was in New York at the Roosevelt Hotel close to Carrel's apartment. John Dewey the organiser was understandably upset and commented sharply in reply that if Einstein could come, so could Carrel.[23]

Cancer Studies

By the late 1920s the Institute's lacklustre performance continued. Frederick Gates, still active as an Institute trustee, gave a talk to the Municipal Club of Brooklyn in November 1927 and starting by saying:

---

[20] R.W.G. Wyckoff (1984) 'Souvenirs d'Alexis Carrel à New-York' *Lyon Chirurgical* 80: 194–6. Wyckoff admired Carrel and was loyal to him later. He particularly liked Carrel's proposals for cultivation of viruses and later Wyckoff was to make one of the earliest anti-viral vaccines using chicken embryos, as Carrel had suggested.

[21] Carrel and Tarbell letters, May 1930, box 97 folder 3, GULBFC (note 2). This allegation of opposition to original thought was a favourite of Carrel, one made regularly against his Lyon medical school or when complaining about Parisian and German medical institutions. The British public, according to Carrel, were also uninterested in new ideas.

[22] Carrel to Bainbridge, 21 November 1925 'folder 3 14-1' GULBFC (note 2).

[23] Dewey to Carrel, box 41 folder 54, GULBFC (note 2).

'A question which is in many of your minds, no doubt, is "What has the Institute done about cancer?"' He was on the defensive, and his reply was unconvincing. Adding to the concern, John D. Rockefeller junior made a rare intervention at the Institute and asked James B. Murphy about what could be done to improve the quality of cancer research.[24]

Flexner was watching what the Carnegie Institute in Washington was doing, and saw they had an emphasis on human cancer studies and eugenics. The Carnegie studies had wrongly concluded that much human disease, including common cancers, were hereditary and could be prevented by eugenic measures. Carrel told Flexner that he believed that diet was also responsible for the emergence of cancer, a view based on some personal data Carrel gathered in Brittany. This suggested a low cancer rate in those rural areas which retained a traditional simple peasant diet. Although this was unimpressively anecdotal, Flexner encouraged Carrel to take this further. Flexner in his studies of epidemics had used large mouse colonies at the Institute, and with this experience, they drew up a larger project to explore any linkage of genetic constitution, diet and cancer in mice. He wrote to Carrel: 'Once you undertook it, I knew you would [do it]. ... We agreed on a sharp concrete experiment and to be discontinued unless a significant lead obtained.'[25] This project would take the Institute far from its traditional strength in reductionist laboratory science. Flexner had faltered and bowed to the new mood. Carrel may not have been a totally enthusiastic supporter of the Loeb mechanistic credo, and now released from it, he could return to studies of the whole body rather than then continue with the unproductive cellular biology. For Carrel, cancer could now be studied not from the cell upwards, but downwards from study in the whole animal.[26]

---

[24] Murphy's response was to suggest research support for James Ewing at New York's Memorial Hospital.
[25] Flexner to Carrel, 2 May 1929, box 2 folder 3, Faculty/Carrel FA 231, RUA RAC (note 12).
[26] Alexis Carrel (1925) 'The future progress of medicine' *The Scientific Monthly* 21: 54–8.

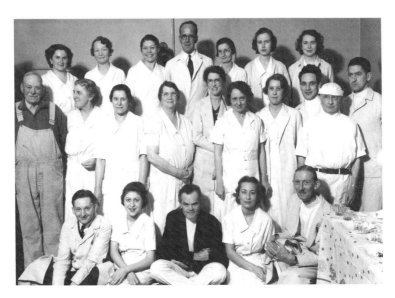

Carrel's large laboratory staff, plus some of the Mousery team, circa 1930, including his long-serving assistant Albert Ebeling, in the middle of the front row, with Lillian Baker, the young chemist, on his left. Carrel's devoted secretary Miss Kathleen Crutcher is the tall figure in the centre of the middle row. (*Courtesy of Yale University Archives.*)

The Project

Accordingly, a grand study named 'The Environmental Effects on Cancer in Mice by Dr. Carrel' was started at the Institute. It was a major three-year project which commenced in October 1928 and which was later extended for a two more years. An extra grant was obtained by Flexner from Rockefeller junior and the Institute constructed a large new experimental area as an extra floor on top of the Power House. It was known officially as 'The Laboratory for Study of the Environment and Physiological Processes' but was soon understandably dubbed 'The Mousery'. The cost of construction of the Mousery was $70,000, with added annual running costs of $20,000. This was a strange episode, one poorly described in any studies of Carrel or the Institute. The historian of the Institute later was puzzled to find that 'the story of this venture is almost wholly undocumented'. The reason for this silence is that there are no substantial reports from Carrel on its work, and the expensive project was eventually terminated, with some embarrassment.[27]

For the study, Carrel turned to newly-available strains of mice, inbred over many generations to give identical animals. Each strain had differing susceptibility to disease, and they were found, surprisingly and intriguingly, to be prone to develop cancer in variable degrees. Carrel suggested that varied diets might increase or decrease these tumour rates. In taking this project on, Carrel had some other less obvious agendas. His affection for France and French science meant that his genetic thinking was Lamarckian; he, like the French geneticists at this time, believed that characteristics acquired during life could be passed on to the next generation. If diet could increase cancer in the mice, then the offspring might have an increased burden of cancer. This linked with Carrel's interest and his peripheral involvement with the 'race betterment' organisations. The mood of the times was eugenic, and there was a scientific need to check these broad assertions about heredity.

Carrel was in overall charge, and he obtained new extra staff, notably Miss Alleyne MacNab plus her deputy Miss Scharfer and another assistant. For the day-to-day work, they appointed five 'college girl' technicians, plus seven 'Bohemian' helper women, and a handyman. The unit had sterilising rooms, offices, an extra lab and a kitchen. Carrel's usual fastidiousness and attention to detail was in evidence, and sterility was important, since there was an ever-present fear of epidemics among the mice, notably of typhoid, which could wreck the project. The unit used a huge number of conventional mouse boxes, but there was an odd extra feature. This was the four large soil-filled pens which allowed free-range living conditions for almost half of the mice, and, running free they made dens in these large soil enclosures. Carrel had added this feature,

[27] George W. Corner, *A History of the Rockefeller Institute 1901–1953: Origins and Growth* (New York: Rockefeller Institute Press, 1964): 228. There is however some information from Dr. McNab in Alexis Carrel Papers, box 2 folders 15, 21, 42, 45 and 48, GULBFC (note 2); in box 10, FA 208, Malinin Collection, RUA RAC (note 12); and a short Carrel report in May 1931 in box 20, FA 137, Business Manager (Mousery 1928–34), RUA RAC (note 12).

unusual for a laboratory, and explained to visitors that 'it re-created real life and the struggle for existence'.[28]

Mouse Supplies

Obtaining enough inbred mice for the start-up was difficult and breeding up sufficient numbers in-house at the Institute was slow.[29] But help came from the Jackson Laboratory in Maine, headed by the controversial geneticist Clarence Cook Little, who had pioneered the development of inbred mice.[30] The Laboratory now produced surplus mice for sale and Little supplied the Institute with lines, notably his inbred 'Dilute Brown' strain which, when adult, had a remarkable cancer incidence of 95%. Numbers built up and soon 12,000 mice, including cancer-prone strains, were held in the Mousery, with the number reaching 15,000 later. In all, about 55,000 mice were eventually studied.

The Studies

The diets studied varied. There were different levels of salt, sugar, and fat. Some diets had added coal tar, copper, manganese, lead, iodine, zinc, aluminium, nickel, cobalt, titanium, arsenic, aniline dyes, iron, potato extracts, raw meat, bone meal, gentian violet, scarlet red, malachite green, phenol, garlic, alcohol and egg yolk.[31] Even boiled faeces were given — influenced by Sir Arbuthnot Lane's view that human disease

---

[28] From David M. Friedman, *The Immortalists: Charles Lindbergh, Dr Alexis Carrel and Their Daring Quest to Live Forever* (New York: HarperCollins, 2007): 9. However, Friedman used invented conversations and hence his text may not be reliable.

[29] For Flexner's earlier mouse epidemic work, the stock of Miss Abbie Lathrop of Holyoke, Massachusetts, the first commercial mouse breeder, became available after her death in 1918, and the Institute made haste to purchase all her animal lines for $3,300; see Hamilton, *Transplantation* (note 8): 46.

[30] C.C. Little pioneered inbreeding of mice at the Carnegie Institute and, taking up the cause of eugenics, he did not survive as a university president and returned to research at the private-funded Jackson Laboratories at Bar Harbor, Maine.

[31] Garlic was added to the diets because folklore in Italy considered it prevented typhoid fever, and in France it was thought to protect dogs from distemper.

resulted from autointoxication from the colon. To these diets, Carrel added a quirky extra, namely depriving some mice by regular periods of starvation, investigating a hunch, derived from his religious background, that it might prolong life. Routine measurements of mouse weight, fertility, health and age at death were made. Autopsies were done and Dr. Santesson, recruited from Stockholm, eventually had data and slides from 23,000 examinations. Blood serum taken from the mice was tested against cells in culture, looking for enhancement or inhibition of cellular growth. There were 'metabolic studies' by Dr. G de Kock, visiting from South Africa, and they also judged the physique of the mice using the pulling strength in the animals' limbs. Carrel wished to look at the linkage of mind, body and diet, since he proposed that 'creative imagination, judgement and other qualities possibly require ... substances introduced into the organism with the food'.[32] Drs. Theiler, Webster, and Saddington at Columbia University assessed mouse intelligence by measuring an animal's ability to learn how to run through a maze to reach food. They made films of 'nervous excitability', one of Carrel's interests, filming the mice in reaction to sudden noises.

The formidable amount of information which accumulated was managed by using the new Hollerith punched card system, and to analyse the data, the Institute rented a 'Powers Accounting Machine', for $780 yearly. The project started in November 1928 and after a delay, Carrel reported briefly to the Scientific Directors in April 1930, but without any major analysis or conclusions. Nevertheless, the next year, Carrel requested and obtained an expansion of the Mousery to enable an even greater number of mice to be studied.

The End

By 1932 there was concern, and the project was reviewed. Flexner had to announce that the Scientific Directors agreed 'that the major work of the Mousery would be discontinued in June'. The main reason would be the lack of data or reports from Carrel, and on his part, it is likely that the

---

[32] Carrel 'Future progress' (note 26).

results failed to support his ideas on the dietary cause of cancer. After this disappointment, he lost interest; as we will see, Carrel's thoughts were perhaps elsewhere. Closing the Mousery helped the Institute at a time when the Wall Street Crash and the Depression were causing financial difficulties. The Institute's investment income had fallen by 6%, and cost-cutting at all New York's academic institutions at this time meant reduced staff numbers and cuts in salaries. The Mousery closure saved the Institute about $30,000 annually. The massive data held on the punched cards awaited analysis, and although the Institute hired the Powers machine for another year, there was still no report from the data gathered, then or later.[33] All that remained of the grand plan came in asides that Carrel made occasionally later in letters and lectures.[34]

The closure of the Mousery was a blow to Flexner, who had suggested it, funded it and supported the expensive un-analysed project from the first. He was now age 70 and in this and other matters, the Scientific Directors were concerned that Flexner had lost his touch. Although he was close to retirement, they took the opportunity to obtain more control of policy decisions at the Institute.

Other Work

Carrel still had his large, well-staffed tissue culture laboratory, but his output of publications fell even further. In 1931 he published only three short, popular articles and three similar followed in the next year. He had no publications in 1933, and the required reports to Flexner almost ceased. However, after his arrival in Carrel's group in 1930, Parker continued to work steadily on his own, publishing two papers on tissue culture each year thereafter, and this made the output from Carrel's large group look more respectable.

---

[33] These data cards are preserved in the Carrel Papers GULBFC (note 2).
[34] Carrel did make a remarkable claim, over dinner, to Ida Tarbell, the distinguished journalist, that the effects of alcohol and fasting on the Mousery mice were passed on, in Lamarckian fashion, to the following untreated generations: see Alexis Carrel Papers, box 97 folder 3, GULBFC (note 2) — this important claim should have been published.

In Carrel's laboratory in 1930, during these difficulties, a new project started in a small way. It was a start on designing and using a pump to perfuse organs, and was perhaps a logical development from his experience in culturing cells. The venture perhaps signalled a further retreat from the earlier mind-set that cellular studies would reveal all; perhaps a whole organ could be of interest after all. Carrel's first attempt was not satisfactory, but soon after, development of a larger organ perfusion pump was going ahead steadily in the capable hands of an unpaid, part-time, celebrity volunteer. When success was announced in 1935, as described later, it would restore Carrel's scientific status and catch the attention of the public yet again.

But in the meantime, Carrel, now in his early 60s, was increasingly preoccupied with broader issues, and began to fret about the state of the world. He shared these views regularly at the meetings of the Philosophers, and his friends there suggested he publish his ideas. Flexner also encouraged him to write a book, and arranged for closure of the laboratory for a while for refurbishment, giving Carrel some time off.

Carrel felt something had to be done about the human race, and that he was the man to lead the way. He knew from the letters he received that he had a public following — now he was going to reach out to them. The book came out in 1935, as did the good news about the organ pump. It was Carrel's *annus mirabilis*, and the book would sell and sell. The writing of *Man, the Unknown*, and its reception, can be considered first.

CHAPTER THIRTEEN

His Book — *Man, the Unknown*

With his tissue culture work stalled, and the disappointments over the Mousery project, Carrel was restive; his output of conventional scientific papers almost ceased by 1933. Another uncertainty was that Simon Flexner's retirement as director of the Institute was due in 1935, and an era was ending. There was national malaise as well. The Wall Street Crash of 1929, followed by the Depression, affected everyone in America, adding to concerns that America was in decline as a nation. As an observer of the French political scene, assisted by his long summer visits to Europe, Carrel was also concerned for France and indeed for the Western world.

In New York, the Philosophers had much to talk about at their Tuesday dinner meetings. 'Cultural despair' was prominent, and Carrel took a leading part. Walter Price, an irregular but enthusiastic attendee, noted two camps in their group over the question of national decline and teased Carrel in one of his friendly letters saying that 'for all your [Carrel] talents and fame, yet you are a misanthrope. You go along in life predicting general disaster, terrifying innocent souls like Boris Bakhmeteff and myself'.[1]

Carrel's friend Frederic Coudert, one of the group, was also watching events in France, and over the years he was particularly sympathetic to Carrel's oft-stated diagnosis of national malaise. Coudert and fellow 'philosopher' Boris Bakhmeteff now urged Carrel to write up his ideas in a book. Simon Flexner, perhaps surprisingly, was also supportive and gave

[1] Price to Carrel, 6 June 1934, Alexis Carrel Papers, box 42 Price folder, Georgetown University Library, Booth Family Center for Special Collections (GULBFC).

335

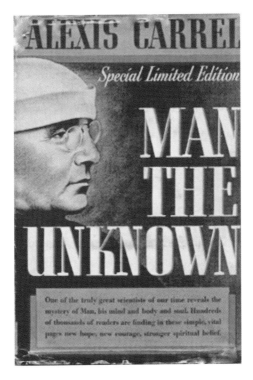

The dust jacket of one of the many editions of Carrel's hugely successful book *Man, the Unknown* (1935).

Carrel time off to write the book. Carrel, in the scientific doldrums, but increasingly convinced that he had something to say to the world, started writing. His *Man, the Unknown* was destined to be a best seller.

Popularising Science

In the 1920s, the public welcomed books explaining the higher mysteries of science and also listened attentively to these scientists' thoughts on broader matters.[2] These books sold well and British science had two stellar, populist authors. Arthur Eddington (1882–1944) was first in the field

---

[2] See Peter J. Bowler (2006) 'Presidential address: experts and publishers: writing popular science in the early twentieth century' *British Journal for the History of Science* 39: 159–87.

with his *The Nature of the Physical World* (1928), which tried to explain Einstein's theories,[3] and James Jeans (1877–1946) followed with his *The Mysterious Universe* (1930). While these savants' books sold well in Britain and France, there were no equivalent popularisers in America, except for the respected Harvard physiologist Bradford Cannon, who published his holistic, optimistic, and readable *The Wisdom of the Body* in 1932.[4]

With the genre well now established, particularly in Europe, Carrel now sought to contribute to it.[5] He was well placed to appeal to the public through his award of a Nobel Prize, and his war work and celebrated immortal cells kept him elevated as a 'visible scientist'. Like Einstein, Carrel's face was familiar to newspaper readers.[6] Carrel was a natural populariser, regularly quoted, and he had talents in simplifying and explaining biological matters. However, writing a popular book had its professional risks. In Britain, Jeans and Eddington had waited to publish until they were members of the Royal Society, and once elected to this high scientific honour, they were safer from the criticism of colleagues. The prospect of such peer disapproval did not trouble Carrel.

Writing the Book

In a letter to his nephew, Carrel made a grand renunciation suggesting that his tissue culture work was now over, announcing: 'I begin a new career ... there are much more important things to achieve than scientific experiments.'[7] The writing occupied much of 1934, and although he

---

[3] Matthew Stanley, *Practical Mystic: Religion, Science and A.S. Eddington* (Chicago: University of Chicago Press, 2007).

[4] S.J. Cross and W.R. Albury (1987) 'Walter B. Cannon, L.J. Henderson and the organic analogy' *Osiris* 3: 165–92.

[5] For a list of popular titles written by French scientists, see Andrés H. Reggiani, *God's Eugenicist: Alexis Carrel and the Sociobiology of Decline* (New York: Berghahn Books, 2007): 60.

[6] Using the Google Ngram viewer to judge celebrity, in France Einstein's fame exceeded Carrel in the 1920s, but they were equal by 1930, with Einstein then pulling ahead again thereafter.

[7] A large batch of letters written by Carrel but lacking a salutation survive in his Georgetown archive. They were earlier thought to be to his brother Joseph. It is more

sought some isolation outside of New York at his country club, the golfers distracted him and he moved to a quieter retreat upstate. In summer that year he worked on the book in France, and on return to New York, showed the draft chapters to friends, including the 'Philosophers'. All gave encouraging responses, although Frederic Coudert considered that some passages were rather dogmatic. Carrel produced both French and English manuscripts, helped by Carrel's resourceful secretary Miss Crutcher, who was now fluent in French.

Entitled *Initiation à la connaissance de nous-memes*, he offered the book first to Plon, the Paris publisher, who turned it down.[8] After the Paris rebuff, Harper & Brothers in New York accepted the English version, but changed the title to *Man, the Unknown*.[9]

Publisher's Caution

Although they accepted the book, and Carrel's career and achievements were well known, the New York publishers were sanguine about potential sales. It was apparently a popular work on biology, but they knew that the text strayed from the topic, and advance orders were poor. Harpers launched the book with a crisp yet rather cautious blurb:

> Dr. Carrel feels we are at a critical period of human development and that the race is to the swift and strong. He suggests ways of developing strong, healthy and complete people and his suggestions will come as a surprise to many. Science tells us what man is and what his limitations are. Incidentally, it tells us that woman is very different from man. ... It

---

likely that they went to Carrel's brother-in-law Attale Gigou, who died in 1934, and that Carrel continued thereafter to write to Gigou's son, Daniel.

[8] James D. Newton, *Uncommon Friends: Life With Thomas Edison, Henry Ford, Harvey Firestone, Alexis Carrel and Charles Lindbergh* (New York: Harvest Books, 1989): 132.

[9] Carrel's *Man, the Unknown* (*MTU*) went to many editions, and the page numbers cited here are those from the popular Blue Ribbon/Halcyon House edition of 1938. For a recent account, see Andrés H. Reggiani 'Drilling Eugenics into Peoples' Minds' in Susan Currell and Christina Cogdell, *Popular Eugenics* (Athens: Ohio University Press, 2006).

is a credo that has surprises for the materialist as well as the spiritualists, for the pessimist as well as the optimist.

This alerted the reader to the book's unusual content. It even hinted that the publishers were distancing themselves from his views.

The Text

Carrel dedicated his book to three of the inner group of the 'Philosophers' — Frederic R. Coudert, Boris A. Bakhmeteff and Cornelius Clifford. Human biology features only in the middle chapters and instead Carrel was keen to enter quite different areas, or rather one area in particular. His arresting agenda in the Preface makes his intentions clear:

> Men cannot follow modern civilisation along its present course, because they are degenerating. ... We are beginning to realise the weakness of our civilisation.

Carrel was coming out as a 'declinist', and the book was largely a declinist agenda. It was a crowded space, but he was soon to emerge as a major spokesman. Carrel considered that mankind, far from evolving and advancing, had gone backwards, and that some restorative action was necessary. To him, this degeneration was a given, a crisis which was self-evident, one well known to the reader. Like others, he blamed the rise of science and technology for creating a world into which man no longer fitted. The sorcerer's apprentice had created something that was out of control. If the reader accepted that there was a crisis, it then followed that 'something had to be done', and Carrel had a unique and personal solution. Mankind must look to scientists for the necessary action to halt and reverse civilisation's decline. For this, new study of man was needed, and a new type of institute was required to support those who would make these studies. This broad approach might be called Carrelism — science has given us the problem, and now a proper scientific study of man will get the human race out of the mess. To this he added a call for spiritual renewal.

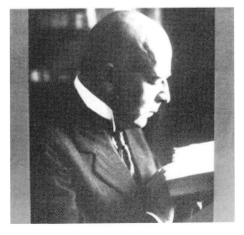

Carrel's diagnosis of the 'cultural decline' of Western civilisation was first suggested by the German philosopher Oswald Spengler. (*Wikipedia*)

The Interwar Declinists

To put the book in context, Carrel was one of many Jeremiahs active in the interwar period announcing an international crisis — political, economic, biological and spiritual:

> Just as a crowd gathers dismayed but fascinated to watch a disastrous fire, so the interwar intelligentsia wanted to be at the front of the throng of onlookers if civilisation crashed. ... One writer after another competed to explain the nature of the current malaise, and publishers and the public colluded with them.[10]

Carrel's book contains an eclectic mix of the views of like-minded doomniks. Early concern had come from the German philosopher Friedrich

---

[10] From Richard Overy, *The Twilight Years* (London: Viking, 2009): 29.

Nietzsche, who, after famously declaring that 'God is dead', concluded that there was no way back and no way forward either — a gloomy impasse. American contributions started with Madison Grant's *The Passing of the Great Race* (1916), and the anxiety was spread by Oswald Spengler's *Decline of the West* (1918), pointing to a natural cycle of national vitality which, turning inexorably, destroyed each civilisation in turn, and hence that the end was nigh for the West. In Britain, T.S. Eliot's celebrated poem *The Waste Land* of 1922 described the post-war 'sense of desolation, of uncertainty, of futility, of the groundlessness of aspirations, of the vanity of endeavour'. In New York, Raymond B. Fosdick, holding a senior position at the Rockefeller Foundation brought out his *The Old Savage in the New Civilisation*, mentioned earlier, making the point again that modern man was lost in the world he had created. Psychiatrists added their gloomy thoughts, and after Freud announced a widespread malaise in his *Civilisation and Its Discontents* (1930), Carl Jung agreed in his *Modern Man in Search for a Soul* (1933), also suggesting that the modern mind was deeply troubled. Since the concern was often for possible biological deterioration as well as political or economic decay, many observers used medical metaphors of illness, diagnosis and treatment — picturing the body politic as under attack from within, and heading for death.[11] Even Harvey Cushing joined the declinist camp, believing that there should be a rethink within the scientific community:

> So let us hope that when some future student of this confused and disconcerting period in our history comes to tell of it, he will be able to say: ... the scientists and engineers of the country temporarily abandoned the investigations dear to their heart in order to concentrate on problems the most difficult of all to solve — those that have to do with the social well-being of the community at large.[12]

To the declinists, the human predicament was considered to be self-evident, and it was seldom necessary to give evidence for the diagnosis

---

[11] For these metaphors, see Robert Nye, *Crime, Madness and Politics in Modern France: the Medical Concept of National Decline* (Princeton, N.J.: Princeton University Press, 1984).
[12] Harvey Cushing (1935) 'The humanising of science' *Science* 82: 70–1.

before urging possible treatments. When any evidence of national decline was offered, it varied from nation to nation. In Britain, where eugenic thinking had its first airing through Galton's teachings, the alarm was over the relative demographic decline of the 'superior classes', who bred less vigorously than the rest of society. In Europe, an overall fall in population numbers was the main concern and in America, the critics pointed to immigration and an increasing presence of the allegedly 'unfit' as holding back the nation.

Optimists were few. Aldous Huxley's *Brave New World* (1932) was not an entirely dystopian vision, since in his imagined world, science had brought both good and bad. Karl Marx (a Prussian who moved to France) believed that mankind was steadily moving on the road to a desirable political triumph. Henri Bergson, the French philosopher known to Carrel, identified an *élan vital* which drove favourable human change, and the Jesuit philosopher and theologian Pierre Teilhard de Chardin also taught that the human race was heading towards a bright end point — his 'Omega Point'. In America, Nobel Prize-winning physicist Robert Millikan was optimistic and in his *Science and the New Civilisation* he confidently considered that man does adapt quickly to new circumstances and new technology.

Carrel's Book

After his gloomy Prologue, some chapters on human biology follow later, but there are no accompanying images, nor any list of sources or suggestions for further reading. He neither mentions scientists by name regularly nor dwells much on individual discoveries. There are the dogmatic statements that his friends knew so well. When Carrel soon returns to his main agenda of decline and degeneration, he uses the urgent language of an evangelist or the rhetoric of a politician. Carrel's writing is assertive, using the French style of short emphatic sentences and the 'piquancy of aphorisms', as an otherwise hostile reviewer remarked.

In examining the book, some additional material can be included from his *Reflections on Life*, written as a sequel immediately after publishing

Man, the Unknown. Reflections covered much the same ground, but with even greater conviction.[13]

Degeneracy Explained

Carrel was convinced that the Western nations were in decline — physical, mental and moral — and he does offer some evidence. In claiming a physical decline in the West, he accepts that people are taller than before but takes the view that this has come at a price. He states that 'the better the physique of children, the worse their state'. 'Increased height', he says, gives a 'lack of resistance of the nervous system, decreased alertness and slow intelligence'. He then points to great men who were small in stature, notably Napoleon and Mussolini.[14] Any gain in general physique he also sees as a problem, since 'athletes have small brains' and 'do not live long'. He adds that the dinosaurs became extinct because their brains were too small for the enlarged body.[15]

The decrease in infant mortality in the developed nations was generally regarded as a good thing, but Carrel did not share this view, taking the stance favoured by 'social Darwinists', namely that weakly infants should not survive, since they are a burden: 'Medicine has extended its beneficent influence to the weak, the defective, those predisposed to microbial infections, to all who formerly could not endure.'[16]

He also considers that living longer might also be in vain. Men were not growing old gracefully, he says, and some new seniors could be

---

[13] *Réflexions sur la conduite de la vie* was eventually published posthumously in France in 1952, with an English translation *Reflections on Life* (London: Hamish Hamilton, 1965), but the book was largely ignored. Some material can be taken here from *Reflections* to assist with displaying Carrel's thinking in the 1930s. In *Reflections* Carrel's views on women are less extreme, the proof of telepathy is emphasised, and there are many more references to God; Mme Carrel may have posthumously adjusted his text.

[14] Mussolini, of short stature like Carrel, is praised three times in *MTU* (note 9): 62, 220–62.

[15] Carrel, *MTU* (note 9): 19, 122.

[16] Carrel, *MTU* (note 9): 16, 268.

344   *The First Transplant Surgeon*

'pseudo-young men, who play tennis and dance as [if] at 20 years, ... [thus they are] liable to softening of the brain'.[17] Nor does the young man of the day please him — 'rude, slovenly, unshaven, slouching about with hands in his pockets and a cigarette in the corner of his mouth'.[18]

Unable to show physical decline, Carrel is clear that average intelligence had declined in America because

> the lower classes of prolific nations, the very 'canaille' [riff-raff] of Europe were imported into this country to satisfy the imperative demands of industry. And the common man became unintelligent, corrupt, incapable of self-government.[19]

Mental Decay

Carrel places great emphasis on an alleged decline in the mental health of the West. He says that the American asylums were overflowing with the 'feebleminded, the morons, and the insane', using the chilling terms 'sub-human' or 'sub-men', and he adds epileptics to his list of those burdening the nation. He then asks the question: 'Is an idiot a human being?'[20] Modern man, says Carrel, still using his non-scientific fuzzy terminology, now has a 'delicate nervous system', one lacking the 'equilibrium' which is needed to prevent 'soft flabby minds'. Carrel has hopes however, since he knows that 'in the communities where moral sense and intelligence are simultaneously developed, criminality and insanity are rare'.[21]

Changes in Food and Drink

However, his criticisms of dietary changes still read well. He notes wryly that in the West 'human beings have never been fed so punctually

---

[17] Carrel, *MTU* (note 9): 178.
[18] Carrel, *Reflections* (note 13): 95.
[19] Carrel's draft for an unpublished book quoted in Joseph T. Durkin, *Hope for Our Time: Alexis Carrel on Man and Society* (New York: Harper and Row, 1965): 77.
[20] Carrel, *Reflections* (note 13): 25.
[21] Carrel, *MTU* (note 9): 146.

and uninterrupted'. He dislikes white bread, sugar, tea, coffee, chemical fertilisers, battery hens, and refined cereals.[22] Children's diets have changed for the worse, and bland diets are bad because the jaws no longer need to work; children, he says, should instead be given stale bread and tough meat. He dislikes smoking and drinking, adding the claim that 'France is the nation which drinks most wine and least often wins Nobel Prizes'.[23] He blames alcohol for much mental illness and agrees with a story that drunkenness on part of either man or woman at the moment of conception causes mental illness in the child.[24] He sensibly comments that people do not exercise or walk enough. But his advice is to avoid the usual sports, and he does not like golf, particularly for women. Instead, he patriotically recommends the outdoor gymnastic exercises of Hébert.[25]

Life is too comfortable and has hidden threats since

> weakened by central heating, heated automobiles, and wind and water-proof clothing, free of hard labour, famine and adverse climate, personal effort and moral discipline has gone. The result is not only weakness but an inability to adapt to adversity, since the lack of stressors had numbed the protective responses.[26]

Disease Mechanisms

In his view of disease he shows a remarkable conversion from medical orthodoxy to become an advocate of constitutional and holistic medicine. He now rejects the Institute's reductionist biology. He deplores that

---

[22] Carrel, *MTU* (note 9): 13, 14, 25, 116; see also Carrel, *Reflections* (note 13): 165.

[23] France had in fact done quite well for Nobel Prizes at this time, with awards for Charles Richet (1913), Charles Nicolle (1928), Marie Curie (1903 and 1911), Irène Curie (1935) and Carrel's philosopher friend Henri Bergson in 1927. Carrel also claimed a dismal French standing as regards philanthropists and athletes.

[24] Carrel, *Reflections* (note 13): 101. This 'bad science' idea and its emergence is amusingly dealt with by De Kruif in *Our Medicine Men* (New York: The Century Co., 1922): 145–9.

[25] *Reflections* (note 13): 97. Hébert opposed static gymnastic exercises, instead favouring 30 minutes training over an varied outdoor course.

[26] Carrel, *MTU* (note 9): 219 and Carrel, *Reflections* (note 13): 41.

we still regard the human being to be a poorly constructed machine, whose parts must be constantly reinforced or repaired. ... [In disease] we must help this whole to perform its functions efficiently rather than intervene ourselves in the work of each organ. Some individuals are immune to infectious and degenerative diseases, and to the decay of senescence. We have to learn their secret.[27]

Carrel considered that the outcome of illness can be predicted by 'a precise analysis of the organic, humoral and psychological personality of the individual'.[28] He invokes susceptibility to disease of the different 'biotypes', the various body habitus classifications in the 1920s — including the asthenic (liable to tuberculosis) and the picnic (liable to diabetes and rheumatism). Holistic medicine at the time emphasised that the mind and body are linked, and hence 'psychosomatic' disease was possible, with organic disease following mental disturbance. Carrel agreed:

The lack of equilibrium and the neuroses of the visceral nervous system [autonomic nervous system] bring about many affections of the stomach and intestines.[29] Colitis and the accompanying infections of the kidneys and bladder are the remote results of mental and moral imbalance, even causing chronic kidney disease. Such diseases are almost unknown in social groups where life is simpler ... .[30]

Social Decay

Family life is in crisis, according to Carrel, since

modern parents know nothing about the psychology of childhood and youth. They are too naïve, too neurotic, too weak or too stern. One could say that the majority of them cultivate the art of producing defects in their children.

---

[27] Carrel, *MTU* (note 9): 313. For criticism of Jaques Loeb, see pp. 4, 40 and 108.
[28] Carrel, *MTU* (note 9): 248.
[29] Carrel, *MTU* (note 9): 115, 313.
[30] Carrel, *MTU* (note 9): 146.

Carrel notes that the nations are also held back by some bad day-to-day habits, like

> endless chattering; card-playing; dancing; rushing about endlessly in motor-cars — all these reduce the intelligence. ... we are helpless against the invasion of our homes by the din of next-door radios or drinking parties.[31]

Carrel even detects moral harm in day-to-day human discourse

> such as the love of denigration and lying; delight in duplicity, a taste for sophistry, verbosity, verbalism and witty backbiting. This spiritual immoderation is almost as dangerous as the ridiculous pleasure of excessive drinking.[32]

His other targets for reform include the 'vulgar' radio, gramophone records and the cinema.[33] In Scrooge mode, he deplores the 'idiotic agitation of Christmas Eve. The people seem struck with folly. They hurl themselves into the shopping-centre'.

Environmental Degeneration

Carrel is on surer ground in his sections on the environment. Like many Frenchmen at the time, he did not like American cities and deplores that:

> The modern city consists of a monstrous edifices, of dark narrow streets full of gasoline fumes, coal dust and toxic gases, torn by the noise of taxicabs, trucks and cars, and thronged ceaselessly by great crowds.[34]... The environment which has moulded the body and soul of our ancestors during many millenniums is now being replaced by another. Science and technology is making life pleasanter but is leaving the body defenceless.[35]

---

[31] Carrel, *Reflections* (note 13): 106.
[32] Carrel, *Reflections* (note 13): 33.
[33] Carrel, *MTU* (note 9): 12, 152, and Carrel, *Reflections* (note 13): 33.
[34] Carrel, *MTU* (note 9): 25.
[35] Carrel, *MTU* (note 9): 27.

Carrel also regrets the grind of factory life and supports regulations on health in the workplace. He has sensible ideas on house and factory design to allow better living and working conditions:

> In the organisation of industrial life, the influence of the factory upon the physiological and mental state of the workers has been completely neglected. Modern industry is based on the conception of the maximum production at lowest cost, in order that an individual or a group of individuals may earn as much money as possible. … Our life is influenced in large measure by commercial advertising. Such publicity is undertaken only in the interest of the advertisers and not to the consumers.[36]

Elsewhere in his writings he was concerned about the growing availability of information:

> Through modern 'gadgets' man is ever in contact with his relatives, his friends, his business associates, with all his affairs, not only of the town, but of the nations and whole world. Such unceasing, painful awareness of an environment infinitely too large to be comprehended by human intelligence has led to dispersion, worry, nervous and mental instability.[37]

Moral Degeneration

'Man is not free to live according to his own fancy,' says Carrel, and the result is degeneracy from this absence of 'moral restraint'.[38] He states that the number of homosexuals is increasing and that churchgoing is falling. Then, perhaps surprisingly, he states that the churches, notably the Roman Catholic Church, have also decayed: 'Ministers have rationalised religion. They have destroyed its mystical basis. In their half-empty churches, they vainly preach a weak morality.' Nor do scientists escape his displeasure, since they are now 'a profession like those of the schoolteacher, the clergyman, and the bank clerk'.

---

[36] Carrel, *MTU* (note 9): 25.
[37] Unpublished draft, Carrel Papers, box 38 folder 65, GULBFC (note 1).
[38] Carrel, *MTU* (note 9): 153.

Those to blame for the decline in the West include politicians, since it is the 'intellectual and moral deficiencies of the political leaders, and their ignorance, which endanger modern nations'.[39] Among this general indictment of politicians, there is one exception — it is Mussolini again — of whose 'strong leadership of a great nation' Carrel approves. In an aside, he says 'democracy has contributed to the collapse of civilisation in opposing the development of an élite ... everywhere the weak are preferred to the strong'.[40]

Racial Factors

In explaining the degeneration he diagnoses, Carrel claims that the West had an increasing proportion of citizens of the wrong sort. Carrel has no time for 'southern Europeans', and instead takes the view that the northern 'blue-eyed, fair-haired' race is naturally superior. Carrel also deplores the rising numbers of black and brown citizens of the world, and warns of the 'yellow peril' as a threat to the West from the Orient. Turning to lessons from the classical world, Carrel sees a warning to the West in the fall of Rome, and he has a confident analysis. The Roman pursuit of luxury, eating, drinking and chariot racing, plus the promotion of yellow, brown and black slaves to positions of power, caused the disaster.

Still looking for explanatory weaknesses and culprits in the West, Carrel identifies women as a problem, and he treats them as a group without any diversity. His complaint is that women are now working, instead of staying at home, having babies, and building up a 'better stock' of offspring. Of women he says:

> Motherhood is the only role in which she excels. In medicine, teaching, science, philosophy, aviation or business, she is nearly always man's inferior.[41]... Mothers abandon children to kindergartens to attend to their careers, their social ambitions, their sexual pleasures, their literary

---

[39] Carrel, *MTU* (note 9): 262.
[40] Carrel, *MTU* (note 9): 271.
[41] Carrel, *Reflections* (note 13): 99.

fancies, or simply play bridge, go to the cinema, and waste their time in busy idleness. … Women voluntarily deteriorate through alcohol and tobacco. They subject themselves to dangerous dietary regimens in order to obtain a conventional slenderness of the figure. Besides, they refuse to bear children. … [who] would, in all probability, be of good quality.[42]

Dating the Decline

Before looking at his remedies for the widespread deterioration he identifies, his chronology of the decay is of interest. Carrel was not, like an evangelist, seeking to rescue man from original sin, nor followed most other declinists who timed the onset of decline to the Industrial Revolution. Carrel has a surprise for the reader: he picks a much earlier point, namely the era when science first started to influence man's world. He holds the Age of Enlightenment as responsible for mankind's woes. Matters, he says, went downhill after Galileo measured things and in particular, when Descartes separated mind from body. Claude Bernard, though admired as a fellow-countryman, 'wrongly reduced man to a machine'.[43] Also responsible were 'the philosophers who enthroned this blind cult of liberty in Europe and America'.[44] The American Declaration of Independence was an error, he considers, as were the Declaration of the Rights of Man and the French Revolution. Carrel indicts the French Revolution on a second count, since the executions got rid of a valuable gene pool belonging to the aristocrats. However, he says, all is not lost — some of these valuable genes are still around and are recoverable.

His Remedies

Having made a confident diagnosis of decline, listed the manifestations and dated the onset, Carrel is equally clear on what has to be done.

---

[42] Carrel, *MTU* (note 9): 299.
[43] Carrel, *MTU* (note 9): 37, 279.
[44] Carrel, *Reflections* (note 13): 17.

'Science' can step in, and by studying man and man's behaviour, can analyse what went wrong:

> For the first time in the history of humanity, a crumbling civilisation is capable of discerning the causes of its decay. For the first time, it has at its disposal the gigantic strength of science.[45]

By 'science' he does not mean laboratory studies but observational (operational) and sociological studies. Once a study of man's activity is completed and the defects identified, then action would follow. It is a technocratic plan. However, Carrel is not prepared to wait and has made up his mind on a large number of issues, and he goes on to list what must be done. Carrel uses the word 'must' a lot.

Physical Remedies

The race, Carrel says, needs to toughen up. Life in the West is too soft. The defects in diet he identified, such as refined cereals, must be reversed. He recalls that, of old, there were two kinds of diet. The great men

> who fought, commanded and conquered, used chiefly meats and fermented drinks, whereas the peaceful, the weak, and the submissive were satisfied with milk, vegetables, fruits and cereals.[46]

To add to this, Carrel says periods of fasting and sexual abstinence are a good thing, although he knows that great men are strongly sexed.[47] Other advice is less clear: 'Man sleeps too much or not enough'. And there are other dangers — 'food too elaborate or too poor' causes mental illness.[48]

---

[45] Carrel, *MTU* (note 9): 321.

[46] Carrel, *MTU* (note 9): 87.

[47] Carrel, *MTU* (note 9): 143, 307.

[48] Carrel, *MTU* (note 9): 158, 229. These are not necessarily Carrelian contradictions, since his new neo-Hippocratic thinking blamed disease on lifestyle excesses in any direction. A holistic physician's consultation looked for a lifestyle excess, and advised their patient to do the opposite, thus restoring the body's 'natural harmony'.

Spiritual Reform

The separation of mind and body has left the human race disadvantaged, Carrel says, and caring for the body alone in health and times of disease had been a mistake. Concerned for man's spiritual health, he supports the religious observance of old:

> Christianity, above all, has given a clear-cut answer to the demands of the human soul. For centuries, it has calmed the restless curiosity that men have always felt about their destiny.

God is only briefly mentioned in his book, but his existence is nowhere denied. Carrel does not exclude a role for other faiths and has no suggestions for reforming the organised religions in the developed nations of the West. However, he does call for a return to the life of mysticism,

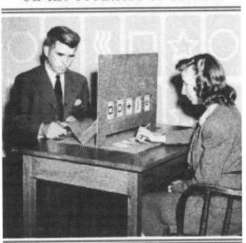

Joseph B. Rhine's parapsychology department at Duke University, admired by Carrel, claimed to have found scientific proof of telepathic mechanisms.

contemplation and personal prayer. Prayer should be repeated during the day, in an area provided in the work place, but it is far from clear where the prayer is directed.[49] In lauding the power of prayer, it is not clear if God is being invoked or whether Carrel merely considered that intense supplication empowers a person toward desired ends. In prescribing a return to this mysticism he says:

> There have been great inspired ones, who, by a phenomenon analogous to telepathy, have put themselves in contact with a force that is one and the same time immanent to and transcending the universe.[50]

In supporting the existence of these transcendental forces, he urges that telepathy and clairvoyance should be further studied with scientific methods. Carrel cites support for these mechanisms from a fellow Nobel Prize winner, the French immunologist Charles Richet.[51] Carrel was also confident that Joseph Rhine at Duke University had succeeded in identifying these phenomena:

> Rhine's now classic experimental and statistical study of telepathy and clairvoyance leaves no doubt that there are mental processes which bear no relation to known mechanisms and which are independent of space and possibly of time.[52]

---

[49] Carrel, *MTU* (note 9): 135.

[50] Carrel, *MTU* (note 9): 133–6.

[51] Carrel, *MTU* (note 9): 124. Richet was active in the Paris Institute Metapsychique International and the British Society for Psychical Research, organisations which credulously reported on the activities of some of the celebrated mediums and psychics of the day, mostly eventually shown to be frauds; see M. Brady Brower, *Unruly Spirits: the Science of Psychic Phenomena in Modern France* (Urbana: University of Illinois Press, 2010).

[52] Carrel, *MTU* (note 9): 123–4 and Carrel, *Reflections* (note 13): 139, 144, 152. Joseph B. Rhine (1895–1980) published his popular *New Frontiers of the Mind* from Duke University's Parapsychology Department in 1937 and described subjects who, under controlled conditions, allegedly demonstrated extra-sensory perception (ESP). This department had initial respectability in academia, but their work was later discredited and the department closed.

To add to the case for the existence of these elusive mechanisms and the power of prayer, Carrel, as always, brings in as evidence the cures he witnessed at Lourdes.[53] Harnessing these powers, he says, is crucial for the future of the West.

More Remedies

Running ahead of future findings from his new 'science of man', he has proposals for changes in marriage law, the family, leisure, criminal punishment, housing, health, public entertainment and the publishing industry. He already has an advance agenda for the future of education. After making international comparisons, he pinpoints the problem as the 'defective educational systems in place in the democracies, and under fascism and communism which all hinder human development'. His new system will start in childhood:

> There must be effective censorship of the cinema and the radio. The majority of dance halls, cinemas and bars should be closed, the periodical article literature which children and young people so eagerly devour needs to be radically transformed. Once this purifying process has been accomplished, it will be necessary to proceed to the education of parents and teachers.[54]

He notes that others had already embarked on reform, and Mussolini's Italy again is admired:

> Unless we emulate certain worthwhile features of fascist education — notably their discipline and utilisation of every waking hour   we shall be no match for the tougher products which result from such education.[55]

Carrel liked the philosopher Bergson's ideas on time and hence proposed that any child's developmental age should be considered as

---

[53] Carrel, *MTU* (note 9): 148 and Carrel, *Reflections* (note 13): 147.
[54] Carrel, *Reflections* (note 13): 172.
[55] Alexis Carrel 'Work in the laboratory of your private life' *Readers Digest*, September 1940.

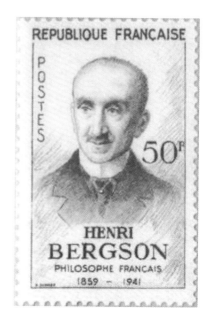

Carrel knew the French philosopher Bergson
and used his views on time and intuition.

different from their chronological age. In boys, he seeks masculine, even
military qualities — 'manliness, and the audacity to fight, to love and to
conquer' — and two years of military national service would follow
school days. Other proposals were directed to producing an elite. He
wants to segregate some bright boys early in life and teach them in special
schools to be leaders.[56] For girls, schooling is instead to be towards the
needs of marriage, childbearing and a life in the home.[57] He has no
interest in higher education, having a low opinion of universities and
their academics.

The successful effects of these educational changes, and his other
reforms, would be passed on because:

> Environment stamps human beings with its mark... . Thus, new
> structural and mental aspects appear in the individual and in the race.
> It seems that environment gradually affects the cells of the sexual

---

[56] Carrel, *MTU* (note 9): 48, 269, 297, 302.
[57] Carrel, *MTU* (note 9): 22, 90, 153, 270 and Carrel, *Reflections* (note 13): 100.

glands. Such modifications are naturally hereditary. ... Opinion today tends to admit that this environmental influence is more or less transmissible ... the children of a man who has cultivated his intelligence will be more intelligent than if the father had remained uneducated.

This is Carrel's hope that acquired characteristics could be transmitted to future generations, revealing again his Lamarckian leanings, a system by then almost abandoned in Western genetics.[58]

Marriage and Women

Carrel's view is that marriage 'should not be for love or sexual attraction but for good heredity' and should produce more children of 'the right sort ... higher types'.[59] He even advocates restoring the dowry system, since 'it brings filial respect'. In his support for these positive eugenic measures, the old elites could be useful, he says, since 'in the aristocratic families of Europe there are also individuals of great vitality'.[60] In his affection for other aspects of a bygone age, Carrel adds a bucolic anti-modern extra vision: 'The family must be rooted once more in the soil. Everyone should be able to have a house, however small, and make himself a garden.'[61]

---

[58] Carrel's leanings towards Lamarckism in *MTU* are clear; see pp. 180, 215. For the French geneticists' unusual acceptance of Lamarckism at the time, see William H. Schneider, *Quality and Quantity: The Quest for Biological Regeneration in Twentieth-Century France* (Cambridge: Cambridge University Press, 1990). The leading American Lamarckian was William McDougall at Harvard, who claimed that maze-running skills learned in rats could be passed on to their progeny.

[59] Carrel, *Reflections* (note 13): 15, 100.

[60] Carrel, *MTU* (note 9): 297.

[61] Carrel, *Reflections* (note 13): 113. Carrel visited Henry Ford at Detroit in 1928, introduced by Roy McClure, the young Hopkins-trained surgeon in charge of Ford's company hospital, and who spent time earlier with Carrel in New York. Carrel at first considered Ford to be 'a mystic, a scientist, a leader of men'. Carrel strangely does not mention Ford in *MTU*, although Ford had constructed villages offering his workers leisure and land to enable self-sufficiency.

Carrel is here approving the agenda of 'anti-modern' movements in the industrialised nations. Claiming that society was over-civilised, they indulged in *nostalgie de la boue*, a longing for a simpler primitive life. This group was ill-defined but within it

> Aesthetes and reformers sought to recover the hard but satisfying life of the medieval craftsmen; militarists urged the rekindling of archaic martial vigour; religious doubters yearned for the fierce convictions of the peasant and the ecstasies of the mystic.[62]

For Carrel, life before the Enlightenment, being science-free, was a 'Golden Age', and there were other blessings. Mediaeval life was overseen by a wise local aristocracy in cooperation with the mother Church:

> The spire which rose above the village was a true symbol of aspiration of the human community towards the divine ... [which] kept our medieval ancestors in a hitherto unparalleled state of spiritual and social stability.[63]

'Isolats'

Carrel suggests that there are still some isolated communities that, having escaped the ills of the modern world, live in Arcadian bliss. He adduces the case of the Doukhobors, who were persecuted in Europe and, exiled to Canada in 1897, settled in Manitoba and Saskatchewan, retaining their ancient lifestyle.[64] However, Carrel also admits that the small Brittany villages which he knew well have their problems, notably inbreeding, alcoholism and feeblemindedness. He predicts that Brittany, unless it reforms, will be 'sooner or later replaced by biologically stronger races. The

---

[62] T. J. Jackson Lears, *No Place of Grace: Antimoderism and the Transformation of American Culture* (New York: Pantheon Books, 1981): xiii.

[63] Carrel, *MTU* (note 9): 295, 298. A more usual view is that in mediaeval times, life for the ordinary people was short and unpleasant.

[64] Carrel's praise for the Doukhobors (*MTU*, note 9 p. 298) proved unfortunate, since shortly after, internal rivalry, including arson and bombing attacks, led to dispersal of their communities.

newer methods of 'swift deportation' would allow eradication to be complete'.[65]

The 'Unfit'

To add to his positive eugenics aimed at increasing the numbers of the right type of humans, he also supports negative eugenics, namely prevention of the birth of 'unfit' children. This strategy is not aimed only at the underclass, since Carrel also aims at dealing with hereditary disease. He still shared the simplistic view of the eugenicists, soon to be discarded, that a raft of serious, common diseases, including cancer, tuberculosis, epilepsy and mental disease, ran in families through inheritance. Carrel suggests:

> Wretchedness is in store for those who marry into families contaminated by syphilis, cancer, tuberculosis, insanity or feeblemindedness. Obviously those who are afflicted … should not marry.[66]

He suggests marriage control since Carrel, like the Catholic Church, did not support sterilisation as a eugenic measure, although it was already in use in some European nations. Denmark used compulsory sterilisation from 1929. In Germany, a late starter, the total sterilised would be about 360,000, and in America, after the Supreme Court *Buck vs Bell* legitimised compulsory sterilisation of the mentally retarded, California's 60,000 was the greatest number of state sterilisations. These American state programmes slowly ceased after World War II.[67]

Euthanasia

Carrel has firm proposals to deal with some forms of criminality, and a return to flogging was one of them. Another appears in the most notorious passage in *Man, the Unknown*:

---

[65] *Reflections* (note 13): 97.
[66] Carrel, *MTU* (note 9): 300.
[67] The 7,600 sterilised in North Carolina from 1929–1974 included criminals, the sexual promiscuous and epileptics. In 2012, the governor brought in a compensation scheme for the 1,500 still living.

Those who have murdered, robbed while armed with automatic pistol or machine gun, kidnapped children, despoiled the poor of their savings, misled the public in important matters, should be humanely and economically disposed of in small euthanasic institutions supplied with proper gases. A similar treatment could be advantageously applied to the insane, guilty of criminal acts.[68]

This was not just another form of capital punishment for serious offences. Instead, he is suggesting that the mentally ill who had committed low-level crime, which ordinarily did not attract a death sentence, should be killed. Chillingly, his extermination units would be an add-on to the usual correctional institutions. Elsewhere Carrel adds to his indications for euthanasia. He suggests that sustained 'dysgenism' (i.e. producing numerous 'undesirable' offsprings) constitutes 'a capital offence'.[69] Elsewhere he floats the idea of culling human babies, 'like puppies, as did the Greeks at the time of Pericles,' but this, he points out, cannot be introduced.[70]

Military Strength

According to Carrel, in man's natural state, 'might is right':

Strength is the only thing that allows man to rise higher. In the eyes of nature, it is the supreme virtue while weakness is the worst vice. The weak are destined to perish, for life loves only the strong.[71]

He then pays tribute to those who sacrificed their lives for their beliefs:

In the noblest, the struggle always ends in submission to that law of life that is peculiar to man. Socrates drank hemlock: St. Paul was beheaded: they burnt Joan of Arc at the stake. Each time a whole level of humanity

---

[68] Carrel, *MTU* (note 9): 318. Death by gassing was pioneered at the Battersea Dog Home in London from 1884. Others at Carrel's time proposing human use of the gas chambers included the British fascist Major-General J.F.C. Fuller in his book, *The Dragon's Teeth: a Study of War and Peace* (London: Constable, 1932).

[69] Carrel, *Reflections* (note 13): 87.

[70] Carrel, *MTU* (note 9): 296.

[71] Carrel, *Reflections* (note 13): 96.

was raised. Today it is the heroes and the martyrs who advance life further along that mysterious way on which it set out from its beginning.[72]

Islam

By this point in *Man, the Unknown*, a comparison with Islamic thought and practice is irresistible. When consolidating Carrel's views, the similarities to Muslim attitudes become quite marked. He favours a return to the mystical and spiritual life, advocates frequent daily prayer and a society under firm control of a non-democratic, learned hierarchy. His view of the role of women is distinctly Muslim. His admiration for martyrdom supporting a cause is jihadist. It is ironic that Carrel's writings and lectures warned that the white races of the West were endangered by various 'yellow perils', yet his agenda for survival was not to strengthen Western culture and democracy. Instead, it was to return to much of the ancient ways of the barbarians who he claimed were at the gate.[73]

His Institute

To deal with degenerate mankind, Carrel seeks to set up an organisation which would study the human race, and after a 'synthesis' of the findings coming from all relevant disciplines, it would work out solutions for the salvation of the Western world. Experts would run the new body, a 'composite Aristotle', as he calls it, and in this Carrel was following a long line of similar worthy proposals, notably by Plato in his *Republic*, Salomon's House as envisaged by Francis Bacon (which led to the foundation of London's Royal Society) and by Thomas Moore in his *Utopia*.[74] In Carrel's plan, the institute would be led by an elite group of 100 'Founders' overseen by a council of seven. These experts would be

---

[72] Carrel, *Reflections* (note 13): 70, 80.
[73] Contemporary Islamists and neo-paganists have noted Carrel's book with interest — see Chapter 19.
[74] For a survey of utopian thinking, see René Dubos, *The Dreams of Reason: Science and Utopias* (New York: Columbia University Press, 1961).

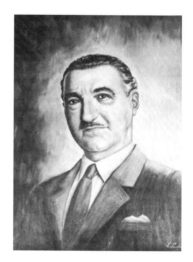

Carrel admired Nicola Pende's proposals for human engineering in fascist Italy. (*Portrait by V. Laudadio.*)

talented 'Renaissance men' capable of synthesising knowledge, and on special issues women might be consulted. The men would work together in monastic seclusion:

> These gifted individuals who dedicate themselves to this work will have to renounce common modes of existence. They will not be able to play golf and bridge, to go to cinemas, to listen to radios, to make speeches at banquets, to serve on committees, to attend meetings of scientific societies, political conventions and academies, or to cross the ocean and take part in international congresses. They must live like the monks of the great contemplative orders, and not like University professors.[75]

Carrel wants study of all

> the subjects pertaining to the physical, chemical, structural, functional and psychological activities of man, and to the relations of those activities with the cosmic and social environment.

---

[75] Carrel, *MTU* (note 9): 285. In Sinclair Lewis's novel *Arrowsmith*, the hero finally retreats to the solitude of the backwoods to obtain proper research conditions.

He perhaps surprisingly additionally praises 'the supreme science, psychology, which needs the methods and concepts of physiology, anatomy, mechanics, chemistry, physical chemistry, physics and mathematics'.[76] This attempt to prioritise psychology is exactly what the Rockefeller Foundation, led by Fosdick, was attempting to do at that time.[77] Carrel felt that human emotions like love and hatred produced physiological changes which could be measured, and hence understood. Added to this he proposes that the human mind had undiscovered capabilities, like telepathy, which could be detected and improved by training, and assist a return to an improved spiritual life.

Administratively, Carrel is unclear about how to fund his institute, but he thinks that some governments might be supportive and even hand over power:

> In Italy, Germany or Russia, if the dictator judged it useful to condition children according to a different type, to modify the adults in their ways of life in a different manner, appropriate institutions would spring up at once. ... [it] would provide knowledge for democratic rulers as well as dictators, but would be able to impose, by either persuasion or force, changes in civilisation.[78]

Carrel had in mind that Mussolini had supported the Italian biologist Nicola Pende, Rector of the University of Bari, who from the mid-1930s ran his Istituto di bonificia umana ed ortogenesi della razza ('Institute for the Study of the Human Individual'). Pende sought racial improvement, and hoped that in this way the greatness of ancient Rome would be restored.[79] Pende, later disgraced, is one of the few contemporary scientists praised in Carrel's book.[80]

---

[76] Carrel, *MTU* (note 9): 290.

[77] Raymond B. Fosdick, *Wanted: an Aristotle* (New York: Elbert Print, 1924).

[78] Carrel, *MTU* (note 9): 286.

[79] Aaron Gillette, *Racial Theories in Fascist Italy* (London: Routledge, 2002).

[80] Carrel, *MTU* (note 9): 288. Nicola Pende (1860–1970) joined the Italian fascists and became a senator in 1932. He later supported antisemitism in fascist Italy and was an (allegedly reluctant) signatory to the notorious 'Manifesto of Racial Scientists' of 1938

In summary, *Man, the Unknown* has some rather ordinary biology content, which is awkwardly mixed into an eclectic collection of the gloomy bio-political ideas then current in the unsettled interwar period. Added to this are many personal prejudices and support for some of the dubious sciences of the day. The tone of the book is serious and assertive: there are no anecdotes or humour.[81] Carrel, like an evangelist, declares that man, or rather the white races, have fallen, but can be saved, and he has proposals for action. Science and technology have given the modern world comforts, but also added defects, and he says that flawed human beings are thriving, deficient in both body and mind. He offers help to reverse the decay by setting up a cadre of monk-like experts who would do a thorough study of man, and who will then tell the Western nations what must be done. Although it is unfair to judge his book without reference to the *zeitgeist* of the times, it remains unappealing.

Publication

The New York publishers had distributed review copies widely. A helpful review appeared quickly in the *New York Herald-Tribune* and Harper and Brothers could include it with their direct mailing of regular customers. It read:

> This is a rich and well-written book, full of information and provocative speculation. It deals in original fashion with matters of unquestionable importance and timely interest. In some ways, it seems almost a work of genius and certainly, it shares the spaciousness, the surprising variety of outlook, and the brave disregard for currently accepted beliefs that distinguish great books. … Dr. Carrel is a scientific Jeremiah, but he is more than that. He has advice to offer that will be hard to follow, but may prove to be right.

---

as described in Carl Ipsen, *Dictating Democracy: the Problem of Population in Fascist Italy* (Cambridge: Cambridge University Press, 1996).

[81] There is one joke in *Reflections* (note 13: 136): 'An explorer set out from the Great Lakes in Canada hoping to reach China: by travelling, he at least discovered Chicago'.

The major medical journals usually noted the book in short polite notices, but *The Lancet* ignored it. Many other reviews appeared in a diversity of publications, and were at first supportive. Raymond Pearl, by then the authority on the biology of ageing, and who had been on the American Breeders' advisory Expert Committee, though cooling in his support for eugenics, spoke well of the book in the *New York Times*. Because of Carrel's wide-ranging themes, many niche organisations found something to interest them. Physical culturists and environmentalists were glad to have his support. The Roman Catholic religious journals were impressed by this call from a scientist to restore spiritual values and prayer, but the *Catholic World* noted the sparsity of references to God. Those supporting psychic phenomena were glad to have the scientist as 'one of us', and hailed the book as bringing in a 'new era in the attitude of scientists'. A Theosophist journal gave a supportive review, but deplored the biologists' need to do laboratory animal experiments, and the Rosicrucians liked the book and its mysticism. The humanists were pleased with his humanism, but disliked his call for a return to religion, and felt that Carrel 'has lent to many current superstitions the sanction of his great name'. The astrologers were unexpectedly unhappy, and their journal *American Astrology* said the text was more appropriate to 'the whoop-la of a civic money-raising campaign dinner'. The secretary of the New Jersey Sterilization League wrote giving their support to his eugenic proposals.

When the more important reviews came in, *Time* magazine suggested that the book might be a practical joke, calling him

> a sly mocker who delights in a wild rant. Whether his thesis of iatocracy [rule by doctors] was meant to be a colossal joke to fool members of his profession or whether he offered them in all seriousness … he alone knew.[82]

Other considered verdicts were usually negative. John F. Fulton, professor of physiology at Yale, in *The Saturday Review* noted 'platitudes

---

[82] *Time* magazine, 16 September 1935.

and extravagant statements'. He also disliked the idea of the new institute and was concerned whether 'men who have spent their lives in the sheltered walls of scientific institutions could ever be entrusted with the destiny of our social order'. Some reviewers used it as an opportunity for wit and sarcasm. A.J. Carlson, from the Hull Physiology Department in Chicago, where Carrel had worked, noticed

> the mysticism of religious cults, the dogmatism of dictators, the showmanship of Hollywood, and the froth of the seasoned raconteur at Greenwich Village cocktail parties. ... The author browses widely and naïvely.[83]

Other cutting comments came from Sir Arthur Keith in the *British Medical Journal* and, although his far-right leanings might have meant a sympathetic review, Carrel's book did not please him. Keith perceptively noticed that the attitudes in the book were similar to those of the misanthrope Alexander Carlyle in his *Sartor Resartus* (1836), since 'both were disgruntled men who suffer from mental astigmatism'. Keith went on that

> He [Carrel] wants to set up a junta of super experts ... aided by a voluntary fascist organisation — of a kind which has been so successful of late in Italy, Germany and Russia... . Those of us who believe that the art of healing can be advanced only by careful observation, clear-cut experiment, and sound reasoning will have Dr. Carrel cast in our teeth by charlatans, Christian Scientists and faith healers, who believe there is a shorter road.[84]

Mary Colum, the distinguished literary critic, acknowledged some insights but, in a long review in *The Literary Magazine*, she noted

---

[83] Anton J. Carlson (1936) 'Entertaining rather than informing' *The Journal of Higher Education* 7: 170–1.

[84] *BMJ*, 30 November 1935, 1057–8. Keith opposed racial mixing, believed that war was 'nature's pruning hook' and supported conspiracy theories about Jewish international plots; see Gavin Shaffer (2005) ''Like a baby with a box of matches': British scientists and the concept of race in the interwar period' *British Journal for the History of Science* 38: 307–24.

'puerilities and platitudes' and that for the rambling text 'a good editor
should have been involved'. She saw the author as a mix of 'a village curé,
a Sinclair Lewis Rotarian, a man of profound insight and a columnist in
a mid-Western farm magazine'.[85] Curiously she did not highlight his
misogyny, nor did anyone else.

Others pointed to the danger when senior scientists took to writing
on cosmic themes. Fritz Wittels, biographer of Freud, wrote in the *New
York Times* that

> some scientists, after a long and glorious lifetime of strict adherence
> to the principles of logic and reliable evidence, retire into mysticism.
> Perhaps they should play the violin or paint or secretly compose poems:
> this would satisfy the demands of the oceanic feelings.

One group who were justifiably annoyed were the sociologists, now
well established as an academic discipline looking at 'the study of man'.
Much of Carrel's analysis was sociological, without calling it such, and
the *Journal of Educational Sociology* warned readers to be 'wary of
biological conjurers who seem to pull ready-made solutions of our social
problems out of glands and genes'.[86] The distinguished editor of The
American Sociological Review attacked the book as 'poppycock, naïve
speculation, opinionated guess, mediaeval-minded mysticism, a kind of
research-foundation fascism and super humanism which sneers at
democracy'.[87] Strangely, Carrel's proposal of sending the criminally
insane to the gas chambers was not picked up by critics at the time, such
were the attitudes of the day, and doubtless because the Nazi extermi-
nations camps were yet to come. Carrel's repeated praise for Mussolini
was hardly noticed, since the book appeared before Mussolini invaded
Abyssinia on 3 October 1935. Alone the *Pan-American Epicure* opined:

> Dr. Carrel's admiration for Mussolini gives us a hint of what he had
> in mind. Dr. Carrel will do better to stick to biology. ... Too long

[85] Mary Colum 'Life and literature' *The Forum*, February 1936, v–vii.
[86] *Journal of Educational Sociology* 9 (1936): 314.
[87] *American Sociological Review* 1 (1936): 814–17.

already has mankind wandered in the wilderness listening to false prophets.[88]

In France, the book was widely noticed, and there was an enthusiastic review in *La Presse Médicale*, which concluded that the book formed 'le roc solide sur lequel reposent les assises de la civilisation [the rock solid foundation of civilisation]'.[89] But Roger Caillois, an influential anti-fascist sociologist, wrote a hostile review in *Nouvelle revue française* noting 'shocking mediocrity' and that it was 'intellectually crude'. A sarcastic review by Emile Chauvelon named Carrel as a 'devenu Yankee', and the book itself was an 'œuvre décadente'. Ominously for Carrel, other reviews by University of Paris academics were hostile; he would need but not obtain these men's support later.

At the Institute, Simon Flexner seems to have genuinely liked the book, as did Peyton Rous, and other letters from friends go beyond the usual pleasantries. Criticism from within the Institute came from Florence Sabin on specific points, which did not include Carrel's misogyny. At the Institute, Henry James, the General Manager, did not like the book, nor did his uncle and, importantly, Herbert Gasser the new director of the Institute, would shortly make it clear that he disliked Carrel's dogmatic style and his high public profile.

Responses

Carrel received many other letters of praise. Bergson the philosopher admired the book, Upton Sinclair approved, and Margaret Sanger wondered if it might make a good film. Letters from the public now increased again, all praising the book, but usually without specifying what had moved them to write, other than its reaffirmation of spiritual values. Few letters came from established scientists. Harvey Cushing wrote a personal note expressing 'admiration that you have done it so well'. But in private he told a friend that the publishers 'phoned me and

---

[88] *Pan-American Epicure*, October 1936.
[89] *La Presse Médicale*, 1 February 1936.

asked me if I would review it. ... It was the sort of book a man might be tempted to write when he reaches our age of maturity, but he had much better resist the temptation'.[90]

Carrel's failure to credit the work of others was noticed. One gentle reproof came from Raymond Fosdick at the Rockefeller Foundation who, years earlier, had taken a similar stance to Carrel in his book *The Old Savage in the New Civilisation* and he had directed the Foundation towards the very studies Carrel described. Fosdick enquired courteously if Carrel, a fellow member of the Century Association club, had read his book. Carrel replied, improbably, that he had not, and that they must have had the same ideas independently. Another complaint came from C. Ward Crampton, director of physical training for New York public schools. He pointed out that it must have escaped Carrel that in 1908, he (Crampton) had introduced the useful idea of physiological or developmental age, which Carrel used as if it were his own.[91] Carrel placated Crampton by offering to write the introduction to Crampton's next book. Another who might have been aggrieved was William Fielding Ogburn, professor of sociology at nearby Columbia University until 1927, before moving to Chicago. Ogburn had introduced the term 'cultural lag' in 1922 for society's problems in adjusting to the challenges of new technology.

Impact

The book was talked about, and it started to sell and sell, with the publishers soon reporting November 1935 sales of 1,000 per day.[92] It was soon into a fifth reprint and continued to sell in 1936 without the usual fall-off. One year later in September 1936, sales were further boosted by a 'condensed' version of the book appearing in the *Reader's Digest*. Carrel was surprised by the success of his book. He wrote to his nephew: 'If I

---

[90] John F. Fulton, *Harvey Cushing: A Biography* (Springfield, Illinois: Charles C. Thomas, 1946): 668.
[91] Carrel, *MTU* (note 9):164–6 and 187–8.
[92] 'Book Notes' *NYT*, 25 November 1935.

had been a wise man, I would not have written it. They accuse me of having written from a love of publicity'.[93]

This remorse, if sincere, was short-lived, and Carrel enjoyed this new involvement with the public. He had already embarked on his book *Reflections on Life*, as a sequel, and explored the idea that a film might be made. He welcomed the audience opened up to him by *Reader's Digest*, and he would later contribute to that magazine again. Shortly after publication, he agreed to give a hugely successful public lecture in New York in December 1935, as described later.

Distant Sales

In Paris, the publisher Plon was lucky to get the French rights after turning it down initially, and their French translation came out in late 1935 as *L'Homme cet inconnu*. Plon also had to reprint quickly, and the book sold 31,000 copies by the end of 1935 in France. It would sell 132,000 more in the following year, settling at 20,000–30,000 annually in subsequent years, and it is still in print in France.[94] It did not sell well in Britain, and the disappointed London publisher Hamish Hamilton reported to Harpers that their costly local publicity for the book had been wasted. Continental European language translations quickly followed in Norway, Denmark, Holland, Czechoslovakia, Poland, Sweden, Portugal, Finland, Estonia, Rumania, Turkey and Spain. The Hungarian edition was reprinted three times in the following years.

The biggest sales of the book in Europe, outside France, were in Germany. For the German translation, the German publisher asked Carrel to add some comment referring to German events, and Carrel obliged promptly, adding extra text:

> The German government has taken energetic measures against the propagation of the defective, the mentally diseased, and the criminal. The

---

[93] Carrel to Gigou, February 1936, Carrel Papers, box 37 folder 8, GULBFC (note 1).
[94] For French sales figures of *MTU*, see Alain Drouard, *Alexis Carrel (1873–1944): De la Mémoire à l'histoire* (Paris: Éditions L'Harmattan, 1995): 174–5. There is full list of national editions in Reggiani, *God's Eugenicist* (note 5): 83.

ideal solution would be suppression of each of these individuals as soon as he is proving himself to be dangerous.[95]

The 'measures' taken in Germany prior to 1935 were compulsory sterilisation of criminals and those with allegedly hereditary disease. Carrel's vague advocacy of 'suppression' may have meant something more than Germany's sterilisation measures.

In Turkey, the Republican People's party, founded by the moderniser Mustafa Kemal Attatürk, bought 200 copies and distributed them to the

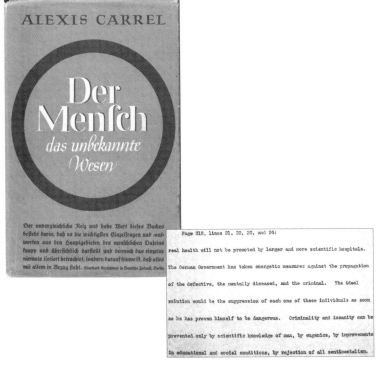

Carrel's German publisher asked him to add to the eugenics section in *Man, the Unknown* by commenting on events in Germany. In reply, Carrel sent this extra paragraph to insert in the text. (*Courtesy of Georgetown University Library, Booth Family Center for Special Collections.*)

---

[95] Pre-war Nazis atrocities also involved the disabled; see Suzanne E. Evans, *Hitler's Forgotten Victims* (London: Tempus, 2007).

People's House, a network of cultural clubs.[96] Japan had an edition in 1936, as did Australia shortly after, where there were four reprints in the coming years.

Sales continued strongly into the late 1930s, and in America, the book reached its 60th printing by 1939, making it the non-fiction bestseller of the 1930s.[97] Later, with war imminent, Carrel wrote a new Introduction to the book in 1939 and, in Cassandra mode, he could indulge in some *schadenfreude*. The European events, he said, were the result of the weakness of the democracies, and this proved his case.

The War did not halt considerable sales in Occupied France, and after the War, as described later, the book was re-issued in many countries. A new English language edition appeared in the late 1940s, with further German editions in 1955 and 1965. Good sales continued in countries with totalitarian or military governments, notably South America, where it was reprinted in Buenos Aires in 1946, and in Spain, where *La Incognita del Hombre* last appeared in 1971.

Earnings

American and French royalties came flooding in, increasing Carrel's already considerable financial security. In the first year of sales, he may have earned $50,000, with substantial annual sums added thereafter.[98] When a foreign publisher obtained the rights, there was an initial payment to both Harper & Brothers and Carrel, and then regular foreign royalties to Carrel. After an interval, Harpers arranged for a cheaper hardcover reprint in 1938 with 52,000 copies issued by the Halcyon House/Blue Ribbon Company. This earned Carrel an additional initial fee of $6,997, and a new burst of sales followed.[99]

---

[96] Rom Landau in his *Search for Tomorrow* (London: Nicolson and Watson, 1938): 267.
[97] These 1930s book sales figures came from the *New York Times* lists; the leading fiction title of the decade was Margaret Mitchell's *Gone with the Wind* (1936).
[98] Carrel's first year royalty earnings would be about $700,000 in purchasing power in 2016, but Carrel's estate after death in 1944 was not substantial. His archives suggest he moved funds to Mme Carrel and that he also supported his own family members in France.
[99] Four large companies, including Harper & Brothers, used Blue Ribbon Books to

Meanwhile, Carrel's tissue culture laboratory work had stalled and his last-ever tissue culture publication, in late 1934, was a short preliminary communication to a Paris journal. The reason was not only the diversion caused by success of *Man, the Unknown* but because at this time in the mid-1930s, there was other excitement in his laboratory. The important laboratory project in the hands of his celebrity volunteer assistant had prospered. By 1935, it was known that Charles Lindbergh, the famous young aviator, was working in Carrel's laboratory on an organ perfusion pump, and, just before *Man, the Unknown* was published, they announced its first successful use. Carrel would now be re-established in the public eye as a scientist.

reprint successful non-fiction titles from their lists. In spite of the huge sales, Carrel was gifted only the traditionally tiny number of free personal copies at the time of publication, and thereafter he nobly purchased further copies for himself, at a 30% discount.

CHAPTER FOURTEEN

The Organ Pump

Carrel's personal laboratory work had faltered after the disappointment of the Mousery, and the writing and publication of *Man, the Unknown* was a new interest. Meanwhile, possibly American's most famous citizen was working steadily in Carrel's laboratory as an unpaid volunteer. He was reviving one of Carrel's pet projects — the culture of organs.

Carrel had obtained lengthy survival of cells in his tissue cultures, and had much experience in making up and improving the complex fluids which sustained cellular life. Now he wanted to venture further. Keeping whole organs alive when isolated outside the body had been an early goal for biologists.[1] The most obvious way was to perfuse an organ with blood, and there had been attempts, even in the mid-1800s, to preserve human organs removed at surgery or after death. Brown-Séquard in Paris in the 1850s used blood to perfuse animal or human limbs obtained after execution by guillotining, and others had perfused human hearts obtained in this way, and had allegedly restored the heart beat. But in these earlier experiments, the blood clotted rapidly in the pumping system. When using 'defibrinated' blood (the fibrin was removed with glass beads), there was some success, but even so, the blood red cells clumped together or

---

[1] For a historical review see W. Boettcher, F. Merkle and H.H. Weitkemper (2003) 'History of extracorporeal circulation' *Journal of Extracorporeal Technology* 35: 172–91, and Robert L. Hewitt and Oscar Creech (1966) 'History of the Pump Oxygenator' *Archives of Surgery* 93: 680–96. Carrel's accounts of their pump have only brief historical reviews.

were damaged by the pump. After hirudin, the first anti-coagulant, became available, there was some success with blood perfusion of whole organs, particularly of the isolated heart by Newell Martin at Johns Hopkins Medical School in 1883. But perfusion of organs with simple salt solutions was more easily accomplished and as these 'physiological' salines became more sophisticated, notably using Sidney Ringer's formulation, reasonable short-term organ function could be obtained. By the 1930s, organ perfusion with saline was widely used by physiologists in their research; isolated heart preparations could survive and show function for up to five hours.[2]

But there were no reports of success with prolonged perfusion. If it was attempted, it failed either through a lack of nutrients in the saline perfusate or because infection soon entered the system. In any case, prolonged survival was of little interest to the physiologists, who could obtain all the data of interest within a few hours' study.

The Plan

Carrel had a more ambitious agenda: as with cells, he now sought long-term survival of organs. Short-term study was of little interest to him since he hoped that with more prolonged survival, there was time for the complexity of an organ's function to be revealed. There was also his goal, from Lyon days, of changing an organ's function via changes in the inflow. In his 1920s tissue culture work he had (wrongly) thought that tissue culture could change one cell type into another — and perhaps more complex organs would be just as malleable. Missing from his hopes for organ perfusion were that the pump itself would be an artificial organ, or could be used to preserve organs for use in transplantation.

In 1929 he made the first moves, and Heinz H. Rosenberger, the Institute's talented instrument maker, supplied Carrel with a simple pump. The organ, in this case an artery, was held in a glass container, and

---

[2] For a typical 1930s organ perfusion study, see I.D. Daly and W.V. Thorpe (1933) 'An isolated mammalian heart preparation capable of performing work for prolonged periods' *Journal of Physiology* 79: 199–217.

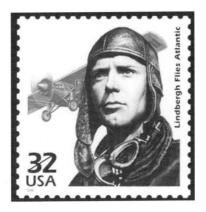

Charles Lindbergh's transatlantic flight in 1927 gave him lasting fame.

external magnets drove the internal pump, but infection soon appeared in the warm perfusion fluid after a few days. Carrel tried adding Dakin's antiseptic fluid to the system, but to no avail. Discouraged, he gave up the study.[3]

Enter Lindbergh

Charles Augustus Lindbergh (1902–1974) was the American hero of the day. In a risky venture three years previously, in 1927 at the age of 25, he had been first to fly across the Atlantic from America to France, gaining the $25,000 Orteig Prize offered by a French hotelier. Instant international fame followed, and the tall, good-looking young man comported himself with dignity during the many national and international tours and receptions which followed, initially accepting his celebrity status. But constant exposure and intrusion by the press made him uncooperative, and his relations with journalists soured. Lindbergh considered that the Hearst newspapers in particular were 'overly sensational, inexcusably inaccurate … '[4]

---

[3] Heinz Rosenberger (1930) 'An electromagnetic pump' *Science* 71: 463–4. Having an electrical device inside precluded sterilisation with heat, and chemicals were used instead.

[4] A. Scott Berg, *Lindbergh* (New York: G.P. Putnam's Sons, 1998): 163.

Earlier Interest

Just after his famous flight, and before he joined Carrel's laboratory, Lindbergh took up his old interest in biology. He purchased simple equipment for a biological laboratory and had visited some laboratories, including a visit to Princeton. Lindbergh's maternal grandfather, Charles H. Land, was an innovative dentist who had gained many patents, and was notable for introducing porcelain crowns to dentistry. Lindbergh had frequently visited the dentist's house where he watched and could tinker with the equipment and tools. At the University of Wisconsin he started to train as an engineer, but had some poor grades and left in his second year, attracted instead to training as a pilot and took on the pioneering risky airmail flights across America. His university training in making engineering 'blueprint' drawings was not wasted, since he regularly proposed detailed improvements in aircraft construction.

When his wife was pregnant with their first child, Lindbergh engaged a prominent New York anaesthetist, Dr. Paluel J. Flagg (1886–1970) to assist with the delivery. Flagg had worked at Carrel's Demonstration Hospital earlier, and thereafter he also did research work at the Rockefeller Institute, with Donald Van Slyke, on measuring oxygen in the blood. Flagg, an innovative man who designed new anaesthetic equipment, had a particular interest in methods of resuscitation.[5] At the time of their baby son's birth, Lindbergh took an interest in Flagg's apparatus, and their discussion turned to Lindbergh's sister-in-law Elizabeth's heart valve disease, which was worsening, and from which she would die four years later. Lindbergh was puzzled at the inability of surgeons to deal with the narrowed valve, which seemed to him to be a solvable engineering problem. He questioned Flagg about possible heart support devices to assist open-heart surgery, but Flagg could not answer the question, and suggested that Carrel was the man to talk to. With his contacts, Flagg arranged a visit by Lindbergh to the Institute.

---

[5] Flagg's well-known works were *The Art of Anaesthesia* (Philadelphia: J.B. Lippincott Company, 1916) — which has an Introduction by Carrel — and *The Art of Resuscitation* (New York, 1944). Flagg, a Roman Catholic, shared Carrel's belief in the rapid healing events at Lourdes.

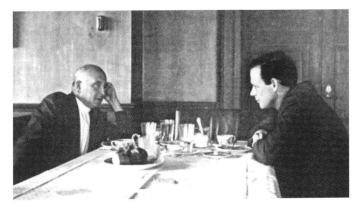

Lindbergh joined Carrel's laboratory at the Rockefeller Institute as a volunteer in 1930. (*Courtesy of the Yale University Manuscripts and Archives.*)

The Visit

Lindbergh arrived on 28 November 1930 at a side entrance to the Rockefeller Institute, having, as usual, travelled through New York disguised with dark glasses and a fedora hat. But somehow word had got out, and the staff watched his arrival from the Institute windows. Lindbergh started a discussion on human heart surgery, but Carrel then discouraged Lindbergh's interest in machines to allow direct heart surgery. Carrel pointed out that blood would clot in any such heart pump, and that pumps could damage blood cells. Carrel was wrong in discouraging Lindbergh's hopes for heart surgery, since there were already some hopeful strategies available. Carrel himself had got round the problem of blood clotting on his rubber aortic patch grafts by using Vaseline coating. Direct person-to-person blood transfusions were quite common at that time and used tubing with an inner lining of sterile paraffin wax. To prevent clotting, anti-coagulants like hirudin and heparin were available, though initially difficult to use.[6] Carrel might have heard of the Soviet studies of perfusion of detached animal heads using citrated blood, since these were highly

---

[6] Pure, safer heparin was not available until 1934. It was difficult to use clinically until 1939, when reversal of its potent action and hence control became possible.

publicised, reaching the *New York Times* in 1929.[7] About this time, John H. Gibbon in Philadelphia was starting to look at a device to bypass the human heart and lungs, which he eventually perfected and which allowed open heart surgery.

In spite of these promising strategies for a pump to bypass the heart, Carrel did not encourage Lindbergh's own hopes. Instead Carrel had a ready-made project for Lindbergh. It was to build a better pump than the earlier Rosenberger device. Lindbergh was flattered to be brought in to work on this pump, and Carrel was pleased to add a celebrity to his group. Lindbergh recalled later that although he was glad to take on Carrel's project, he still had hopes of returning to work on devices to assist heart surgery. This was never realised, but he wrote later:

> Of course, the perfusion pumps were not artificial hearts but it was obvious that they were a step in that direction. ... If I could build a satisfactory perfusion pump, I felt, a mechanical heart might follow.[8]

Carrel now had a famous assistant, one who proved to have the talents and determination that Carrel needed. Lindbergh was impressed with the resources at the Institute and was impressed by Carrel. But he was unimpressed with the simplicity of the laboratory equipment, and felt confident that with his engineering skills he had something to offer.

Pump Work

Lindbergh got to work and at one point moved into an apartment nearer the Institute to assist with his studies. He had many other activities at this time, mainly assisting the embryonic commercial airlines by exploring new routes and locating useful air fields across America. He told the American Museum of Natural History that exploration by air could be

---

[7] Nikolai Krementsov (2009) 'Off with your heads: isolated organs in early Soviet science and fiction' *Studies in the History and Philosophy of Biology and Biomedical Science* 40: 87–100. Sustained perfusion of isolated hearts with blood was claimed by the Russian Sergei Briukhonenko in the later 1920s.

[8] Lindbergh to Durkin, 20 May 1966, box 447 folder 2, Charles A. Lindbergh Papers, MS 325, Yale University Library, Manuscripts and Archives (YULMA).

useful and on doing it, he discovered some ancient settlements. On his flights he was first to collect air samples at altitude with his 'sky hook', and this showed for the first time that there was high altitude movements of spores and bacteria.

Between these ventures, at the Institute, he relished the solitude of the laboratory, often working alone at night. Carrel, ever the publicist, perhaps surprisingly did not make Lindbergh's presence known for some time, doubtless at Lindbergh's request. The other Institute scientific staff had been wary at first of the celebrated aviator's presence, but were impressed by his serious-minded application to his task.[9] In Carrel's laboratory, Lindbergh made improvements to their equipment and even redesigned the Institute's newly-arrived, expensive, high-speed centrifuge. He devised a quicker method to obtain serum when separating red cells from blood, and as described later, he designed a continuous circulation flask for the lab's tissue culture work.[10]

For the main project, Lindbergh first made a simple, enclosed, spiral glass device which, driven from outside, rocked to and fro on the base and gave low-pressure perfusion of an isolated artery. It was not large enough to study organs. Details of this pump were published in 1931, and the article was unusual in not having an author, being merely published 'From the Institute', such was Lindbergh's desire for seclusion.[11] A journalist heard a rumour that the aviator might be involved and contacted the Institute. Carrel and the Institute management discouraged this speculation and replied rather piously:

Publicity about political, economic, and scientific events is one thing. But publicity about the men who are expected to make discoveries is another thing. An indispensable condition for intellectual creation is the uninterrupted concentration of the mind on one subject and such

---

[9] Lindbergh was entitled to subsidised lunches at the Institute, and the serving staff kept his signed meal chits as souvenirs.

[10] C.A. Lindbergh (1932) 'A method for washing corpuscles in suspension' *Science* 75: 415–6.

[11] The anonymous article was titled 'Apparatus to circulate liquid under constant pressure in a closed system' *Science* 73 (1931): 566. Only later was Lindbergh's name attached to this citation.

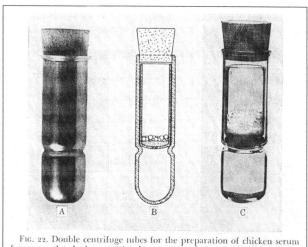

FIG. 22. Double centrifuge tubes for the preparation of chicken serum from coagulated plasma: (A) tube constructed from sterling silver; (B) cross-sectional diagram; (c) tube constructed from pyrex glass. For complete description, see text. (C. A. Lindbergh, unpublished experiments.)

Lindbergh's engineering skills led him to make changes in Carrel's laboratory equipment, including constructing this simple centrifuge tube for rapid production of serum from whole blood. (*From Raymond C. Parker Methods of Tissue Culture, 1938.*)

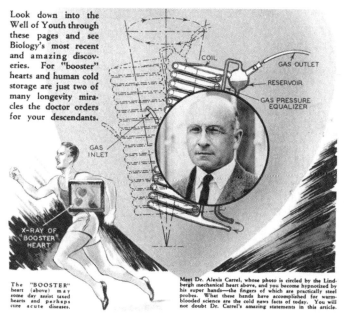

Lindbergh's first version of his organ pump was later claimed to be an artificial heart in *Modern Mechanix and Inventions Magazine* June 1936.

concentration absolutely requires solitude and silence. Men of science should not attract the curiosity of the public.[12]

Lindbergh acknowledged that in his unusual position in the Institute, he also had to be careful:

In the research I'm doing, publicity of any kind is bound to create jealousy among just enough people to make it more difficult to accomplish anything. ... I can do a great deal more if I can avoid notice.[13]

One of Lindbergh's other reasons to avoid publicity was a curious one: he had a fastidious approach to the written word, and he knew that journalists did not. After his historic flight to Paris, he was accompanied back on the boat to America by a ghost-writer serving a contract with a publisher for a book, if he survived. The manuscript was ready for printing on arrival in New York, and the bookshops were waiting. After reading the text, Lindbergh prevented the book's publication and slowly rewrote much of it in less dramatic prose, removing the factual inaccuracies; the bookshops had to wait.

The Team

Carrel and Lindbergh were now an oddly-matched pair.[14] Considerably different in height, there was a 32-year age difference, and perhaps Carrel saw Lindbergh as the son he never had. On his part, Lindbergh perhaps

---

[12] Carrel to *New York Herald Tribune*, 22 September 1931, box 14–5 folder 3, Alexis Carrel Papers, Georgetown University Library Booth Family Center for Special Collections (GULBFC).

[13] Lindbergh to Breckinridge, 2 April 1936, box 5 folder 5, Charles A. Lindbergh Papers, MS 325, YULMA (note 8).

[14] Carrel's work with Lindbergh is presented in a dramatic way in David M. Friedman, *The Immortalists: Charles Lindbergh, Dr. Alexis Carrel and their Daring Quest to Live Forever* (New York: HarperCollins, 2007). For other descriptions of Carrel's influence on Lindbergh, see Anne Morrow Lindbergh, *War Within and Without: Diaries and Letters of Anne Morrow Lindbergh 1939–1944* (Orlando: Florida, Mariner Books, 1980) and the more controversial account in Max Wallace, *The American Axis: Henry Ford, Charles Lindbergh, and the Rise of the Third Reich* (New York: St Martin's Press, 2003).

sought a father figure, since his father lived apart from the family in a failed marriage. The attitude of the two men to the press and public differed greatly, but they shared some puritanical attitudes and both shunned cigarettes and alcohol.[15] Lindbergh was impressed by Carrel's scientific status and was soon in thrall to the older man, as a willing listener to Carrel's intense discourse and his wide-ranging, confident pronouncements. Years later, when Lindbergh took on a prominent place in national politics, some of Carrel's ideas on nationalism, race and eugenics feature in Lindbergh's writings and speeches.

The Lindberghs' family life was settling to near normality, when on 27 February 1932, an evening when Carrel was expecting the couple to dine with him, their baby boy was kidnapped from their home. America's largest ever man-hunt followed, and the events were followed with international interest. Although a ransom was paid, the murdered baby's body was found on 12 May. No further leads appeared, and it was not until over two years later, in September 1934, that an arrest was made.

By this time that autumn, Lindbergh had delivered what Carrel hoped for, and with most of the engineering work on the pump done,

Dr. Carrel Home From France.

Dr. Alexis Carrel of the Rockefeller Institute returned on the Ile de France yesterday after three months in France. During his visit in Paris it was reported here that he had spoken of Colonel Charles A. Lindbergh as one of his ablest pupils in biological research. He denied it yesterday and was annoyed when told that the story had been widely circ lated here.

Lindbergh's presence at the Institute was kept secret, until Carrel revealed it in France, soon confirmed in the *New York Times* on 26 September 1934.

---

[15] However, it is now known that, from the 1950s, Lindbergh fathered a number of children in Europe outside his marriage and made provision for them.

Lindbergh was less often in the lab.[16] The news got out, at last, to the American newspapers that Lindbergh had indeed been working in the laboratory, since Carrel let it be known to friends in France that year that Lindbergh was an aide and a 'brilliant student of biology'.[17]

To use the pump, an improved composition of the perfusion fluid was required, and Carrel's assistant Lillian Baker, who worked with him since 1922, had developed an increasingly complex perfusion fluid.

Lindbergh's Design

The elegant, one-piece Pyrex glass pump was made by the Institute's legendary glass-blower Otto Hopf, who came from a family of master

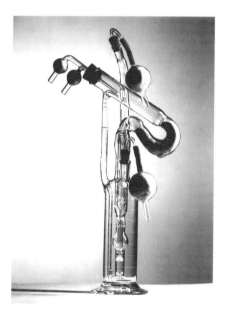

The carefully-taken prize-winning image of Lindbergh's complex organ pump. (*Courtesy of the Rockefeller University Archives.*)

---

[16] See Richard J. Bing (1987) 'Lindbergh and the biological sciences' *Historical Perspectives in Cardiovascular Medicine & Surgery* 14: 231–7 and R.J. Bing (1983) 'Carrel: a personal reminiscence' *JAMA* 250: 3297–8.

[17] 'Lindbergh Praised For Biological Work' *NYT*, 28 August 1934, quoting the Paris newspaper *Jour*; Carrel initially denied the story.

glass-blowers in Europe.[18] Inside the pump was a small chamber for the organ and, attached to the pump by its artery, it was perfused by recirculating oxygenated fluid at body temperature. The organ chamber was very small and could permit study only of small organs like the heart or kidney from newborn small animals. A single thyroid lobe from a cat or rabbit connected to a segment of carotid artery was regularly used. Pulsatile perfusion was used rather than continuous flow, being a more 'natural' approach.[19] The bacterial infection found in the earlier pump after prolonged use was now prevented when Lindbergh found that simple cotton filters in the air inlets solved the problem. The device was connected by rubber tubing to a rather ordinary air pump which was usually missing from the famous images of the photogenic glass device.

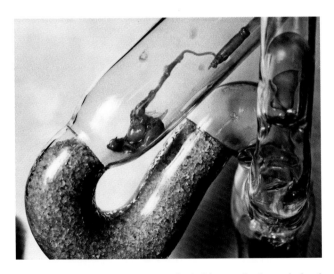

The small central chamber of the pump usually held a single thyroid gland or occasionally a tiny organ from a neonate. (*Courtesy of the Georgetown University Library, Booth Family Center for Special Collections.*)

---

[18] Hopf left the Institute in 1940 to form his own company in Upper Black Eddy, Pennsylvania; see 'Glass blowing at the Institute' *Rockefeller Institute Review* March/April 1965: 14–16.

[19] Later, the improved heart–lung machines and organ perfusion systems developed in the 1970s initially used pulsatile perfusion, but this 'natural' addition was soon shown to be unnecessary.

For longer perfusions, the organ was transferred after some days to another pump containing fresh fluid.[20]

The studies on the use of the pump continued over the winter of 1934, and into 1935. The trial of Hauptmann, the suspect in the kidnapping, justifiably named 'the trial of the century', took place in January. Although all the evidence was circumstantial, he was found guilty and sentenced to death.[21] He appealed and the proceedings hung over the Lindberghs throughout the rest of the year. Conspiracy theories arose which suggested that Lindbergh, still unpopular with the tabloid press, had assisted in getting a false conviction.

First Results

The first results from using the pump were published in the summer of 1935, which was eventful and busy for both Carrel and the Lindberghs. Carrel's *Man, the Unknown* would appear that autumn, as described earlier. Anne Lindbergh also published a book, *North to the Orient* which, describing their pioneering flight to Japan, was the non-fiction bestseller of 1935.

The first news of the organ pump came in a short account in the generalist journal *Science* on 21 June 1935.[22] But this was no ordinary publication. The journal also ran 'Science News', a press agency which supplied newspapers with science stories, and was delighted to have the Lindbergh–Carrel story coming up. The agency issued the pump paper

---

[20]The perfusion solution devised by Dr. Lillian E. Baker was Tyrode's or Ringer's saline plus many extras, usually 'protein-split products', hemin, cysteine, insulin, thyroxine, glutathione, vitamin A, ascorbic acid, and blood serum'. Phenol red was added to detect any undesirable pH change during perfusion.

[21]Only the court action against John Scopes in 1925 for teaching evolution in a Tennessee school rivalled the fame of the Hauptmann trial in 20th century America.

[22]There was also a popular account in *Science Newsletter*, 29 June 1935, 411–2; much later the *Science* article was accorded 'landmark' status in *Science News*, 30 June 2005.

text to the press, embargoed until publication, plus some added briefing and comment:

> Editors — This is one of the best stories of the year. ... consider it for page one play. Herewith our image of Carrel, pick up a photo of Lindbergh from your morgue.[23]

The article was only two pages in length, and had few results — full details of the design were promised in later publications.[24] The article largely dealt with the possibilities for the device, and Carrel said of their pump that

> its ultimate purposes are the manufacture *in vitro* of the secretions of endocrine glands, the isolation of the substances essential to the growth, differentiation and functional activity of those glands, the discovery of the laws of the association of organs, and the treatment of organic and arterial diseases, etc.

This was an ambitious list, verging on science-fiction, rather than a cautious biological agenda. The paper said that there had been 26 experiments with the final model of the pump with runs of up to 20 days without infection or blockages in the system. The organ most studied was the thyroid gland, and Carrel said perfusion could have gone on much longer than 20 days, since 'there was no reason why they could not keep organs alive indefinitely'.

Publicity

The newspapers, alerted by the press agency, were ready, and with Lindbergh involved, it was a major story throughout America. The *New York*

---

[23] Press release from Science Service, Alexis Carrel Papers, box 74 folder 422, GULBFC (note 12).

[24] Lindbergh later described the pump carefully in C.A. Lindbergh (1935) 'An apparatus for the culture of whole organs' *JEM* 62: 409–33, as did Carrel two years later in *JEM* 65 (1937): 515–26. Neither of these papers gave any results, and any data are found only in their 1938 book, Alexis Carrel and Charles A. Lindbergh, *The Culture of Organs* (New York: Paul B. Hoeber, 1938).

Times headline was 'Carrel, Lindbergh Develop Device to Keep Organs Alive Outside Body', and there were further articles in the next three days, including the thoughts of the *Times'* other science correspondent William L. Lawrence.[25] The *Los Angeles Times* considered that 'whole parts of the body can be made to grow and live indefinitely'. The *Baltimore Sun* considered that the pump was an artificial heart, as did the *Chicago Tribune*, but the *Boston Globe* soon preferred 'robot heart'. Some journalists understandably conflated the new pump with the allegedly still-beating chicken heart cells, and announced 'Immortal Hearts in Glass', and *Time* magazine went further and claimed that human immortality was being sought. The historian of the Institute later concluded that the 'newspapers recklessly exaggerated' the results and uses of the pump.[26] But the blame did not lie with the press. Carrel had raised expectations and was, as ever, unconcerned at the journalists' dramatic accounts. About this time, the newspapers added a new folksy story about Carrel's surgical skill, reporting that he could tie knots with one hand inside a matchbox.[27]

Soon, the elegant multi-chambered glass pump achieved iconic status, and was dubbed the 'saxophone on top of a wine bottle'. The carefully-taken images by the talented Rockefeller Institute photographer were widely used, and the striking images won prizes in the world of medical illustration.[28] Film-makers saw potential in the device and the story of

---

[25] Carrel received $100 from the *New York Times* at this time for his help with the articles.

[26] George W. Corner, *A History of the Rockefeller Institute 1901–1953: Origins and Growth* (New York: Rockefeller Institute Press, 1964): 234. In October 1935, Carrel hosted a journalist from *Harper's Magazine* at the Institute, and he provided non-attributable briefing about the pump.

[27] This story of surgical skill first appeared in *Time* magazine 16 September 1935 then in *Today* March 1936 and, now being on file, was repeated by others, including the *New Yorker* in December 1937. A similar story appearing later was that Carrel could put '50 stitches into the edge of a cigarette paper'; Friedman's *Immortalists* (note 14) recently agreed the stitch tally at 500.

[28] The striking images of the pump made by the Institute photographer Louis Schmidt won a national award. His skills are remembered now through the Louis Schmidt Award given annually by the Biological Photographic Society.

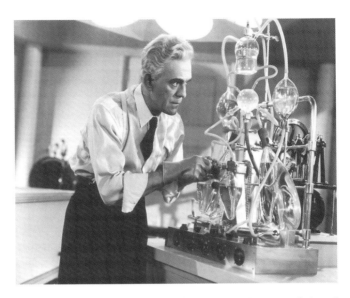

Boris Karloff's science-fiction films included the *Walking Dead* (1936) and *The Man They Could Not Hang* (1939), both using Carrelian pumps to revive the dead. (*thelastdrivein.com*)

organ revival, and next year, Boris Karloff in the *Walking Dead* used a similar pump to revive a dead, unfairly executed man.

There was another burst of letters to Carrel from the public, now asking about the possibilities of heart surgery. As ever, he wrote back explaining what the pump could and could not do.[29] Many letters also reached Lindbergh from sufferers looking for help with their heart disease, and Lindbergh, as ever, disliking press involvement was concerned at the raised public expectations, noting the 'sickly sentimentality of favourable publicity'.[30] Lindbergh's wife Anne however commented approvingly in her diary that his scientific work was a helpful antidote to the bad press he had suffered and showed him in good light; 'the right values are being

---

[29] Carrel's Georgetown archive (note 12) has about 200 such 'fan mail' letters arriving in the following year of 1936, and they were, as always, a mixture of requests for surgical advice, responses to *Man, the Unknown*, advice on sexual problems, long personal statements, begging letters and the long, single-spaced, much capitalised, incoherent views of cranks.

[30] Friedman, *Immortalists* (note 14): 139.

set,' she said. With the news about the pump, the press now renewed their watch for Lindbergh when entering and leaving the Institute.

A scientific description of the design and use of the pump by Lindbergh appeared shortly afterwards, but the full results were slow to appear. The pump was more difficult to use than was supposed. In spite of the claims for general success, function was poor with the kidney and heart. After this disappointment, only the thyroid gland was studied, and even then there were problems. Not until three years later did the detailed results appear in a book published by the two men. These final results and concerns about Carrel's claims are discussed in the next chapter.

Carrel's Lecture

The work with the pump meant that Carrel was back involved doing what he did best. It was a new method, one that others could develop, and it was something to show to the admiring world. After mid-1935, as a result of the announcement of the pump and then the publication of *Man, the Unknown* in the autumn, Carrel was back in favour as the nation's favourite biologist. He was now invited by the New York Academy of Medicine to give a public lecture later that year in one of their 'Lectures to the Laity' series. Public lectures by philosophers and literary figures were becoming less common at the time, but the appearance by a surgical scientist was a novelty, and his title 'The Mystery of Death' caught the public's attention. The lecture at New York's Hoosick Hall on 12 December was planned to start at 8.15 p.m., but the 700-seat hall was full by 7 p.m. Those then arriving outside caused a traffic jam and the police were required to restore order. Inside, an over-flow to other rooms in the building was arranged with loudspeakers conveying Carrel's address.[31]

Carrel, as ever, could hold the attention of an audience. Some of the lecture still reads well, and he skilfully brought in a range of ideas related

---

[31] Carrel's lecture appears in full in Eugene H. Pool, *Medicine and Mankind* (New York: D. Appleton, 1936): 195–217. Some accounts say that the lecture was also transmitted to the crowd outside the building.

to his provocative theme. He told of how the tissues of the body die at variable rates, and that death was not an event, but a process. Carrel explained that resuscitation of the body was possible after the heart stopped, but if delayed by 20 minutes, there was brain damage. He brought in the evidence from his eternal cells to suggest that death and decay were caused by other non-cellular factors. He discussed philosophers' views on death and his own belief in an everlasting soul. He claimed that telepathic and clairvoyance mechanisms were well established and pointed out that some believed that communication with the dead in this way was possible. Then, using his eugenic views, he saw death in earlier eras as getting rid of 'fools, the diseased and weak', and that this useful culling of the race was now prevented by medical care.

The newspapers carried accounts of the lecture next day and were generally supportive.[32] The *New York Herald Tribune* commented on Carrel's status and that 'the man of science is now enthroned where poets and theologians once were'. Not everyone in the audience had been impressed, and another newspaper reported that

> The Academy's doctors were stirring uneasily in their seats. And when the lecture was over, the comments in the corridors were very similar — 'unscientific.'

But otherwise the Academy speech was a public success and was published in abstract in *Vital Speeches of the Day 1935–36*.

Pressure on the Lindberghs

From summer of 1935 onwards, and with the appeal by Bruno Hauptmann against his death sentence dragging on, the Lindberghs endured continued press intrusion and regular death and kidnap threats. The burst of publicity for the pump was an unwelcome addition. Lindbergh felt that America was an increasingly unpleasant place for his family because 'between the politician, the tabloid press, and the criminal,

---

[32] 'Carrel Sees Life Extended For Ages' *NYT*, 13 December 1935.

a condition exists which is intolerable for us'.[33] The Lindberghs concluded that the pressure was too great, and, with their other children at risk, they decided to leave and move to Britain. Although they had little knowledge of that country, Lindbergh felt that they would be safer and their privacy would be respected. One of Lindbergh's few English contacts was Harold Nicolson, the politician and writer, who stayed with them earlier in New York while working on a biography of Anne's father, Dwight Whitney Morrow, the American ambassador to Mexico. From the Nicolsons, the Lindberghs rented 'Long Barn', a venerable and substantial dwelling in the grounds of the Nicolsons' Sissinghurst Castle in Kent to the south of London.

The Lindberghs sailed secretly from New York at midnight on 21 December 1935. One trusted journalist at the *New York Times* had been informed about the imminent dramatic move and though met by the press on arrival in Britain, the Lindberghs soon managed to live relatively unharassed. In the new home, they hired a secretary and employed two English nannies to look after their children during their frequent absences abroad on air explorations.

Hauptmann lost his appeal and was executed next year on 3 April 1936. With this closure, many expected the Lindberghs would return to America, but they did not, and were to stay in Britain until 1939. In exile, Lindbergh kept in close touch with Carrel's staff and advised on the pump experiments, now in others' hands. He tried to start personal laboratory work and though lacking conventional back-up, he managed some pump-related studies. The two men also met up each summer when Carrel was in France, and they managed to finish and publish their book *The Culture of Whole Organs* in 1938.

Meanwhile, in 1937, in New York, Carrel's group continued slowly with the pump work, and Carrel had other matters to attend to. He was working on a sequel to *Man, the Unknown*, and he had many invitations to give important lectures. His summer breaks in France were getting longer, and he and his wife would be involved in European politics, as would Lindbergh.

---

[33] Berg, *Lindbergh* (note 4): 340.

CHAPTER FIFTEEN

Wider Involvement

In Lindbergh's absence, Carrel's pump experiments were still proceeding, but there were difficulties. These concerns were reported to Lindbergh, and he kept in close touch with the unit and was ready with suggestions and solutions. Carrel published nothing else that year, in spite of having a large, well-staffed unit.[1] One reason for his low scientific output was that, in spite of the cool reception to *Man, the Unknown* from his peers, he was writing a sequel, *Reflections on Life*, which was a more assertive version of the same themes. To add to this, he had increasing numbers of invitations to give lectures, and other routine academic obligations included writing Introductions to other scientists' books. These he provided quickly, and they are usually brief and conventional.[2] During this time, Carrel was also increasingly concerned about events in Europe. He made use of his long summer break to travel widely and to take an interest in the political movements and ideas in France. When in Europe, he could also catch up with Lindbergh.

Carrel was increasingly detached from the life of the Institute, and on arrival new staff were told of this isolation. His celebrity status and *Man,*

---

[1] Carrel's only scientific publication in 1936 was an entry on 'Tissue Culture' for the 14th edition of the *Encyclopaedia Britannica*. Raymond C. Parker (1903–1974) had joined Carrel's unit, but worked and published independently on tissue culture.

[2] These Introductions were to works by André Missenard, James M.D. Olmsted (on Claude Bernard), Arthur Vernes, Raymond Parker and Étienne Destot. In Carrel's introduction to Robert Fowler's 1937 book on tonsil surgery coming from his specialist Tonsil Hospital in New York, Carrel pointed out that 'concentrated study of a limited subject generally brings about true progress'.

393

the Unknown had offended many; in return, Carrel let it be known that he considered the Institute to be 'as dead as the Pasteur Institute'. He added enigmatically that 'the bureaucratic spirit of this country is as sterilising as the war spirit of Europe'.[3] Simon Flexner had retired in the previous year, and with Carrel's main supporter gone, only Rous and Wyckoff in the Institute remained as close friends. His personal letters to relatives in Lyon are increasingly gloomy, and being less interested in joining his old friends at the Philosophers' meetings, they chided him for his absence.

Lectures

Academic invitations increased, and became so numerous that Carrel had to be selective and eventually routinely turned down most of these approaches. Various strategies were used to lure him, including personal visits and pleas by senior university staff who pointed out the age and prestige of their institute or the occasion, and emphasised the quality of the previous lecturers. His refusal letters could be gracious and well-crafted. Declining to give the Commencement Address at Duke University, he complimented the faculty on having 'the boldness of youth, particularly in supporting Dr. Rhine and his parapsychology studies'. Declining an offer of an honorary degree from Rollins College in Florida, he wrote:

> I cannot secure the leisure to prepare an address for so important an occasion. It is not an indifferent matter to speak to young people and an address on the subject you mentioned would require most careful preparation. I hope someday to have the leisure to do it.

Rollins College was so charmed by his letter that they promptly invited him, well ahead, to come the following year and give their William Ayres Lecture, which had an honorarium of $200 attached. This time Carrel declined more abruptly. A similar sum was offered with New York University's 1938 James Arthur Lecture on 'Time and Its Mysteries',

---

[3] Carrel to Gigou, 16 December 1938, Malinin Collection of the Papers of Alexis Carrel and Charles Lindbergh, box 14 folder 30, FA 208, Rockefeller University Archives, Rockefeller Archives Centre (RUA RAC).

delivered on a previous occasion by the Nobel Prize winner Robert A. Millikan, but although it was a very suitable Carrelian theme, he turned it down, and instead John Dewey agreed to speak. Carrel also, perhaps reluctantly, declined to give Harvard's Ingersoll Lecture on 'Human Immortality'. He turned down the Trimble Lecture at Detroit and said he could not address the William Harvey Society at Tufts. He avoided the chance of radio broadcasts, and declined an offer of $200 for a 5 p.m. Sunday address at the First Presbyterian Church in Buffalo. A Northwestern University lecture fee of $400 did not tempt him, nor did the Erie Council of Catholic Women's promise of an audience of 2,000 or more, should he join them. He also turned down offers from agencies to place him on the lucrative lecture circuits, and hence could not oblige The Yale Club in New York who asked for the name of his agent to arrange a fee for an appearance there. A pushy literary agent, Gertrude Algase, unsuccessfuly pestered him to write a book on the 'Significance of Life', eventually offering him an advance of $25,000.[4]

However, in March that year he did agree to give the 1936 Hitchcock Lectures at the University of California, the prestigious award endowed and well-funded from 1885 to 'encourage highest distinction in scholarly thought', and during this time he stayed in residence at Berkeley. Previous lecturers in this series were Jules Bordet, Max Born, J.B.S. Haldane and Walter Cannon. Carrel's titles for his four lectures were 'The Life of Cells Outside of the Body', 'The Lindbergh Apparatus and the Cultivation of Entire Organs', 'Fluidity of the Body' and 'Cells, Blood, and Mind'. In these lectures, as was customary, he could emphasise his own scientific work and, as his use of 'fluidity' suggests, he proposed a general plasticity of cells and organs and described his attempts to control them. In one of the lectures, he gave for the first, and last time, brief details of the results from the Mousery work, and he suggested that diet affected lifespan, fecundity and cancer incidence. At Berkeley, he occasionally ventured into the matters of eugenics and public policy stating that: 'In man,

---

[4] Gertrude Algase (died 1962) had fame soon after by arranging for the young John F. Kennedy's Harvard thesis, *Why England Slept*, to be published as a book in 1939.

natural selection has ceased to play its role. ... The weak and defective are encouraged to live.' But he dismissed serious negative eugenic measures:

> The sterilisation of the criminal, the insane, and the weak-minded would have purely negative significance. It could not lead to a real improvement of the race, to the production of more highly endowed individuals. Compulsory eugenics alone could accomplish such progress, but compulsory eugenics is unthinkable in a free nation.[5]

But even with this disclaimer, his Berkeley audience may have been unimpressed. By now, Carrel's views on 'the unfit' and eugenics, positive or negative, were becoming rapidly unpopular in liberal academic circles.

This may explain why, in that summer, there was a prestigious academic event to which Carrel was not invited. The Harvard University Tercentenary celebrations, held in August 1936, awarded 37 honorary degrees, and among the recipients were Ross Granville Harrison, whose methods Carrel had used decades earlier, and Karl Landsteiner from the

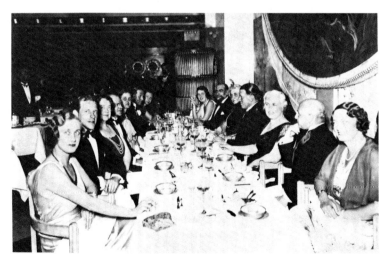

Carrel at dinner during his transatlantic travel. (From *Jean-Jaques Antier*, Alexis Carrel, 1986.)

---

[5] The text of some of Carrel's Californian lectures are in Malinin Collection 650-5, box 6 folder 16, RUA RAC (note 3).

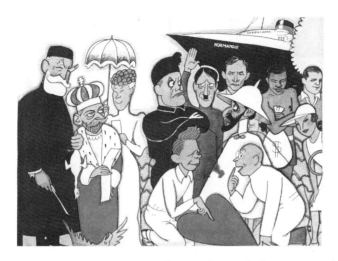

A *Cosmopolitan* magazine cartoon in 1936 fantasised over which international celebrities would use the new fashionable *S.S. Normandie* liner. These include the British King and Queen, Joe Louis, Hitler, Mussolini, Carrel and Lindbergh. (*Courtesy of Georgetown University Library Booth Family Center for Special Collections.*)

Rockefeller Institute. Sir Arthur Eddington, the British astrophysicist, was also favoured, suggesting that scientific popularisers were not excluded. Carrel was a Nobel Prize winner, and his absence from the list might suggest some coolness in East Coast academia towards him. The Harvard event was organised by Jerome Greene who, since 1910, had been involved at a high level with the Rockefeller Institute and Foundation, and would have known Carrel well.

French Politics

Carrel travelled to France as usual that summer. As a celebrity passenger, he was offered an upgrade if he booked with a French Line company ship, but he instead booked a first-class cabin on the new fast, luxurious *SS Normandie*, which had entered service in the previous year. Travelling on it gave acknowledgement of international fame, and when the magazine *Cosmopolitan* carried a cartoon with an array of celebrities who might use the *Normandie*, both Carrel and Lindbergh featured.

Back at his island base, Carrel had a busy summer in 1936, and this included attending the inaugural meeting of a new French political party. French politics were increasingly unstable at this time, and from the early 1930s, quarrelsome political groups produced rival analysis and solutions for the post-war malaise. The political parties of the left and right held meetings featuring their paramilitary wings, and after a rally and near-invasion of the Chamber of Deputies in 1934, many of these French organisations and political parties were banned. The same groups then reorganised more peaceably under new names, and some stability returned to the government.[6]

Carrel was watching events closely and he attended, together with his wife, the inaugural meeting of one of the newly re-formed right-wing parties, the Parti Populaire Française (PPF), which emerged out of the Croix-de-Feu, an older, now-banned, fascist-style party. Led by Jacques Doriot, the PPF policies were rightist, patriotic and eventually anti-Semitic, and the party successfully asked for financial support from Mussolini and the Nazis. To many, particularly the middle classes, fascism seemed the only alternative to communism. Although Carrel was present at the PPF's start-up meeting, it seems that he never joined the party.[7] However, his wife was a member, as she had been of its predecessor, the Croix-de-Feu, and had then been the only woman to parade with the Croix-de-Feu's uniformed paramilitary wing. Carrel's secretary admired Mme Carrel's courage in joining these 'storm troops' and knew 'that she would stay in the thick of things, regardless of her own danger'.[8] Another new right-wing party was the more moderate Parti Social Français (PSF), and although Carrel expressed sympathies for the PSF in letters to

---

[6] In May 1936, an alliance of left-wing parties led by Léon Blum won the elections, but did not last long after bringing in radical legislation favourable to workers and trade unions, including a 40-hour week, increased salaries and paid holidays.

[7] See Andrés H. Reggiani, *God's Eugenicist: Alexis Carrel and the Sociobiology of Decline* (New York: Berghahn Books, 2007): 96.

[8] Crutcher to Carrel, 25 July 1935, box 9 folder 11, Alexis Carrel Papers, Georgetown University Library, Booth Family Center for Special Collections (GULBFC).

relatives, he did not join them. Later, after the French defeat in World War II, both these parties would support the French collaborationist Vichy government for a while.

Carrel at this time also took an interest in some other French organisations. With his American friends Frederic Coudert and first lady Eleanor Roosevelt, he was on the board of directors of *La France*, a magazine designed to improve relations between France and America. Carrel additionally assisted the Office Française de Renseignements aux Etats-Unis, which also aimed to foster links between France and America, and the invitation to join it had come from its director, Marshal Pétain the World War I military hero. Pétain also invited Columbia's Nicolas Murray Butler, one of the Philosophers, to join. Carrel, like all Frenchmen, admired Petain, who was in and out of politics at this time. Pétain's invitation meant that the Marshal was aware of Carrel's interest in France's future, and a few years later they would be linked together in a major project.

Pontigny Meeting

After this launch of the PPF, Carrel travelled south to join a small gathering, starting on 26 July, organised by Jean Coutrot, the French engineer-sociologist, to discuss 'a complete knowledge of man', a project close to Carrel's own interests.[9] Coutrot had invited a group of about 20, including writers, economists, businessmen, architects and historians, to meet for four days at the abbaye de Pontigny, a Cistercian monastery in Burgundy used for cultural meetings. The venue made a virtue of being far from Paris, and liked to be seen as a modern counterpart of Aristotle's Lyceum or Plato's Academy. As a result, a new 'think-tank' emerged from the meeting — the Centre d'études des problems humains

---

[9] Marjorie A. Beale, *The Modernist Enterprise: French Elites and the Threat of Modernity, 1900–1940* (Stanford: Stanford University Press, 1999); see also Jackie Clarke (2001) 'Engineering the new order in the 1930s: the case of Jean Coutrot' *French Historical Studies* 24: 63–86.

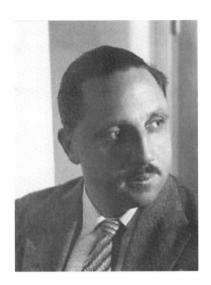

Jean Coutrot's conferences from the mid-1930s
on the French interwar problems were attended
by Carrel.

(CEPH) — which Coutrot hoped would encourage like-minded
'engineers of the science of man' to use science to re-align man within a
world changed by technology and industrialisation. The Centre was
thereafter run by Coutrot, assisted by a four-person executive committee
which included Carrel and Aldous Huxley.[10] There were additional
counseillers, including Pierre Teilhard de Chardin (1881–1955), the
Jesuit theologian, philosopher and palaeontologist,[11] adding in
psychoanalysts and representatives from labour and employers'
organisations.[12] A small administrative office was set up, and more
seminars of the same kind were held at Pontigny before the War with

---

[10] The other members of the executive were art historian Henri Focillon and the Swiss
economist Georges Guillaume. Aldous Huxley's fiction and his essays in *Ends and Means*
(1937) show some overlap with Carrel's own ideas, and a shared belief in the paranormal. Huxley's brother Julian's writings were initially closer to Carrel's position.
[11] De Chardin's acceptance of Darwinian evolution meant that his works were banned
by the Roman Catholic Church; his later books sold well, notably his *The Phenomenon
of Man* (1955).
[12] The Groupe X-Crise, another French 'technocratic' movement, was well-represented,
and it favoured central planning and government in which experts replaced politicians.

some publications resulting. Like some other French organisations at the time, they also looked for a possible political 'third way' between fascism and socialism. To add to this modernising agenda, there was some 'anti-modern' input showing nostalgia and support for traditional values and lifestyles.

Although Carrel was on the executive committee of the CEPH, he had, as always, little interest in such outside administrative work. He did not attend any further meetings at Pontigny and served on the committee for only two years, pleading that distance and lack of time prevented his closer involvement. Privately, he labelled it 'a clumsy and weak organisation'. Though this seems like typical Carrelian disdain, on this occasion he was instead watching the CEPH carefully from a distance; he was to use some of its ideas later.

Lindbergh's Activities

The Lindberghs had arrived in England from New York in January earlier that year and they had settled in the country south of London with their staff and a fierce Alsatian dog called Thor, gifted by Carrel. Lindbergh was keen to keep up his research and explored ways to restart experiments. He brought a letter of introduction from Carrel to Lord Moynihan, but the eminent surgeon was on a long trip abroad. He instead met and talked about his projects with Professor A.V. Hill, the distinguished British physiologist, but did not obtain laboratory space. Lindbergh corresponded regularly with the staff at the Rockefeller Institute, particularly John Zwick, one of Carrel's 'skilled helpers', who dealt with any problems or modifications to the pump. A plan was agreed to add an 'artificial kidney' to the circuit during organ perfusion hoping to remove waste products from the pump's circulating fluid, but no progress was made with this ambitious addition. A more immediate challenge was that, in spite of Carrel's claims for the pump's reliability, infection could occur, and a more regular problem was death of parts of the thyroid gland due to debris in the perfusion fluid blocking the small arteries. Lindbergh sent modifications which added a filter inside the pump. Even so, the laboratory data shows that problems continued with patchy death of the gland.[13] By the summer, Lillian Baker in the laboratory wrote to Carrel that 'lots of glands were 'dead as a door nail' particularly in the centre'.[14] The variable amount of dead gland tissue meant that trying to measure any hormone production by the gland was problematic, particularly as the gland normally had large stores of the iodine-containing hormone, which would leak out after cell death. Baker discouraged any idea that hormone production had been detected and told Carrel 'personally I would not mention iodine [hormone production] at this time'.

Lindbergh's Other Projects

Lindbergh in England no longer had his work for the U.S. aviation industry and with more time on his hands, he expanded his other interests. He encouraged the work of Robert H. Goddard, the American rocketry pioneer, then unknown, and obtained financial support for him. Keen to point out new roles for aviation, even in matters of health, Lindbergh wrote to the U.S. Surgeon General presciently pointing out that international air travel would bring new health hazards, notably the spread of infectious disease, and that new immunisation policies would be necessary. He kept up a correspondence with Paluel Flagg, the anaesthetist who had introduced him to Carrel, and they made plans for the supply of oxygen to pressurised aircraft cabins.

Summer 1936

Carrel and Lindbergh had an invitation to demonstrate the organ pump in action at the third meeting of the International Congress of Experimental Cytology that summer in Copenhagen. Both men made European visits before joining up in Denmark in August. Lindbergh's

---

[13] Carrel's laboratory records from December 1937 to January 1938 are in the Malinin Collection, Experimental Notebooks, box 10, FA 208, RUA RAC (note 3).

[14] Baker to Lindbergh, 5 July 1936, Malinin Collection, box 4 folder 25, FA 208, RUA RAC (note 3). Although the necrosis problem continued, these iodine experiments were published in late 1938; see note 56.

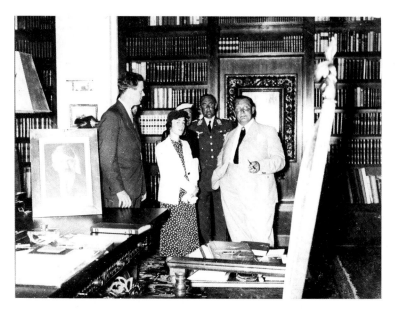

Lindbergh and his wife met Göring during his visits to Germany from 1936. (*Courtesy of the Bavarian State Library*.)

journey into Europe in July was in accepting an invitation from the American embassy to visit Germany. After years of secrecy, Germany had surprisingly agreed to reveal details of their new military aircraft to American diplomats. The Lindberghs visited Germany for 10 days and, given a welcome and protection from the press, they were escorted round factories and airfields. Charles was impressed not only with the design of the new Heinkel and Junkers aircraft, but also with the significance of their capabilities. In an address given to a German aviation society during the visit, he pointed out that World War I military assumptions no longer held, and that a future war would not be fought from the trenches. He added that

> we who are in aviation carry a heavy responsibility on our shoulders … we have stripped the armour of every nation in war. It is no longer possible to shield the heart of the country with its army. Our libraries, art museums, every institution we value most, are laid bare to our bombardment.

The Lindberghs had a seat at the opening ceremony of the Berlin Olympics, and soon after were photographed in the office of the air minister Hermann Göring. They were impressed with everything they saw. Anne wrote to her mother that 'Hitler is a very great man ... not scheming, not selfish, not greedy for power, but a mystic ... '.[15] Charles noted that 'Germany is facing up to a number of fundamental problems which other nations are rolling up for the future'. He was impressed with the post-war revival of Germany, and also considered that Hitler had 'character and vision' and this excused 'a certain amount of fanaticism'.[16] They were told by their hosts that the actions against the Jews in Germany in the previous year were necessary since the Jews were behind the Bolshevik Revolution and backed the communists in Europe. Lindbergh's hosts in Berlin added that American press criticism of Germany was 'Jewish propaganda in Jewish-owned [American] papers'.[17]

After this carefully guided tour, Lindbergh then helped the American Embassy in Berlin to prepare what was to be a famous and influential

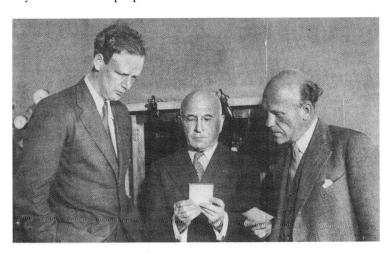

Carrel and Lindbergh attended the Copenhagen Experimental Cytology conference in 1936, hosted by the local tissue culturist Albert Fischer. (*Courtesy of Georgetown University Library, Booth Family Center for Special Collections.*)

---

[15] A. Scott Berg, *Lindbergh* (New York, G.P. Putnam's Sons, 1998): 361.

[16] Berg, *Lindbergh* (note 15): 361.

[17] Berg, *Lindbergh* (note 15): 361.

report on German air power. His assessment was that if any European war were to occur soon, German air power would be dominant and irresistible. From Berlin he flew to Copenhagen.

Copenhagen Meeting

After Pontigny, Carrel met up with Lindbergh in Copenhagen. Lindbergh had characteristically arrived early in case of any problems setting up the pumps, notably with the gas and electricity supply. He had prudently arranged for three pumps, plus their associated equipment, to be crated and shipped from New York to the meeting, in case of damage, and only one had survived the long journey. The survivor was exhibited in a special stall and Carrel, with typical showmanship, provided sterile outer garments for the visitors to be admitted, 10 at a time, to view the pump in action. Carrel spoke at the opening session, and to the press, but Lindbergh hid away, avoiding the photographers and autograph hunters seeking sight of him — 'Danish Crowds Worry Lindbergh', reported Baltimore's *Sun*.

To help Lindbergh and Carrel during the meeting, particularly with translation, the organiser, Albert Fischer of Copenhagen's Carlsberg Biological Institute, gave them the assistance of Richard J. Bing (1909–2010), a young visiting German then on his staff. Bing was half-Jewish, and at the meeting he made it clear to the visitors that he wished to leave Germany. Carrel, soon after, arranged a short-term post for him as a visiting worker at the Rockefeller Institute.[18] Bing gave them an account of his experiences in Germany, and Carrel knew by this time that the German universities were dismissing Jewish staff. Adding to this, the Leopoldina, the important German scientific society to which Carrel belonged, was now headed by Emil Abderhalden, a committed Nazi party member, and it was also steadily expelling its Jewish members, which included Albert Einstein. Carrel and Lindbergh therefore had direct knowledge in 1936 of the growth of the darker side of the Nazi regime.

---

[18] Bing, after a short attachment at the Rockefeller Institute, then moved elsewhere in New York to work as a cardiologist; see R.J. Bing (1987) 'Lindbergh and the biological sciences' *Texas Heart Journal* 14: 231–7.

Back to the Island

It had been a busy summer in Europe in 1936 for both men. After their travels, the two couples settled back on Carrel's island in August. Mme Carrel was a gracious and energetic hostess, and keen to show her interest in the paranormal. She demonstrated water-divining and showed her guests the successful use of a pendulum to find lost objects. She told of local inhabitants with unusual powers, and when an itinerant mesmeriser appeared near the island, Carrel paid him well and studied him for a week. But Carrel could be sceptical and was not always impressed by Jeanne Laplace, the psychic patronised by his wife in Paris.[19] From 1926, Laplace had made herself available to the Institut Métapsychique International in Paris, where she demonstrated her alleged powers.[20]

On the island, Mme Carrel was also developing an interest in herbal medicine and grew a variety of plants from which she made tinctures and gave them out to friends and family. Carrel was impressed with her 'No. 48' remedy for his own intermittent digestive upsets, and of its use for migraine. The Lindberghs also noticed Mme Carrel's own bouts of unexplained sudden prostration which caused temporary alarm, but from which she recovered quickly.

European Report

On Saint-Gildas, Carrel and Lindbergh reported to each other on their travels. Lindbergh told Carrel about the situation in Germany and talked about the new German national confidence, their new roads, social security, their encouragement of sport, their youth movement, and that national planning seemed to work. Carrel, always attracted to strong

---

[19] See Anne Morrow Lindbergh, *The Flower and the Nettle: Diaries and Letters of Ann Morrow Lindbergh* (New York: Harcourt Brace Jovanovich, 1976): 70.
[20] For Jeanne Laplace, see *Journal of Scientific Exploration* 25 (2011): 479. She was also investigated sympathetically by Britain's credulous and short-lived National Laboratory of Psychical Research.

leadership, including Mussolini's regime in Italy, might not have disagreed with Lindbergh's enthusiasm, in spite of the ancient French antipathy to Germany. Carrel wrote to his nephew soon after that 'Germany and Italy must save the world wounded by mechanical civilisation and Russian communism'.[21]

Lindbergh was unimpressed with the dilatory attitudes he found in France. But Carrel, though regularly despairing of France, had hopes for the future and could report to Lindbergh that he had done something towards strengthening France and reversing the decadence he detected, since he had joined the group at Pontigny and supported the inaugural meeting of the PPF.

But when Lindbergh passed on to the Carrels what they were told in Germany regarding the alleged Jewish plots, this may have been a new idea to Carrel, one which he resisted at the time. There is no anti-Semitism in *Man, the Unknown*, and Carrel was close to a number of Jewish doctors in New York and knew many Jewish scientists at the Institute.

Carrel had more European visits in this busy summer before returning to America. He caught up with his family in Lyon and then went on to Italy, where he visited Nicola Pende, one of his favourite biologists. Carrel had praised him and his 'biotypology' in *Man, the Unknown*, and Pende, now a senator in the Italian government, ran the Genoa Instituto de Biotipologia individual y Ortogénesis and was in favour with Mussolini. Biotypology involved the measurement of human physical and psychological features leading to classification of humans, and it further taught that these various types correlated with health and attainments in life. Hence the early allocation of a biotype could direct people towards success, particularly in specific occupations.[22] Carrel was impressed with

---

[21] Carrel to Gigou, 18 January 1937, Malinin Collection, box 14 folder 6. FA 208, RUA RAC (note 3).

[22] For inter-war French biotypology, see William H. Schneider (1991) 'The scientific study of labour in interwar France' *French Historical Studies* 17: 410–46.

what he saw during his visit.[23] Pende's Institute was moving from Genoa to Rome in that year of 1936, and Pende invited Carrel to return later and speak at the formal opening of his new Institute. Another Italian honour came to Carrel, this time from the Pope, to be a founder member of the Pontificia academia delle scienze — the Pontifical Academy of Sciences.[24] This society had an ancient lineage but had lost prestige and, hoping to restore its authority, Pope Pius XI reconstituted it that year, with a new remit to seek a reconciliation between science and religion. Seventy scientists with links to the international Roman Catholic church were elected as members of the revived Academy, and Carrel was an obvious choice. The inaugural meeting was planned for late 1936.

Back to New York

After his summer stay at Saint-Gildas, Carrel returned to New York, awaiting a return within a few months to Italy for both the meetings. But the illness of the Pope in the autumn meant that the Academy re-launch was postponed until next year. Pende's invitation was still awaited, but meantime Carrel sought advice from others. The word was that Pende was poorly regarded by scientists in Rome, notably for his overbearing manner and fondness for publicity, and Pende was also soon linked to the Italian government's anti-Semitism. In the end, Pende's invitation to Carrel never came through.

Reader's Digest

In New York, on his return, there was more good news for Carrel about *Man, the Unknown*. Before publication in the previous year, Harper & Brothers had been privately concerned that sales of the book might be low and that it was worth considering a new publishing strategy. This was to accept an offer from *Reader's Digest* for publication of a condensed

---

[23] Carrel to Lindbergh, 12 September 1936, Charles Augustus Lindbergh Papers, box 7 folio 0178, MS 325, Yale University Library Manuscripts and Archives (YULMA).
[24] 'Foundation of the Pontifical Academy of Sciences' *Science*, 19 November 1937, 470–2. Carrel may have written this lively and informative article.

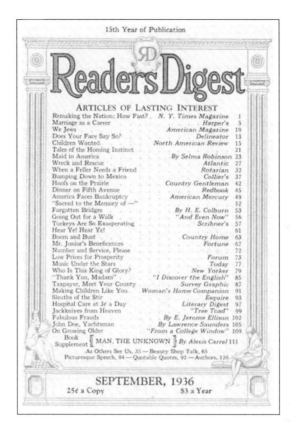

The *Reader's Digest* carried a condensed version of Carrel's book.

version of the book. This pocket-sized monthly magazine, then and later, had a middlebrow readership holding conservative and traditional views. Founded in 1922, it had been hugely successful and by the 1930s had reached a circulation of 1.8 million.[25] Its articles were taken from other published sources but before use underwent considerable editorial revision and compaction towards the required *Digest* style. DeWitt Wallace, the co-founder and editor, considered that most writers were verbose, and accordingly from 1934 brought in his 'condensed book' feature, in which the magazine carried much-shortened versions of the

---

[25] James Playsted Wood, *Of Lasting Interest: The Story of the Reader's Digest* (New York: Doubleday, 1967): 56.

chosen work. The format was to be very successful thereafter. *Man, the Unknown* was the second of the *Digest's* experiments with condensation.[26]

A Harper & Brothers editor later recalled the events, and their initial assessment of the manuscript of *Man, the Unknown*:

> [The book] was by no means a light popularisation and the advance sales of about 3,500 bore this out. Harper's feeling was that the book was destined to reach an intelligent but limited audience. With considerable misgivings, we sold condensation rights in the book to the *Digest* and … demanded a guarantee against loss.[27]

The *Digest's* editor Wallace agreed with the publisher that if the magazine's condensed version adversely affected the sales of the book, then the *Digest* would compensate Harpers with $5,000. Contrary to Harper's expectation, *Man, the Unknown* had sold astonishingly well, and when the condensed book then appeared in the *Digest* of September 1936, about a year after publication, book sales then rose again. The *Digest* did not have to pay out.

After this involvement, Carrel and DeWitt Wallace were to meet later, and took to each other; Carrel was then to write for the *Digest*.

Visitors and Contacts

Carrel continued to host distinguished visitors at the Institute and these included Pasteur Vallery-Radot (head of the Pasteur Institute in Paris), Lord Dawson, the London physician, and Aldous Huxley, known to Carrel from the Pontigny meetings. As mentioned earlier, Huxley had already used Carrel's tissue culture as a theme in a 1927 short story, and in Huxley's 1939 novel *After Many a Summer*, there would be Carrelian influences.

---

[26] The *Digest's* first condensed book was Arnold Bennett's *How to Live on Twentyfour Hours a Day* (1910).

[27] Cass Canfield, *Up Down and Around: A Publisher's Recollections* (New York: Harper's Magazine Press, 1971), an account confirmed in Wood, *Lasting Interest* (note 25). Canfield wrongly dated the use of the condensed version of *Man, the Unknown* to immediately after the book's release in 1935, hence exaggerating the *Digest's* influence on the book's success.

Edward Moore, a businessman involved in natural gas exploration, had been impressed by Carrel's book and had drawn up his own plans for an 'Institute of Man'. He wrote to Carrel and met him at the Institute, and they stayed in contact; Moore would thereafter support Carrel's own hopes for such a venture.

One other new and lasting acquaintance was James 'Jim' Newton, introduced to Carrel by Ed Moore. Newton was an activist in the Moral Rearmament movement, an evangelical but rather mysterious organisation which recruited wealthy and influential supporters and sought 'God-control' at all levels of society and government. Carrel was impressed with the movement's successful rallies, notably in Washington and California, and Carrel assisted by sending a supportive message. He attended one of their fundraising and confessional 'house party' meetings at Stockbridge, Mass. Newton was publisher of the MRA's manifesto *Rising Tide* in 1937, and he was one of the few invited to visit Saint-Gildas. Although Newton became part of Carrel's small inner circle, Carrel characteristically remained detached from the MRA movement even though it shared much of Carrel's agenda for spiritual reform.[28] About this time, Carrel exchanged letters of mutual admiration with J. Edgar Hoover, head of America's Federal Bureau of Investigation. Carrel complimented Hoover on his robust drive for law and order, and in return, Hoover regularly sent Carrel copies of his books and the text of his hard-line lectures, in which he complained of the 'weakening of moral principles, extinction of civic consciousness, country club prisons and their recidivist clientele'.

Lindbergh Activities

Returning to Long Barn after their Saint-Gildas stay and the Copenhagen Congress in the summer of 1936, Lindbergh was developing a new interest. As always, Carrel's wide-ranging discourse was an influence — he recalled later that:

---

[28] James Newton, *Uncommon Friends: Life with Thomas Edison, Henry Ford, Harvey Firestone, Alexis Carrel and Charles Lindbergh* (New York: Harcourt Brace Jovanovich, 1978): 121–206. Newton had talents in befriending celebrities — the *NYT* review of his book said it was 'a weak broth of biography, spiritual uplift and environmental concerns'.

With Doctor Carrel, on Saint-Gildas, conversation shifted from scientific subjects to phenomena as yet unexplained by mind, to accounts of a Breton peasant hypnotising animals, to miraculous cures that had been credited at Lourdes. Was there any reality to ghosts? What circumstances were most stimulating to supernatural perception?[29]

Mme Carrel had impressed Charles with her dowsing and demonstration of the use of a pendulum, and Lindbergh had returned home with a pendulum as a gift. True to Carrel's insistence on proper scientific observation, Lindbergh did some experiments in which he carefully recorded his searches for hidden objects using his pendulum and considered that they were more successful than explained by chance. Carrel's belief in the paranormal encouraged him to look for physical explanations of telepathy and Lindbergh purchased an infra-red light detector, planning to test if invisible radiation might be the transfer mechanism involved. Lindbergh extended his interest to other even more mystical matters. Carrel had told him about Indian holy men who could walk on fire or were unaffected by poisons, and there were those who could enter trances and be buried for days, yet emerge unharmed. Carrel had seen such men in action in New York, and had also studied Eileen Garrett, a well-known American medium, who entered trances. He, ever the scientist, advised her to have physiological measurements made during these altered states.[30] Lindbergh in England decided to take this approach further and

> spent many hours in the library of the College of Physicians, in London, reading reports about rhythmic breathing, controlling pulse rate, and walking on live coals in Asia. Between the trickery of the fakir and the asceticism of the saint, it seems obvious that a wide border zone existed.[31]

---

[29] Charles A. Lindbergh, *Autobiography of Values* (New York: Harcourt Brace Jovanovich, 1976): 367.

[30] See Garrett's autobiography, *Adventures in the Supernormal* (New York: Creative Edge Press, 1949): 169.

[31] Lindbergh, *Autobiography* (note 29): 368.

Taught by Carrel to seek a physiological explanation, Lindbergh wondered if during their trances these men slowed their heart and breathing. Lindbergh wanted to hear testimony from travellers in India and introduced himself to Francis Younghusband (1863–1942), known as 'the Empire's last great explorer', an adventurer like himself, who lived near him in Kent. But Younghusband had little specific information to offer. However, he told Lindbergh about a religious conference in Calcutta planned for the following spring to which the Lindberghs were welcome, and that on the visit, they could investigate further. Charles now had a newly-built British plane, and needed little encouragement to plan another aerial adventure of the type for which they were both now famous. As a result, the Lindberghs decided to attend this International Parliament of Religions, in March 1937, in Calcutta.

They set off in February for India, making the necessary multiple stops on the way. Flying over and staying in Rome, Greece, Egypt and the site of Babylon, and then on to India, they repeatedly encountered and studied the remains of ancient cities.

The conference proved to be a disappointment, and engine troubles limited their further explorations. Lindbergh had hoped to study the holy men and uncover secrets unknown to Western science, but these practitioners proved to be elusive, and when the Lindberghs returned they were little further forward. However, their tour of the ancient civilisations was an epiphany for them both. Their inspection on the ground and from the air of the impressive antiquities led Lindbergh to reflect on the rise and fall of empires, as did Carrel frequently. Lindbergh concluded that the British Empire was similarly doomed, and said so to their host, the politician Harold Nicolson, when they were back in England. Lindbergh told him that Britain wrongly assumed that her powerful Navy and the barrier of the English Channel would be sufficient protection from a war in Europe. Lindbergh told Nicolson and others that air power instead would be the dominant factor in any war, and Britain should be aware of the danger from resurgent Germany. Nicolson was not impressed with Lindbergh's stance nor his patriotism, and recorded in his diary that 'Lindbergh believes in Nazi theology, all tied up with his hatred of degeneracy and his hatred of democracy as represented by the Free Press in the American public'.[32]

Pump Projects

Back from India, Lindbergh caught up with the letters and the news from the Institute. The pump experiments were not extending into new territory. The thyroid glands certainly appeared to survive when looked under the microscope, but detecting hormone production from the glands was proving to be elusive. Attempts to obtain heart and kidney survival on the pump had been given up. Carrel accepted this and reminded Lindbergh in May 1937 that 'as you know kidneys and testicles degenerate rapidly when cultivated'.

There were two new visiting workers in Carrel's laboratories. Richard Bing, who Carrel and Lindbergh had met in Copenhagen, moved to New York before Christmas, and he was joined some months later in early 1937 by Harald Okkels (1898–1970), also from Copenhagen. These two new arrivals seemed concerned, unlike Carrel, at the failure of kidneys and hearts to survive.[33] They both felt that, since the circulating fluid carried less oxygen than did blood, the low oxygen supply might explain the failure with kidney and heart. Bing had the reasonable idea of adding oxygen-carrying haemocyanin, the invertebrate's version of haemoglobin, to the circulating fluid, but found no benefit.[34] Okkels, also concerned about the vitality, even of the thyroid glands, asked Lindbergh to modify the pump to allow studies of oxygen uptake by the organs, to see if they were alive.

---

[32] From Nigel Nicolson (ed.), *The Harold Nicolson Diaries 1907–1963* (London: Weidenfeld and Nicolson, reprint 2004): 126. On publication, Lindbergh proposed suing for libel, but lawyers advised that this quotation could be defended using Lindbergh's known published views. See also Charles A. Lindbergh, *The Wartime Diaries* (New York, Harcourt Brace Jovanovich, 1970): 28.

[33] H. Okkels (1942) 'Culture of whole organs' *Journal of the Microscopical Society* 62: 103–11. He noted the problem with patchy death of the glands and disloyally raised the idea that the pump was a 'white elephant'.

[34] Richard Bing (1938) 'The perfusion of whole organs in the Lindbergh apparatus with fluids containing hemocyanin as respiratory pigment' *Science* 87: 554–5. In this brief article he described improved kidney perfusion using the pigment and that he had detected insulin coming from a perfused pancreas; neither claim was ever confirmed.

Lindbergh agreed to do this, and sent detailed instructions to Zwick. Lindbergh agreed that it was desirable to increase the oxygen supply and to do this, he acted decisively and proposed that the pump should be placed in a high-pressure chamber. At Long Barn, he got to work on the design and did the necessary engineering drawings for a 2×3 foot steel compression chamber to hold the pump, fitted with glass observation panels.[35] He handed over its development and construction to Siebe Gorman and Co. in London, the British experts on diving equipment, but with the company involved in urgent military work, the chamber was not delivered until later that year.[36]

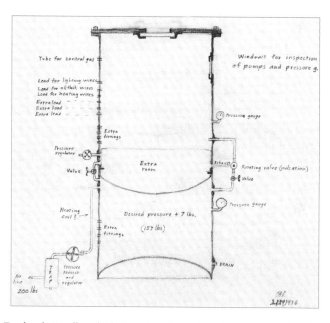

In exile in England, Lindbergh designed and purchased a pressure chamber to increase the oxygenation of the tissue in the organ pump. (*Courtesy of the Yale University Library Manuscripts and Archives.*)

After Bing left the Institute, Carrel asked him for the insulin data, but it was not forthcoming; see Alexis Carrel Papers, box 40 folder 6, GULBFC (note 8).

[35] Drawings for the chamber are in Charles Augustus Lindbergh Papers, box 34 folder, MS 325, YULMA (note 23).

[36] Lindbergh, always aware of his volunteer status at the Rockefeller Institute, personally paid for this and other apparatus, and even for the reprints of his articles arising from his Institute work.

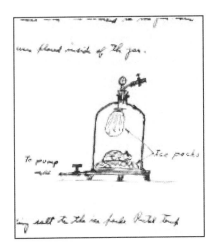

Lindbergh also did simple experiments on hypothermia using guinea pigs. (*Courtesy of the Yale University Library Manuscripts and Archives.*)

Meanwhile, he put together a simple device which delivered air at increased pressure into a glass bell jar chamber containing guinea pigs. These studies showed no ill effects.

Lowering the Temperature

Though the Indian trip had been disappointing, Lindbergh still wished to continue work on states of altered consciousness, and he now wondered if the slow heartbeat and suspended respiration said to occur in the Indian holy men in their trances was caused by a lowered body temperature. He knew from Carrel that low temperatures successfully preserved the life of tissues, work which Carrel had pioneered decades before, and to take up this idea, Lindbergh's bell jar was in use again. This time he used salt and ice packs to cool down the chamber with guinea pigs inside. The observations were inconclusive and no recoverable coma was obtained. Instead, there was the expected fatal outcome when the temperature fell below about 15° centigrade.

Lindbergh was not discouraged. He still wondered if humans could lower their temperatures and routinely recover. If so, and if pain was not felt in this state, low temperature might aid human anaesthesia and surgery. Lindbergh wrote enthusiastically to Carrel about this possible use of hypothermia, and made a remarkable suggestion that

are there not likely to be both medical and surgical uses for such a procedure [hypothermia]? For instance, might we not be able to construct an apparatus to maintain circulation during operations on the heart. You will remember that I did some preliminary work on such a grand apparatus at the Institute two or three years ago. One of the main problems seemed to be coagulability of blood at body temperature … a reduction in body temperature and a corresponding reduction in coagulability and circulation might make such apparatus feasible.[37]

This was an important letter. It shows that Lindbergh, after he first met Carrel in 1930, had indeed made moves at the Institute towards making a heart bypass pump to allow heart surgery, but was discouraged, either because Carrel said it was futile or because Lindbergh attempted it and encountered blood clotting. Lindbergh had clearly not forgotten this episode and was now showing interest in reviving his original project. He now had this suggestion to deal with the clotting problem. Still unaware that anticoagulants were available, Lindbergh reasoned that in using hypothermia in human surgery, the cooled blood might not clot, and hence a pump could be used to maintain circulation during heart surgery. But he had also realised something else. During hypothermia the body metabolism is lowered and the consequent 'reduction in … circulation' would make less demands on a bypass pump.

Carrel should have pondered this suggestion. He had pioneered the techniques of cardiac surgery in dogs earlier, but had only five minutes operating time during suspension of cardiac output before the brain was damaged. Carrel was also first to show the biological value of cold in protecting cells from death. Lindbergh's suggestion to Carrel that there were 'uses' for hypothermia in heart surgery had the answer to Carrel's lack of time for his operations. This strategy of hypothermia was indeed brought in 15 years later as the first method of allowing human open-heart surgery. Only later was it overtaken by the development of the heart–lung bypass machines, which had already commenced, unknown to Lindbergh.

---

[37] Lindbergh to Carrel, 24 July 1937, Charles Augustus Lindbergh Papers, box 35 folder 1075, MS 325, YULMA (note 23).

But Carrel was not listening and did not respond to Lindbergh's new ideas for heart surgery. When Carrel did reply to Lindbergh's prescient letter, he was instead only interested in telling Lindbergh about his plans for a 'Psychobiology Institute' to study mankind's problems, and he enclosed a 10-page proposal.[38] Lindbergh dutifully wrote back with detailed comments; the perceptive ideas for the use of hypothermia were put aside.

Lectures and Awards

Diversions for Carrel from his laboratory work included acceptance of more invited lectures.[39] In that year of 1937, the first was the Cardinal Newman Award given by the Newman Foundation at the University of Illinois at Urbana-Champaign, a college which largely enrolled Catholic students and offered them suitable instruction. The Award went to an individual who had 'made an outstanding contribution to the enrichment of American life in the fields of science, literature, art or statesmanship'. When giving his lecture on 21 February, Carrel pleased the local theologians by deploring 'society's decline and the separation of the soul from the body'. But to their disappointment, his solution was that 'more science' was needed and that particularly 'biotypology is in its infancy'.[40] Supportive of positive eugenics, he suggested 'propagation by the best strains only, under age of 30'.

Summer 1937 Visits

Back in Europe again in summer, Carrel attended the much-postponed inaugural meeting of the Pontifical Academy in Rome. Afterwards,

---

[38] Carrel had copied this title from the Groupe d'études psycho-biologiques, a French organisation linked to the CEPH.

[39] Earlier, less prominent Carrel lectures were to the women's Cosmopolitan Club of Philadelphia, the Lewis Linn McArthur Lecture to the Institute of Medicine in Chicago, and later an address to the Council of the Life Association Presidents in December 1937.

[40] 'Sees Man As A Whole' *NYT,* 22 Feb 1937, and published as 'For a new knowledge of man' *Commonweal* 26 (1937): 12–13. Founded in 1924, it is the oldest U.S. Catholic journal of opinion.

writing to Lindbergh, he was characteristically sour, noting that the Vatican people were 'childish, sly and assured. ... The Academy is a failure. The idea of the Pope was a great idea. But a strange sabotage took place'. When in Rome, Carrel called in on Pende, the biotypology expert, and reported that he 'loves money, a clever politician hated by his colleagues. ... Mussolini is going to build for him a large hospital and laboratories for the study and development of human personality'.[41]

Carrel returned to his island, and Lindbergh flew over from England a number of times to confer. Lindbergh brought with him the glass bell jar and simple hypothermia apparatus and, landing at a small airfield on the French mainland, he and the equipment were noticed. A British reporter got word of Lindbergh's movements and the resulting *Sunday Express* 11 July story was vivid, even by Carrelian standards.[42] The article described a secret machine being assembled on the island to revive dead organs, including the brain, and the island was easily portrayed as a remote and mysterious place suitable for magic and sorcery. Lindbergh was displeased. Carrel, for once, chided the press for their attention, but in doing so, he kept the interest up, and his statement to the Associated Press agency confirmed the idea that there was something afoot on his island:

> You know that for scientific work peace is a requisite. The attention of the public should not be attracted to this spot where we are working and on us. At this time silence is the necessity.[43]

Carrel travelled back on the *Normandie*. The press noted his departure and arrival, and in New York, he spoke to journalists and wondered, disingenuously, why the press was so interested in his work with Lindbergh.[44]

---

[41] Carrel to Lindbergh, 11 June 1937, box 7, folders 0178 and 0179, MS 325, YULMA (note 23).

[42] The *NYT* had articles on Lindbergh's visit on July 5, 6, 7, 11 and 18, 1937. The Baltimore *Sun* reported on 5 July that 'Lindbergh Paddles To Island At Night In Collapsible Boat'. There were further Saint-Gildas island stories on 30 July and 9 August.

[43] 'Carrel And Lindbergh Work On New Experiment' *NYT*, 18 September 1937.

[44] 'Carrel Back: Says We Talk Too Much' *NYT*, 1 October 1937.

Phi Beta Kappa

After his return, Carrel visited his old acquaintance John Harvey Kellogg at his Battle Creek Sanitarium in September, and they talked about matters of mutual interest, notably race betterment. Carrel's next prestigious lecture followed soon after and at Dartmouth University on 11 October 1937 he gave the 'Oration' at the 150th Anniversary of the Foundation of Alpha of Phi Beta Kappa. This highly-respected academic honour society dates from 1776 and, founded 'to celebrate excellence in liberal arts and sciences', it inducts a small number of outstanding students each year. In his lecture, Carrel returned to familiar theme, but adding some ominous extras, telling the audience that

> nervous fragility, intellectual weakness, moral corruption are more dangerous for the future than yellow fever, typhus and cancer. ... The civilised races seem to be losing the courage to live ... happiness eludes us ... propagation of the best strains of the race is needed ... those who have given their lives to the search for the prevention and cure of disease are keenly disappointed in observing that their efforts have resulted in a large number of healthy defectives, healthy lunatics and healthy criminals.

To these now-familiar themes, he added more detail of his thinking in *Man, the Unknown* for a solution to the problems he perceived. It was to construct a new institute. He had given his project a variety of names previously, and he now called for the establishment of an 'Institute for the Construction of the Civilised Man'.[45]

Lindbergh's Return Visit

Fairly soon after the lecture, Lindbergh returned to America in December 1937 for a short visit, and he had a number of reasons. He had made two

---

[45] Alexis Carrel (1937) 'The making of civilised men' *Dartmouth Alumni Magazine* 30: 6–10. In Carrel's lecture, Mussolini was no longer on his list of great men. It was reported as 'Calls On Science To Save Humanity' *NYT*, 12 October, 1937; Carrel's honorarium for the lecture was $225.

more low-key trips to Germany and wanted to report directly to the American military leaders and impress on them again his findings about the power of the German air force. Lindbergh also wanted to catch up with Institute's pump work and to talk to Carrel about hypothermia, and he had shipped the new metal and glass high-pressure chamber back to New York. To add to this, he and his wife were out of touch with their families.

Lindbergh intended the pressure chamber for use either to give a higher oxygen supply in the pump or for hypothermia experiments on animals larger than guinea pigs. It seems no better results were obtained with the pump in use inside. Carrel did start experiments on hypothermia using small monkeys, but these were inconclusive and Carrel was uninterested in carrying on. One understandable distraction for them both was that the publisher Paul Hoeber, who had published Carrel's World War I text on infected wounds, had now joined Harper & Brothers, Carrel's publisher, and Hoeber had responsibility for the firm's list of medical texts. He approached Carrel in November 1937, suggesting that he and Lindbergh write a book on the organ pump and its uses. They agreed to do it, and it would be published in June of the following year.

Biography Suggested

Another matter to divert Carrel were some early moves towards writing his biography. The first move came from Arthur Train Jr., son of his old friend from the Fencing Club days. Train did some reading and interviewed Carrel, and then submitted the draft biography to Carrel for his approval. Carrel showed it to friends, including Coudert and Lindbergh. Coudert liked the text, but Lindbergh was not impressed, in particular by the 'invented' conversations throughout the text. Lindbergh was not placated when Train explained that 'imaginary conversation is necessary in this type of literature'. Others in Carrel's group discouraged the project. Boris Bakhmeteff was concerned it would be seen as publicity-seeking. Train instead published an account of Carrel's life in the *Saturday Evening Post*.[46]

---

[46] Arthur Train Jr. 'More will live' *The Saturday Evening Post*, 23 July 1938; Train annoyed Lindbergh by dropping in Lindbergh's name as having assisted with the article.

A draft for another biographical article arrived later from Emil Ludwig.[47] He was known for his biographies of Napoleon, Goethe, Bismarck, Beethoven and others, and he had famously been granted interviews with Stalin and Mussolini. Carrel was displeased with the way he was portrayed, but Ludwig defended his approach by saying that 'my New York friends warned me you were a fascist. I answered I don't care, I am portraying the eminent scientist'.[48]

Winter 1937

The Lindberghs stayed in New York for three months before returning to England, and Mme Carrel, for once, also settled in New York for a while that winter. Lindbergh had enjoyed the visit to Saint-Gildas in the summer, and when Mme Carrel told him that an island close to Saint-Gildas was for sale, Lindbergh purchased it almost unseen. Though it lacked plumbing, heating and electricity, Anne, as ever, bravely agreed to the purchase to have this summer home for the family, and it offered the seclusion they needed. French citizenship was required when purchasing a maritime property, and Mme Carrel obliged by making all the legal arrangements.

Lindbergh's four acre Île Illiec was small compared with Carrel's 100 acre island, but it had a large mansion house, big enough for the Lindberghs, their sons age five and one, and their staff, and there was a cottage for a caretaker. They now had a cook. The two islands were connected by a sand bar at low water. The house had earlier been built by Ambroise Thomas (1811–1896), head of the Paris Conservatory, and he had composed the opera *Mignon* there in the 1860s.

Into 1938

After their short stay in New York, the Lindberghs returned to Long Barn, and they would take possession of their island in the summer. With the launch of their book *The Culture of Organs* coming up, Carrel spoke

---

[47] Carrel later appeared in Ludwig's *Galerie de portraits* (Paris: Fayard, 1948).
[48] Ludwig to Carrel, box 42 June–August 1940, GULBFC (note 8).

about it at the American Philosophical Society meeting on 21 April in Philadelphia. He was in a confident mood and enthused about the pump and spoke of its ability to keep organs alive for prolonged periods, and that infection had occurred in less than 1% of the runs. He said that practically every important organ had been studied, and that although most experiments were terminated to allow study of the tissues, there was no reason not to keep organs alive indefinitely. He claimed that 11½ years of life had been gained for the organs used in the 100,000 hours of perfusion. He even suggested 'test-tube baby' production was possible since guinea pig uterus and ovaries had been used in some experiments. He said that insulin and thyroid hormone had been produced by the glands. Carrel misled the audience and was, not for the first time, blurring

THE CULTURE

OF ORGANS

by

ALEXIS CARREL

and

CHARLES A. LINDBERGH

WITH 111 ILLUSTRATIONS

1938

HAMISH HAMILTON MEDICAL BOOKS

90 GREAT RUSSELL STREET,

LONDON, W.C.1.

Carrel and Lindbergh's book on 'Organ Culture' appeared in 1938.

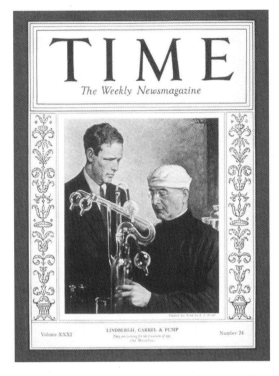

The cover of *Time* magazine 13 June 1938 showed Carrel and Lindbergh with the pump.

what might be achieved with what had been found thus far. Next day the *New York Times* carried an editorial, and although detecting a hint of science-fiction, concluded that 'here is a feat of the laboratory which dwarfs anything that [Edgar Allan] Poe ever conceived'.[49]

Their book was published in June 1938 and was announced well ahead by Hoeber, the publisher. *Time* magazine approached Hoeber and asked to be given exclusive coverage of the launch, but when Lindbergh in England was contacted he was not happy. He told Carrel that '*Time* is not the magazine I would select to cooperate with ... they are not as

---

[49] 'Organs Live Days In Lindbergh Pump' *NYT*, 22 April 1938 and 'Medical Engineering' [Editorial], 23 April 1938. His lecture was never published in full. The American Philosophical Society welcomed journalists and assisted their coverage of the meetings; see David Dietz (1937) 'Science and the American Press' *Science* 85: 107–12.

much interested in fact, as in sensation'. However when *Time* agreed that their journalist's text could be checked ahead, and that the two men would appear on the magazine's cover, the package was irresistible to the publisher, and Lindbergh gave in.

On 13 June 1938, Carrel, for the second time in two years, was on the cover of *Time* magazine, joined this time by the reticent, but absent, Lindbergh. The cover used a curious commissioned oil painting which placed Lindbergh on one side behind Carrel, looking down as if in awe of the serious older scientist, who is holding, even posessing, Lindbergh's iconic glass pump.[50] On this occasion, the newspapers were even keener on the pump than three years previously when the first news of organ perfusion broke. Waldemar Kaempffert, the *New York Times* science correspondent, a member at the Century Association, and always enthusiastic about Carrel's work, wrote a series of three articles on the pump, assisted by an interview with Carrel given over dinner. The articles described how

> 1,000 organs have been kept alive within its stylish glass bulbs from 2 to 30 days — hearts, lungs, livers, spleens, reproductive organs. The hearts beat on, the glands secrete hormones, organs function just as they do within the bodies from which they were dissected.[51]

Kaempffert added that organs would now be removed to Carrel's glass 'organ hospital' to be repaired and then replaced in the body. A diabetic's defective pancreas could be removed and revived by feeding in the missing chemical.

The respected *New York Times* journalist also included a vivid update on the immortal tissue cultured cells:

> The culture has its microscopic ailments. Perhaps it needs a bath; perhaps a change of diet; perhaps a period of fasting. The Vestal virgins who guard the living flame know. 100 years hence their descendents

---

[50] The painting by Samuel Johnson Wood is now held in the National Portrait Gallery in Washington.

[51] 'Carrel, At 65, Deep In New Studies' *NYT*, 26 June 1938.

may also be starting over the culture, performing the same surgical and aseptic rites.

The analogy with the Roman eternal flame was apt. Carrel's technicians, like the attendants in Rome, knew the consequences of letting the 'living flame' go out.

Next year there was release of another Boris Karloff film, *The Man They Could Not Hang*, and yet again it showed a Carrel-like pump in use to revive an executed man. The run of low-budget Boris Karloff science-fiction films of the late 1930s continued and other Carrelian themes were used — transplantation, reversal of aging and the paranormal.[52] The pump had been on show in Paris at the 1937 Exposition Internationale, and in 1939, at the New York World Fair, a working pump was the chief attraction in the Hall of Medicine.[53]

The Book

In spite of the excellent publicity, and the fame of the authors, the public realised that *The Culture of Organs* was a technical work, and the first year sales were only 927, hardly even a creditable figure for a scientific work. Only 82 were sold in the second year.[54] The greater part of the book was devoted to Lindbergh's design and the fluids in use, with little on the results. It fitted the pattern of Carrel's scientific style, introducing methods for others to follow and develop. But, as always, his results have to be looked at with care.

The results showed again that only the thyroid gland was studied regularly over the years. The failure to sustain heart or kidney and other

---

[52] The Karloff films were *The Man who Changed his Mind*, 1936 (mind transplant), *Black Friday*, 1940 (brain-switching), *The Man with Nine Lives*, 1940 (resuscitation from frozen), *Before I Hang*, 1940 (rejuvenation by serum), *The Ape*, 1940 (serum for polio cases), and *The Devil Commands*, 1941 (contacting the dead by telepathy).

[53] 'Carrel Explains Mechanical Heart' *NYT*, 6 May 1939, had an interview with Carrel at the World Fair.

[54] Hoeber's contract with Carrel and Lindbergh for *The Culture of Organs* only paid royalties after 1,000 copies were sold, and hence they received only small cheques. The book was later translated into French, Czech and Swedish.

tissues was noted only briefly. The earlier claim for insulin production from a pancreas was dropped.[55] When perfusing the thyroid gland, there certainly was iodine coming out into the fluid, but the gland had considerable stores of iodine-containing hormone which might simply have leaked out.[56] On the fundamental question of whether or not his thyroid glands were alive, Carrel's tests for survival have to be looked at closely — it is odd that thyroid could apparently survive so well when all other organs did not.

His tests of thyroid vitality were indirect and are only briefly described. He relied on microscopy of the gland after perfusion, which is risky, since tissue can be dead but cellular architecture remains normal for a while. Small fragments taken for tissue culture from three- or six-day cultured organs gave colonies of fibroblasts, which Carrel took as a test of survival of the gland's secretory cells. But the most convincing way to show that his long-perfused glands had survived, indeed the only test, would have been to re-transplant a slice of the perfused tissue back into the original donor and study the graft's survival. There are some suggestions that this was done. The verdict is carefully worded: the results of re-transplantation were 'inconsistent'.[57]

Carrel may have obtained prolonged thyroid survival or he may not — firm evidence is lacking. Carrel's intuition, ever active, suggested that eventually such organ perfusion machines would succeed in obtaining long-term organ survival, and he could ignore any short-term setbacks. Similar premature Carrelian enthusiasms had been noticed before, notably in his pre-WWI claims for tissue culture success, and he had been eventually vindicated. But this time, as with his announcement of the immortal cells, he was wrong about the general use of the pump, at least

---

[55] Carrel could not get the data from Bing about Bing's claims for insulin production (note 34).

[56] Lillian E. Baker (1938) 'The secretion of iodine by thyroid glands cultivated in the Lindbergh pump' *Science* 88: 479–80 and *JEM* 70 (1939): 29–38 and 39–51.

[57] David M. Friedman, *The Immortalists: Charles Lindbergh, Dr Alexis Carrel and Their Daring Quest to Live Forever* (New York: HarperCollins, 2007): 132, quotes this re-transplantation attempt, but gives no reference. I failed to find any re-transplantation data at Georgetown or at Yale, and it is not given in the Carrel–Lindbergh book.

so far. By the 1960s, with revived interest in perfusion of kidneys for transplantation, only about seven hours' survival was obtained. Well into the 21st century, long-term organ culture has still not been achieved, the best survival with kidney preservation being about 60 hours. Leaving the organ in chilled preservative fluids can be just as effective.[58]

Nevertheless the Carrel pump became famous, but not for its original purpose of long-term organ study, and later admirers were hazy about its usage in Carrel's hands. Instead the elegant photogenic device is now claimed to be the forerunner of organ transplant perfusion pumps, or to be the first attempt at a heart–lung machine for cardiac surgery, or even as a first step towards an implantable artificial heart.

Pump Use Spreads

Because of the celebrity of the pump, other scientists made haste to buy or borrow one, and the Rockefeller Institute allowed Hopf their glassblower to make pumps and sell them for $330. Carrel's laboratory

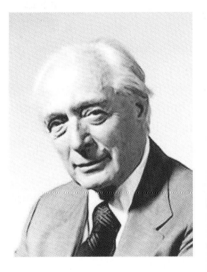

Richard Bing left Germany in 1936 and worked briefly with Carrel on the organ pump.

---

[58] Judah Folkman, Peter Cole and Shirley Zimmerman (1966) 'Tumour behaviour in isolated organs' *Annals of Surgery* 164: 491–501 pointedly mentions that 'no one has approached Carrel's perfusions of three weeks'.

also gave training in its use, and in 1937, J.J. Hayes from California's Alta Bates Hospital was an early arrival for instruction. Cornell University's Dr. Foot also obtained a pump, and Dr. Shorr at the New York Hospital borrowed two. Richard Bing in Carrel's lab annoyed Carrel by secretly obtaining a special pump to take with him to Columbia University but later described his failures to obtain any significant results with it.[59] A German version was patented by Karl Bauer at the Kaiser-Wilhelm-Gesellschaft institute, and one was delivered to the Pasteur Institute's distinguished biologist Emmanuel Fauré-Fremiet.

The most determined attempt to use it successfully was by Leon C. Chesley (1908–2000), the distinguished obstetrician-gynaecologist at the Margaret Hague Maternity Hospital in Jersey City who borrowed a pump for seven years and used it to perfuse human placentas in the hope of finding something coming out which would raise blood pressure, thus explaining the pregnancy condition of pre-eclampsia. He also looked at the output of hormone — the gonadotropins — from the placenta.

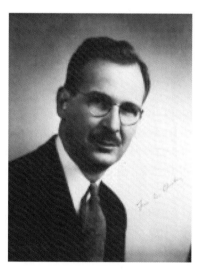

Leon Chesley, the talented New Jersey obstetrician, persevered with organ perfusion studies in the 1940s using Carrel's pump, but without success. (*Courtesy of the National Library of Medicine.*)

---

[59] Bing (note 34) said that thereafter he only used the pump to carry out simple isolated blood vessel perfusion.

Chesley, for a while, shrewdly employed Miss McFaul, Carrel's assistant, after Carrel retired, but they eventually concluded that nothing affecting blood pressure came out in the circulating fluid.[60] Their finding on hormone output was revealing. Gonadotropins did indeed appear in the fluid, but when they ran the pump with nitrogen instead of oxygen, thus killing the tissue, hormone release continued, showing that it was simple leakage from dead tissue.[61]

Although many other investigators started work on organ perfusion, only one scientific publication — Chesley's negative report — can be traced which resulted from the use of these dispersed gifts, purchases and loans. These experienced scientists published regularly, and their silence on their experience with this expensive piece of apparatus is striking. The unavoidable conclusion is that they found that the pump could not sustain the vitality of organs. Replication is at the core of good science, and in normal circumstances even difficult new technology is mastered in time and becomes routinely used and improved. For the pump, this essential scientific test of replication failed, and it sheds serious doubts on Carrel's claims.

Legacy

Discarded and neglected bits of scientific equipment are not usually highly regarded, and devices which do not work are usually scrapped. But although Carrel's pumps gave no reportable results in others' hands, many survived, doubtless because of their mystique, elegance and complexity, and these found their way into historical collections. There are pumps on display at the National Museum of American History in Washington, the Hall of Fame of The International Museum of Surgical Science in

---

[60] Chesley was the American authority on the eclampsia of pregnancy. The negative placenta perfusion findings are in Leon C. Chesley and I. E. McFaul (1949) 'Studies on surviving placental tissue' *American Journal of Obstetrics and Gynecology* 58: 159–65.
[61] Leon C. Chesley (1949) 'Studies on surviving human placental tissue. II. The placental production of gonadotrophin' *Bulletin of the Margaret Hague Maternity Hospital* 2: 71–73.

Chicago, the Mütter Museum of the College of Physicians of Philadelphia, and in Harvard's Collection of Historical Scientific Instruments. The description is usually reverential but unclear about what the pumps were for, or how they worked, particularly as all are displayed without the crucial but unsightly air pump and rubber tubing.

By autumn 1938, Carrel was at the height of his fame, and was now age 65. Normally, senior Rockefeller Institute scientists could have expected to go on working after this conventional retirement age, and Simon Flexner had taken a relaxed attitude to the matter. But Flexner was gone, having retired in 1935, age 72. And Gasser, the new director, was not an admirer of Carrel.

CHAPTER SIXTEEN

Retirement Nears

Simon Flexner, who had been Carrel's greatest supporter, retired as director of the Institute in 1935. In appointing Carrel 30 years previously, Flexner made a bold decision in choosing and nurturing a surgeon as a full-time scientist, and he was pleased to watch Carrel rise to fame and a Nobel Prize. Carrel repaid Flexner by playing a major role in establishing the reputation of the Rockefeller Institute in its early days, thus also pleasing the Institute's founder and funder John D. Rockefeller senior.

By the late 1930s, Carrel was one of the best-known scientists of the day and his book *Man, the Unknown* had been a remarkable popular success. The world now also knew about his organ pump and the input from Charles Lindbergh. But the conventional scientific output from Carrel's department had fallen off badly, in spite of having a very large staff — three scientists, 10 technicians, two 'skilled helpers' and three 'helpers'. Carrel was less interested in the laboratory work, and his mind seemed to be on other things. Gasser, the new director, was well aware of this. Flexner had been grateful to Carrel and was ever-tolerant of his flamboyant scientific style, but Flexner's successor had no such investment in Carrel.

The Lecture

After the success of *Man, the Unknown*, published in mid-1935, and at a time of added publicity from the announcement of success with the organ pump, Carrel gave the lecture on 12 December 1935 at the New York

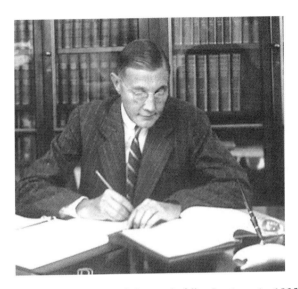

Herbert Gasser, appointed director of the Rockefeller Institute in 1935, made many changes, and was not an admirer of Carrel. (*Courtesy of the   Rockefeller University Archives.*)

Academy of Medicine, described in the previous chapter. Gasser knew of the event from the newspaper accounts, and afterwards read the full text of the address. Finding some parts distasteful, Gasser decided to make his views clear to Carrel. Although newly in post as director, Gasser wrote formally and firmly to Carrel about the lecture's content, in a letter marked 'Confidential':

> Had I seen the manuscript before it was read, I should have counselled caution with regard to the statements on page 14 and on pages 19 and 20. ... The exactions which the world places on science make me hold a most conservative attitude about the making of statements. ... Without the rigorous precaution which is exerted in one's own experimental field, they create in the rebound the possibility of raising doubt with respect to the correctness of conclusions about which the expected scientific care is exerted.[1]

---

[1] Gasser to Carrel, 6 February 1936, Malinin Collection of the Papers of Alexis Carrel and Charles Lindbergh, Carrel files, box 4 folder 34, FA 208, Rockefeller University Archives, Rockefeller Archives Centre (RUA RAC).

Gasser was generally displeased, even hinting that a public lecture of this kind might have been cleared ahead with him as director, but the particular items Gasser highlighted on the pages were Carrel's support for transcendental mechanisms such as telepathy. Gasser was also giving Carrel an extra, coded warning. It was that if Carrel was later found to be wrong in supporting the existence of these supposed phenomena, then belief in the rest of Carrel's work would be undermined. Gasser was perhaps suggesting that this was already the case.

This was a serious rebuke to a senior staff member, and there were other hints of Gasser's displeasure at the time. Just after he arrived as director, Gasser drew up a list of the Institute's strengths, and this did not include Carrel's work. Soon after, Gasser declined to raise the salaries of Ebeling and Parker in Carrel's unit, and did not support the promotion

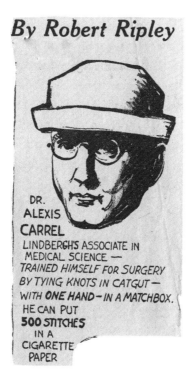

Belief in Carrel's exceptional surgical skills aided his public acclaim. (*Courtesy of the Georgetown University Library, Booth Family Center for Special Collections.*)

of one of Carrel's skilled technicians. An added change at the Institute was that the summer vacation break for the scientists was reduced from two months to one. Carrel might reasonably have thought that his prolonged absences in France were the target.

But Carrel showed no willingness to change the pattern of his scientific life. He remained obstinately unproductive in the following year of 1936, and in 1937 he published no scientific papers. But, judged by his newspaper cuttings, he was at a new peak in his fame in 1937.[2] Only Albert Einstein exceeded him in scientific public fame.[3]

Gasser's Agenda

Gasser and those who appointed him, knew that changes were needed at the Institute; Flexner had lost focus from the late 1920s onwards. Gasser faced a number of problems. The first was that the Institute faced, for the first time, some scientific competition. The second difficulty was that the Wall Street Crash and the Depression which followed had reduced the value and income from the Institute's endowment, and the third challenge was that the Institute was top-heavy with senior staff.

The new scientific competition came from a rather unfriendly change in policy by the Rockefeller Foundation, the family's other charity, which had thus far been careful not to overlap with the Institute's role in America's basic medical research sector.[4] The Foundation had been content in its earliest days with an international role, notably in public

---

[2] The Georgetown University archives show that Carrel's yearly press cuttings at this time were 33 (1936), 65 (1937), 49 (1938), 37 (1939), 45 (1940) and 55 (1941): GULBFC (note 19).

[3] In the *New York Times* in the five-year period 1935–40, articles on Einstein are double the number on Carrel. However, although much photographed, Einstein never spoke to the press; see David Dietz (1937) 'Science and the American press' *Science* 85: 107–12.

[4] The Rockefeller Foundation had evolved from the Rockefeller Sanitary Commission, instituted in 1909, which had initially investigated hookworm, first in the Philippines and then in the southern American states.

health, to which it added some domestic projects to assist agriculture, and it also provided a few fellowships for scientific research. In the late 1920s, the Foundation entered the holistic phase described earlier, announcing a study of man

> considered as a conceiving, child-bearing, thinking, behaving, growing and finally dying organism. … Can we develop so sound and extensive a genetics that we can hope to breed a superior race of men? … In short, can we rationalise human behaviour and create a new science of man?[5]

With the Foundation putting substantial funds into psychology, psychiatry, and even psychoanalysis, it was no rival to the Institute's traditional basic biological science interests. And only Carrel, and perhaps Flexner briefly, were attracted to the Foundation's 'study of man'.

But Warren Weaver, the new director of the Foundation's Division of Natural Sciences from 1932, changed its grants policy after disenchantment with the poor scientific returns, particularly from the studies of the mind. He re-adopted the reductionist gospel preached at the Institute earlier by Jacques Loeb, namely that the body was a machine, made up of component parts, which could be separated and understood. Weaver started to approve fellowships and project grants for basic biological research but which would apply the methods of physics and chemistry to cellular mechanisms. For this, the Foundation encouraged the use of new investigative tools, notably the ultracentrifuge, electron microscope and electrophoresis. Insights emerged from these grants, notably at the new West Coast institutes like the California Institute of Technology. Soon, Weaver famously called these projects 'molecular biology', a name which stuck. The Foundation had stolen the Institute's birthright.

Further competition for the Rockefeller Institute emerged when, after complex political negotiations, the U.S. government's own fledgling National Institutes of Health was established in 1930. Starting as a small organisation, it was to grow hugely. Nearer home, to add to the Institute's discomfort, in poliomyelitis research, an area of research that Flexner had

---

[5] *The Rockefeller Foundation Annual Report* 1933: 198–9.

jealously regarded as his own, others were claiming progress with understanding and preventing the disease.[6]

To sustain the status of the Institute, Gasser needed new initiatives and new people. Gasser's own work was ultra-reductionist, looking at electrical currents in nerves isolated from the body, and for him this was the way forward in understanding the workings of the nervous system. Carrel's reflections on the state of man and his mind were of no interest to him.

Retirements Proposed

The obvious staff imbalance had arisen because Flexner had made a number of appointments, decades before, of staff in middle life and who were now in their late 60s. Florence Sabin was 66 years old, Winthrop Osterhout was 66, and Pheobus Levene and Karl Landsteiner were both 68. Earlier, Theobald Smith, the distinguished head of the Division of Animal Pathology had been in post until he was 70, and Flexner himself was 72 years of age when he left the directorship. William Welch, the patriarch, had stayed on as President of the Institute until the age of 83 years and six months. Until this time, retirement at the Institute had been tolerantly left as a matter for personal decision, but in American life outside, retirement at age 65 was being slowly accepted.[7]

Gasser and the directors knew that this new mood gave opportunities for a restructuring within the Institute. New rules on retirement would not only deal with the unbalanced age structure, but also save money at this difficult time, and give a chance for an influx of new, younger staff. While these moves may not have been targeted at Carrel in particular, Carrel and his high profile featured prominently in Gasser's thinking. Carrel had a

[6] For the tensions see David Oshinsky, *Polio: an American Story* (New York: Oxford University Press, 1905): 56–8. William H. Park, the director of New York's public health service, with whom Flexner had clashed in the past, announced (wrongly) in 1935 that he had developed a vaccine for poliomyelitis.

[7] Starting in 1934, U.S. state and private pension schemes brought in retirement at age 65.

staff of 20, and the group were not productive — and the Lindbergh pump, its one apparent success, was perhaps too well-known for Gasser's liking. The Mousery debacle, and its cost, would also be known to Gasser. Though Carrel's retirement was part of a more general change in policy, Carrel was the youngest to be affected, and Carrel soon concluded that he was being unfairly treated.

In 1937, the Institute directors announced a new policy for staff retirement at age 65, which would come into force two years later in 1939 — when in Carrel's case he would then be 66 years of age. The conditions were generous. After 15 years service, an annual pension of three-quarters salary was offered, up to a limit of $10,000. In addition, those retiring could stay on in a reduced role, with the Institute generously offering personal laboratory space and supplies, plus some limited staff support. Letters were sent out to the senior staff in June 1937 with details of the new scheme. Gasser discussed the new retirement date informally with Carrel and asked if Carrel was minded to take up the offer of continuing with a small laboratory after June 1939. Carrel replied that he had not yet decided.

Next year, in March 1938, with a year or so to go, Gasser raised the matter of Carrel's retirement again, but got no response. It was a familiar scenario, in which a new director was facing up to an older, proud, longer-established staff member. On 1 January 1938, Carrel had grumbled about the new leader in a letter to the now-retired Flexner:

> Is it not strange that, such a short time after your departure and after the deaths of Mr. Gates and Doctor Welch, the Institute is already failing to play the very role for which it was intended by its founders?

The newspapers somehow got an indication of Carrel's displeasure with the new retirement scheme. Later that year, Carrel's friend, the science editor of the *New York Times* commented:

> The [pump] work must be finished. Carrel is at the height of his intellectual powers and technical skill. Retire just when he has broken down

some of the barriers that have concealed the mystery of living and dying from the inquisitiveness of man? Impossible.[8]

Summer 1938

Before leaving, as usual, for his island from New York, Carrel gave a short press conference, and again spoke to journalists when he disembarked from the *Queen Mary* at Cherbourg on 27 June. Most of the questions were about Lindbergh, his new island neighbour, and the hopes for the organ pump. He corrected a story that Lindbergh would be first to have it implanted, and also denied that Lindbergh might run for president of the United States.[9]

During his summer sojourns in France from 1937 onwards, Carrel had developed a friendship with a local priest, Dom Alexis Presse (1883–1965), who had left a conventional position at a Benedictine monastery and, seeking a simpler life, found a ruined chapel at Boquen on the mainland near Saint-Gildas. Sustained by help from local supporters, he started to rebuild it, and the shrine soon attracted other monks. Carrel enjoyed the company of Father Clifford in New York, but Clifford died that year, and Dom Alexis perhaps entered the same role, offering the theological jousting which Carrel enjoyed. He would share Carrel's criticism of the Catholic Church. Carrel also involved Dom Alexis in discussions about his future plans, notably for an 'Institute of Man'. While at the island, Carrel took an interest in two local mainland Catholic youth organisations — the Jeunesse ouvrière chrétienne and L'Action Catholique des Enfants.

In that summer of 1938, the Lindberghs also arrived to move into their springtime purchase. While the extensive renovation of their large house was going on, they stayed with the Carrels and would later spend much time with them by walking over the causeway between the islands when the tide allowed. Reporters were still a nuisance, and one group rowing out to the island were warned off by the Lindberghs. But in the following week,

---

[8] 'Carrel, At 65, Is Deep In New Studies' *NYT*, 26 June 1938.
[9] 'Carrel Discredits 'Guinea Pig' Tales' *NYT*, 28 June 1938.

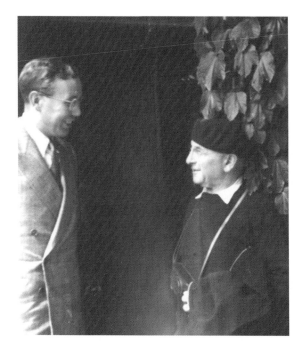

James 'Jim' Newton, active in the Moral Rearmament movement, was close to Carrel and visited at his French island in 1938. (*Courtesy of the Uncommon Friends Foundation.*)

Carrel gave an interview to a reporter from the important Paris daily newspaper *Paris Soir*, which was passed to the American press, possibly as a consolation for Lindbergh's refusal to see the journalists. Carrel said that they were making no further experiments on the island, and Carrel asked that he and Lindbergh be left in peace.[10] Jim Newton, travelling in Europe on Moral Rearmament business in that year of 1938, also stayed for a while with the Carrels that summer.

Lindbergh's Mission

Lindbergh's summer stay in France was interrupted by another request from the U.S. Embassy in London, this time to fly to Russia to assess the Soviet Air Force. He and his wife set off in mid-August, as usual in their

---

[10] 'Carrel And Lindbergh Writing Book On Island' *NYT*, 14 July 1938.

own plane. Their hosts were more secretive than the Germans had been, but Lindbergh thought the Soviet Air Force, though quite impressive, was no match for the Luftwaffe. Nor were they impressed with Soviet life under communism. On their way back, Lindbergh had a meeting in Czechoslovakia with President Beneš and encountered a worried man who was expecting a German invasion. Lindbergh reported on his mission, first to the French military and politicians, and then to Ambassador Kennedy and others in London.

Lindbergh returned to his island well briefed, and increasingly expert, on the European situation. His remarkable travels and his visits to secret places and contacts with politicians and military men also meant that, while previously Lindbergh had listened attentively to Carrel's world view, their roles were now reversing. Lindbergh was uniquely aware of what was going on, and he was forming a clear view of his own about what should be done and what should not be done.

Lindbergh was summoned to London on 21 September by Ambassador Joseph Kennedy, and after their meeting, Lindbergh prepared and handed over his report on German airpower. Lindbergh was perhaps over-impressed with German strength and may have been unaware that the German bombers then in service could barely reach Britain from German bases — the bigger Junkers Ju 88 was still to come. Kennedy may have passed on Lindbergh's gloomy assessment to Prime Minister Chamberlain before he flew to meet Hitler next day, and Britain started the moves towards appeasement at Munich on 28 September.

Return to Germany

In October of that year 1938, Lindbergh was in the air again, this time to attend a meeting of a German aeronautical society. He was again permitted to inspect new military aircraft and joined a private dinner at the American ambassador's house which included industry guests, notably the aviation experts Willy Messerschmitt and Ernst Heinkel, whose company and technical conversation Lindbergh enjoyed. As the host had hoped, Hermann Göring also accepted an invitation, and the Reichsmarshall was perhaps attracted by Lindbergh's presence. Prior to the meal, Göring unexpectedly rose, spoke, and with little ceremony presented Lindbergh with a high honour — the Service Cross of the German Eagle — given, Göring added, 'by order of the Führer'. There was applause, no photographs were taken, and the dinner continued, after which Göring had a few words in private with Lindbergh about the Russian situation.

Soon after the evening event, Lindbergh wrote his usual polite letters of thanks to the long list of hosts, including one to Göring thanking him for the medal, and asking that his thanks be conveyed to Hitler. During their stay, Lindbergh and his wife were again impressed not only with the potential of the Luftwaffe but with life in Germany. To enable a longer and closer study of the nation, the Lindberghs made moves to rent a house in Berlin over the winter.

However on 13 November 1938 came *Kristallnacht*, during which there was a pogrom of synchronised attacks on Jewish property in many German cities. International protests followed, and the event was a tipping point for public opinion in America, leading to the recall of the American ambassador from Berlin. Lindbergh's acceptance of his medal three weeks previously and his admiration for Germany were noted. In the new political climate, he was attacked by the American administration, and they briefed against him to journalists. The *New Yorker* on 26 November 1938 could write of the now-controversial American national hero:

> We say goodbye to Colonel Charles A. Lindbergh who wants to go to live in Berlin, presumably occupying a house that once belonged to Jews. … If he wants to experiment further with the artificial heart, his surroundings should be ideal.[11]

Lindbergh, as ever, declined to respond, but was privately concerned, and after *Kristallnacht* wrote in his journal that 'my admiration for the Germans is constantly being dashed against some rock like this'.[12] Carrel, now back in America, warned Lindbergh that because of ill feeling

---

[11] A. Scott Berg, *Lindbergh* (New York: G.P. Putnam & Sons, 1998): 379.

[12] Berg, *Lindbergh* (note 11): 379.

towards him, he should not stay in Germany any longer. Carrel added for the first time that, in America, opposition to the Nazis was the result of 'Jewish and Russian propaganda'.[13]

Concerned at the news, the Lindberghs moved instead to spend the winter in Paris, and there he met and briefed France's Prime Minister Daladier. He made some further low-key visits to Germany, and on return to London he met with British military staff and told the U.S. ambassador again that

> Germany, on account of her military strength, is now inseparable from the welfare of our civilisation for either to preserve or destroy it is in her power … it would be wise to permit Germany's eastward expansion than to throw England and France, unprepared, into war.[14]

Lindbergh would return to America next year to urge again that America stay out of European affairs.

Lindbergh's Influence

Lindbergh in England kept up a close involvement, at a distance, with the work in Carrel's unit. He kept in touch with news of the pump work, notably in responding to concerns about the low oxygen supply to the perfused organs. Lindbergh also corresponded with Carrel's staff member Raymond Parker about his tissue culture work. One long-standing goal at the Institute was to grow large amounts of viruses using cultured cells as hosts, and Lindbergh took up the challenge, designing a 'circulating' flow culture flask for Parker. It allowed harvesting of virus produced by the cells, and Parker was pleased and started to use it. He urged Lindbergh to publish a description of the flask, but Lindbergh, still unhappy about the publicity over the organ pump, declined, since 'there would be an unfortunate amount and type of newspaper publicity attached'. Lindbergh

[13] See David M. Friedman, *The Immortalists: Charles Lindbergh, Dr Alexis Carrel and their Daring Quest to Live Forever* (New York: HarperCollins, 2007): 160.
[14] Charles A. Lindbergh, *The Wartime Journals of Charles A. Lindbergh* (New York: Harcourt Brace Jovanovich, 1970): 203, 213, 216 and 230.

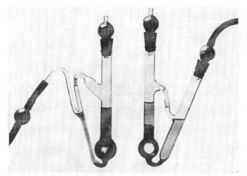

FIG. 32. Lindbergh gas-lift flasks for the continuous circulation of fluid media. (C. A. Lindbergh, unpublished experiments.)

In 1936 Lindbergh designed and produced a flask for allowing prolonged culture of cells infected with viruses, hoping to harvest the virus in quantity. (*From Raymond C. Parker* Methods of Tissue Culture, 1938.)

instead encouraged Parker to write about the new device under Parker's own name.

There were also letters to Lindbergh from Ebeling and Miss McFaul, Carrel's nurse in charge of the operating room. All the letter writers confided in Lindbergh in their letters, clearly trusting his discretion, and because of Carrel's imminent retirement, the situation in the laboratory was fraught, particularly as all the staff needed to find other positions. Ebeling's letters passed on the news and gossip that Carrel's friend Ralph Wyckoff was not favoured by Gasser and just before Wyckoff managed to move to the Lederle company, Ebeling noted that 'Wyckoff has not been able to land a job. ... things have been made very disagreeable for him — to say the least ...' Ebeling complained about Parker's 'tantrums', adding that 'Parker is working on his [tissue culture] book quite actively ... his troubles are by no means over'.[15] Parker's letters explained these 'troubles' to Lindbergh. Parker was also under pressure from Gasser to leave, and as an inducement, Gasser offered Parker a one-year 'portable' salary if he could find an unpaid place at another institution. Parker understandably

---

[15] Ebeling to Lindbergh, 28 October 1937, box 24 file 0750, Charles Augustus Lindbergh Papers, MS 325, Yale University Library Manuscripts and Archives (YULMA).

was not in a charitable mood, and referred in his letters to the senior Institute staff as 'men of measured merriment'. Parker also passed on to Lindbergh an unsympathetic verdict on Carrel:

> He [Carrel] really doesn't understand American scientists. He has never entered their little ways and vanities (as we have to cater to his) and without realising it he has a special knack of insulting the wrong people at the wrong time. From long observation on the sidelines, I have concluded that his greatest handicap has been Crutcher and Ebeling. They both consider him something between God and the Saint and try in their foolish way to protect him from everything and everyone. They also impress on him constantly that no one is to be trusted. His best friend in the department is Miss McFaul. In fact he will never know how much she has done for him and how many messes she has patched up for him. Over the past year he has treated her like a dog … in spite of it all she comes through. Instead of resigning (as I would) she comes back the next morning because she realises how alone he is and how much she could do for him.[16]

Parker then added a friendly compliment — 'you [Lindbergh] could teach Carrel a lot'.

The loyal Miss McFaul recalled later that Carrel at this time was 'petty, querulous, and nursing injured vanity'.[17] Ebeling, as we will see later, was less supportive of Carrel than it seemed. With this exchange of letters with the staff, and his many suggestions, Lindbergh had taken over some of the leadership from the now-detached Carrel.

Carrel's Plans

With a year to go to his retirement date, Carrel looked at possible post-retirement projects. One was to set up a new research unit for more organ pump and tissue culture work, and Wyckoff, at Lederle, offered to

---

[16] Parker to Lindbergh, 20 June 1938, box 24 folder 0751, Lindbergh Papers MS 325, YULMA (note 15).

[17] MacFaul quoted in Joseph T. Durkin, *Hope for Our Time: Alexis Carrel on Man and Society* (New York: Harper and Row, 1965): 130.

support Carrel in this way. At the Institute, Wyckoff had admired Carrel's insights, and took up Carrel's suggestion that viruses could grow in chicken eggs. In this way, Wyckoff made a commercially successful vaccine against the western encephalitis virus, then causing a major problem for horse breeders. Another offer came from Henry Ford's chief surgeon Roy D. McClure, who had earlier worked with Carrel at the Institute, and he suggested that Carrel move and continue his work at his Ford Hospital in Detroit.

However, rather than a new laboratory, Carrel was also considering a different kind of project. It was for a foundation of the kind he had trailed in *Man, the Unknown* and proposed again as an 'Institute of Man' in his Dartmouth lecture one year earlier. This new Institute would carry out a study of man and man's problems. Some of Carrel's friends and admirers in America warmed to these proposals and started to look for funds, and Carrel offered a prospectus for the venture. The text started optimistically, praising man's ingenuity but, as always, announcing that man 'has built a world that does not fit him'. Carrel's plans were that the mind and body would be considered together and that the Institute would look at voluntary eugenics, natural resistance, moral and spiritual growth, longevity, 'metapsychics', the raising of intelligence and factors in the genesis of great leaders. In spite of the lack of conclusions from the Mousery experiments, he proposed further similar work, but using dogs, raising generation after generation in environments controlled for temperature, light, electric fields, carbon dioxide levels and exposure to 'city air'. He clearly believed that any change made in one generation would be transmitted in Lamarckian fashion to the next.[18]

Steadily the 'Institute of Man' became the priority in his thinking, rather than continuing his tissue culture and organ pump in a new location. Charles Lindbergh, still in Europe, offered to place Carrel's institute in his 400-acre family estate at High Fields, New Jersey. Edward C. Moore had kept in touch with Carrel and, encouraged by Boris Bakhmeteff and Jim Newton, Moore now acted as fundraiser and

---

[18] 'Manifesto' Lindbergh Papers, box 7 folder 0178, MS 325, YULMA (note 15).

hoped to enrol 100 'Founders Group' donors who would contribute $25,000 each. John D. Rockefeller junior, DeWitt Wallace of *Reader's Digest* and John Harvey Kellogg were said to be willing to participate. The Macy Foundation seemed interested for a while, and there were preliminary offers of accommodation from Duke University and the University of Michigan.[19] Carrel did make some moves over the winter of 1938 to recruit staff for his proposed institute, but nothing came of it, and fund-raising was slow.[20]

Unknown to his supporters, Carrel had an alternative plan: he had hopes that his institute might be set up in France.

European Possibilities

As described earlier, Carrel was a supporter of Jean Coutrot's Centre d'études des problèmes humains (CEPH) and its aspiration to 'study man'. From 1936 onwards, as one of its four directors, though usually far from France, Carrel was watching its activities closely. André Missenard (1901–1989) a young member of the small CEPH head-quarter staff, kept up a correspondence with Carrel, and in 1937 Carrel wrote the Introduction to Missenard's book *L'homme et le climat*. This work dealt with effects of the environment on the human body in health and disease, but he more controversially linked temperature and climate with the theory of racial achievement.[21] Carrel, when writing back to Missenard, proposed forming his own institute in France, one not unlike the CEPH, and suggested to Missenard that it be called the Institut

[19] Moore to Carrel, 14 March 1939, box 42 file 'Edward F. Moore', Alexis Carrel Papers, Georgetown University Library, Booth Family Center for Special Collections (GULBFC).
[20] The recruitment attempt is mentioned in James D. Newton, *Uncommon Friends; Life with Thomas Edison, Henry Ford, Harvey Firestone, Alexis Carrel and Charles Lindbergh* (New York: Harvest Books, 1989): 172.
[21] For the background to Missenard's book see David N. Livingstone (2012) 'Changing climate, human evolution, and the revival of environmental determinism' *Bulletin of the History of Medicine* 86: 564–95. Carrel also wrote the Introduction to Missenard's *A la recherche du temps et du rythme* (Paris: Plon, 1940).

national pour la rénovation de la Française. Carrel told Missenard to seek possible staff in France and report back.[22] Missenard found that a senior scientist, André Siegfried (1875–1959), was interested and Carrel was pleased to get the news. Siegfried was author of a Carrelian declinist book *La crise de l'Europe*, which urged that a rescue of the white races was required.[23]

In Europe, Carrel now had possible staff, but no funding; in America, there was encouragement and perhaps money, but no staff had emerged. Though the French venture would go no further at this time, Carrel would link up with Missenard later, and reward him for his support.

The Lindberghs Return

By early 1939, the Lindberghs made the decision to return to America. He now felt that, with his insight into the German military preparations, he should offer fresh briefing and advice to the American administration. Added to this, they both had family in America, and Lindbergh was still keen to catch up with the pump and tissue culture work which he had followed so closely from abroad. He could also help Carrel with his plans for an institute.

On 14 April 1939, Lindbergh arrived back in America, ending his exile, with his wife and children following later. Mme Carrel was again staying in New York, and the Carrels and Jim Newton had permission to go out with the pilot boat to the *Aquitania* to greet Lindbergh on the liner, ahead of the journalists gathered in force at the New York docks. But a photographer bribed a steward on the liner and obtained the exclusive first photograph of the returning Lindbergh — and the Carrels are included in the picture.[24]

---

[22] See Philip Nord, *France's New Deal: From the Thirties to the Postwar Era* (Princeton: Princeton University Press, 2010): 59–60.

[23] Sean Kennedy (2004) 'Situating France: the career of André Siegfried' *Historical Reflections* 30: 179–203.

[24] The *Daily Mirror* front page news and picture is reproduced in Newton, *Friends* (note 20): 150.

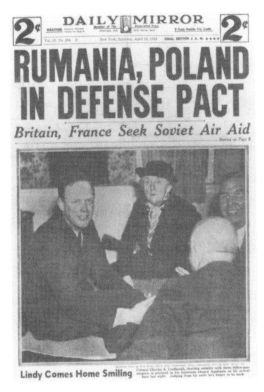

DAILY MIRROR

RUMANIA, POLAND IN DEFENSE PACT

Britain, France Seek Soviet Air Aid

Lindy Comes Home Smiling

Carrel and his wife, surprised by a photographer when welcoming Lindbergh back to America on the *Aquitania*.

Lindbergh, now a reservist colonel in the United States Army Air Corps, met soon after with President Roosevelt and again gave his view that Germany could do anything it wanted in Europe because of superior air power. Lindbergh added that there was also a threat from Russia, which he considered to be a semi-Asiatic power and hence part of the 'yellow peril'. Lindbergh's view was that 'we [the West] should fight yellow, black and brown, not ourselves'. Soon after, U.S. military spending sharply increased and $300 million was allocated for re-equipping. Lindbergh made a three-week tour of American Air Force bases, and, regaining favourable coverage, he was forgiven for his earlier German sympathies. Lindbergh appeared on the cover of *Time* magazine, his third time, on 19 June 1939.

In spite of these military commitments and his personal deep engagement with the rapidly worsening situation, Lindbergh managed to spend time back at Carrel's laboratory among his old friends.[25] He heard, with pleasure, that 30 of the flasks he had designed for Parker to grow viruses were in action. Parker had earlier unsuccessfully urged Lindbergh to publish details of the flask, and Lindbergh now felt that, with all the other dramas unfolding in his life, a scientific paper from him would, for once, be unnoticed. This was not quite the case when the paper, with him as the only author, was published in the Rockefeller Institute's *Journal of Experimental Medicine* in August 1939. But with war likely, the newspapers' interest in Lindbergh as a scientist was transient.[26] Lindbergh also met formally with Carrel, Wyckoff and Newton to discuss plans for an institute for Carrel, but they all agreed that the times were not propitious for further action.

Carrel and Europe

Carrel was increasingly concerned about the events in Europe and his views differed from those of Lindbergh. Lindbergh felt that if Germany was not provoked, Hitler might attack Russia and the two nations would damage themselves in a fight to the death. Carrel's view, in his private letters, was characteristically contradictory. He knew that France was in danger, and that militarily only America could save France. At other times he admired the strong fascist leadership and he could on occasions, admire the Nazi programme:

> The combination within the German youth of enthusiastic faith and absolute submission to competent chiefs gives to National Socialism an

---

[25] Lindbergh, *Wartime Journals* (note 14): 203 describes his conferences at the Institute with Carrel's staff.

[26] 'Lindbergh Widens His Aid To Science' *NYT*, 3 September 1939. The article is C.A. Lindbergh (1939) 'A culture flask for the circulation of a large quantity of fluid medium' *JEM* 70: 231–8. Lindbergh describes his work on the design while in England in *Wartime Journals* (note 14): 230. Lindbergh's many biographers have failed to notice this important incident.

immense conquering strength. On its truly formidable power depends the fate of the world revolution launched by Hitler.[27]

But at the same time he could deplore that 'National Socialism [in Germany] rejects classical culture, Christianity and the sacredness of human personality and liberty'.[28] Carrel agreed that the fascist countries had a right to expand and conquer and in 1937 wrote that 'Hitler, Salazar and Mussolini express the defensive reaction of nations that wish to go on living'. Of Hitler's aggressions he took the view that 'treaties have not an absolute value'.[29] Later, after Britain declared war, he wrote: 'The English are idiots ... they should have allowed Germany to do what she wished in the East [of Europe].'

He also opined: 'How little intelligence the English have. One thus arrives at the wish that Europe be dominated by the Germans.'[30] He again said that German dominance was needed since 'Germany and Italy must save the world wounded by mechanical civilisation'.[31] However, at other times he took a different stance:

England and France can rightly be considered as fighting for the salvation of western, that is, of Christian civilisation. The triumph of Germany, Russia and Italy would mean the failure of an effort made by civilised men during two thousand years.[32]

On Hitler, he was equally ambivalent:

A prodigious phenomenon in the history of humanity — an uncanny and gigantic power, a conqueror more audacious than Tamerlane and Genghis Khan, a mystical teacher through whom the innermost soul of the people manifest itself, a clairvoyant who senses the future.

---

[27] Carrel memorandum, Malinin Collection FA 208, box 14 folder 3, RUA RAC (note 1).

[28] Carrel, *Memorandum* (note 27).

[29] Carrel, *Memorandum*, box 38 folder 37, GULBFC (note 19).

[30] Carrel to Gigou, Malinin Collection, box 14 folder 30, FA 208, RUA RAC (note 1).

[31] Carrel memorandum, Alexis Carrel Papers, box 38 folder 37, GULBFC (note 19).

[32] Carrel to Scoval, 6 May 1939, Malinin Collection, box 15 folder 28, FA 208, RUA RAC (note 1).

Carrel then added, in the same private diary entry, that Hitler 'reaches his goal through cunning, crime and bloodshed with somnambulistic cruelty'.[33]

There was some consistency on other occasions when he took a more detached and resigned view of the European conflict, returning to his declinist diagnosis of a weakness in Western society:

> The crisis is due neither to the presence of Mr. Roosevelt in the White House, nor to that of Hitler in Germany nor of Mussolini in Rome. It comes from the very structure of civilisation. It is a crisis of man …. . The democratic ideology itself, unless reconstructed upon a scientific basis, has no more chance of surviving than the fascist or Marxist ideologies. In Europe, democracy has already succumbed … not because of the superior power of its enemies, but also because of its own weakness. Democracies will crumble when short of youth and encumbered with the old.[34]

The Jews

He now took the view that there was Jewish influence at work in America to turn the world against the Nazis, and that 'we are being pushed into this war by the Soviets and the Jews'.[35] He detected the same influence in France:

> One will not pardon here the Jews for having pushed the war. It is very evident that they are the slaves of Moscow and imbeciles who follow them are pushing French into war.[36]

---

[33] Carrel memorandum, Malinin Collection 208, box 14 folder 3, FA 208, RUA RAC (note 1).

[34] Carrel's new 'Introduction' to *Man, the Unknown* (New York: Harper & Brothers, 1939).

[35] For Carrel's variable views on the Jews, see Philip Nord, *France's New Deal: From the Thirties to the Postwar Era* (Princeton: Princeton University Press, 2010): 61 and Andrés H. Reggiani, *God's Eugenicist: Alexis Carrel and the Sociobiology of Decline* (New York: Berghahn Books, 2007): 159.

[36] Carrel to Gigou, 17 September 1938, Malinin Collection, box 14 folder 8, FA 208, RUA RAC (note 1).

Earlier, no Carrelian antisemitism was evident. At the Century Association, Carrel could be called on by other club members to vote for Jews applying for membership, when opposition was likely. At a meeting in honour of his friend Emanuel Libman, the eminent New York Jewish physician, Carrel spoke with feeling about the Jewish contribution to science and medicine.[37] Carrel could write to his friend Rabbi Wise of New York at this time in 1938 that

> We Christians will always respect the Jews who are proud of being Jews, who recognise that they are profoundly different from us, that they are a people and a great people.[38]

Carrel's various dogmatic views on these matters can hardly be reconciled, and they fit other evidence of his contradictory and enigmatic stances. His many and varied utterances allow, and still allow, supporters and detractors to select from his writings and support radically different analyses. He can be depicted as a Nazi supporter, or a critic of Germany, or that he had rejected France or that he was a French patriot; in addition, antisemitism can be alleged and denied.

Retirement Date Nears

Over the winter of 1938, Mme Carrel had been back in New York, and accompanied her husband to some of his engagements. They did not use his penthouse home but stayed in a hotel and they had time together in Florida visiting Kellogg's Sanitarium and experiencing its Spartan regimen. On 4 May, Mme Carrel had left early for France on the *Ile de France* taking three boxes of belongings with her, together with her three poodles. Her mother, almost 100 years old, was ill after breaking her leg in a fall at the Brittany family home at Angers to the south of

---

[37] Carrel contributed to a celebratory volume on Libman; see '*The Physiological Substratum of Malignancy*' in *Contributions to the Medical Sciences: In Honor of Dr. Emanuel Libman* (New York, 1932): 289–295.

[38] Carrel to Wise, 14 June 1938, Malinin Collection, box 14 folder 28, FA 208, RUA RAC (note 1).

Saint-Gildas, and died soon after. At Saint-Gildas in the previous summer of 1938, the Carrels had buried their silver at a secret spot on the island, a prudent and ancient survival strategy in perilous times.

Gasser wrote to Carrel again on 4 January 1939 saying that a final decision about his retirement later that year was now needed for consideration at the spring meeting of the Institute's Board. Carrel again failed to respond. On 16 May, after the Board had met, Gasser pointed out cautiously to Carrel that 'you have not made a request for a laboratory organisation to continue after July 1st'. Carrel procrastinated and asked for more time to consider, but meanwhile decided to organise support for his cause. On 17 March 1939 he wrote to Harvey Cushing, now in retirement, saying that

> as I am being forced out of science by the Board of Directors of the Rockefeller Institute, I shall have to take up some kind of commercial work. It is the very first time, I believe, that a man who has received the Nobel Prize has been compelled to give up scientific research when the research is most promising. Lindbergh is being stopped at the time when he is developing apparatus of the greatest importance for the culture of viruses and of whole organs.[39]

Carrel's friend Coudert took up his cause and wrote to Rockefeller junior saying that the scientist's departure 'terminates experiments which are considered to be, and I am confidently assured are, of utmost importance'.[40] Rockefeller replied diplomatically saying 'the more valuable the service, the greater the regret at its termination'. Rockefeller also pointed out that he was stepping down, age 65, from his various posts, and that the other Rockefeller philanthropies now had the same policy. Carrel also complained in similar terms to William Sherman, his surgeon friend involved in the World War I wound treatment debate, writing

---

[39] Carrel to Cushing, 17 March 1939, Malinin Collection, Carrel Files Correspondence, box 2 folder 5, FA 208, RUA RAC (note 1).
[40] Coudert to Rockefeller, box 14-2 folder 36, GULBFC (note 19).

that the very important and promising experiments which we are making on the cultivation of viruses, especially poliomyelitis virus, and the cultivation of organs, have come to an end. I am being forced out.[41]

Sherman decided to try to help, and passed on Carrel's letter to Rockefeller junior. But Sherman added some extra new information. This was an added private complaint by Carrel to Sherman that the pressure for his retirement had been 'stirred up by Bolshevik and Jewish propaganda'.[42] Rockefeller promptly brought in the Institute's lawyer who, asked to investigate, found no evidence for the claim. In his report, the lawyer pointed out that, while there were Jews among the Institute scientists, the senior administration made the decision on retirement age, and none of them were Jews. He added, as an aside, that 'the allegations would hurt no-one but himself [Carrel]'.[43]

Countdown

Carrel had gained no significant support. The journal *Science* for 21 April 1939 carried a press release from the Rockefeller Institute stating that five senior members were retiring and that 'every laboratory facility will be provided to enable those who retired to continue their research work on their own responsibility, if they desire to do so'. The following day the *New York Daily News* carried an article saying that the Institute was to 'oust four great scientists' and highlighted Carrel's case. The newspapers thereafter backed off and no significant press backing for Carrel emerged. The leadership at the Institute was relieved, and Gasser wrote to his legal assistant about the Carrel affair: 'On the whole, I suppose we came out of

---

[41] Carrel to Sherman 13 March 1939, Malinin Collection, Carrel Files, Correspondence, box 4 folder 35, FA 208, RUA RAC (note 1).
[42] Alain Drouard, *Une inconnue des sciences sociales: la Fondation Alexis Carrel 1941–1945* (Paris: Editions de la Maison des sciences de l'homme, 1992): 504.
[43] Debevoise to Dodge, 12 May 1938, Herbert Spenser Gasser, Subject Files, Series 4, box 1, FA 813, RUA RAC (note 1); for a commentary, see Leon Sokoloff (1995) 'Alexis Carrel and the Jews at the Rockefeller Institute' *Korot* 11: 66–81.

a tight place pretty well'.[44] In retrospect, Gasser had shrewdly handled the challenge of Carrel's retirement.

Lindbergh's Flask

The unsuccessful chorus of complaint, orchestrated by Carrel, included the claim that he was on the verge of gaining new insights from the organ pump perfusion work; this was, in hindsight, incorrect. His claim for an important on-going development in tissue culture is of more interest. He was referring to Lindbergh's new flask, as used by Parker, which was an important move towards cultivation of viruses on a large scale. Carrel even mentions that they were attempting to grow the polio virus, one of the great challenges of the time. Parker may have been unlucky in not succeeding, and moved into other work when he left the Institute shortly after. In 1949 came the dramatic accidental finding by Enders that the polio virus would unexpectedly thrive in kidney cells in a roller-pump tissue culture chamber not unlike the Parker–Lindbergh device. Enders' finding immediately opened the way to large-scale cultivation of the virus and the prompt appearance of the rival Salk (attenuated) and Sabin (heat killed) vaccines, which gained Nobel Prize fame and fortune for those involved. Parker in Carrel's laboratory may have been close to participating in this success. In retrospect, he had used the wrong cells — nerve cells.[45]

Winding Down

Carrel never replied to Gasser, and Carrel's retirement went ahead without formal agreement. Gasser deemed that Carrel had accepted the post-retirement laboratory support. This gave Carrel the continuing assistance of Ebeling, plus a $2,000 budget for supplies, and he retained the

---

[44] Gasser to Debevoise, 15 April 1939 (note 43).

[45] Polio researchers were shackled with the view that the virus would grow only in nerve cells, an *idée fixe* supported by Simon Flexner at the Institute. Parker probably used only neural tissue in his flask when trying to grow the polio virus.

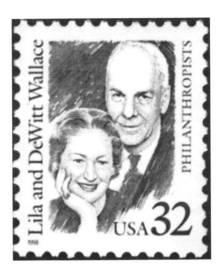

DeWitt Wallace, editor of the *Reader's Digest*, encouraged Carrel to write for his magazine.

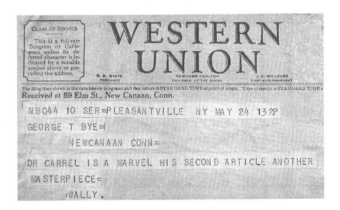

Telegram from the *Digest's* editor DeWitt Wallace to Carrel's agent, enthusing over Carrel's article. (*Courtesy of the Georgetown University Library, Booth Family Center for Special Collections.*)

services of his long-serving secretary Miss Crutcher. On 10 June 1939 the Board of Scientific Directors thanked Carrel for his 33 years work on the staff and made him a 'member emeritus'. In the eulogy covering his considerable achievements, it intriguingly again mentions that 'his tissue culture would provide a viable means for the growing of viruses and the preparation of vaccines'.

As the June retirement day approached, Carrel kept busy. On 14 April 1939 when receiving the Gold Medal of the Rotary Club of New York, he told them: 'We have failed. We are not all equal,' and he alluded to society's burden of 'misfits and the feeble-minded'. Invited by Coudert, he addressed the Annual Meeting of the American Society of International Law, and he wrote a new Introduction for another printing of *Man, the Unknown*, published in June 1939. He saw himself as a Cassandra, who had predicted that degeneration in the West would allow the German attack on weaker neighbours.

The owner of *Reader's Digest* had not forgotten him. Carrel now had a literary agent, George Bye, found by Jim Newton, and Carrel, Bye and Newton had lunch at the Institute with *Digest* editor DeWitt Wallace. They agreed that Carrel would write a series of commissioned articles for the magazine.[46] Carrel got to work quickly, although his summer break was imminent, with his first article appearing in the *Digest* of June 1939. It was, improbably, on breast feeding. The article still reads well, notably in supporting breast feeding, rather than using other milks, and advocating it as emotionally fulfilling for mother and child.[47]

Carrel was paid $450 for this *Digest* article. Wallace had been so pleased with the manuscript that he had already offered the even larger and remarkable fee of $2,250 each for future articles by Carrel, and they agreed that Carrel would contribute a monthly series, if possible. These first two contributions appeared soon after Carrel had left in summer for France. 'Married Love' was published in July and 'Do You Know How To Live' in September, and there were two more *Digest* contributions by Carrel in the following years.[48] The 'Married Love' article is remarkable for its detail about sexual relationships, particularly from the woman's

---

[46] The *Saturday Evening Post* turned down Carrel's proposed articles earlier, as being in the 'inspirational' genre.

[47] Carrel may have followed the unconventional enthusiasm for breast-feeding of Margaret Mead, another 'visible scientist'.

[48] 'Work in the Laboratory of your Private Life' *Reader's Digest* September 1940 and 'Prayer is Power' March 1941. His archives at Georgetown University show draft notes prepared for other articles, or chapters for a new book, including 'Sleep', 'Prevention of War', 'Positive Thinking', 'Intuition' and 'Civilization and Temperature'.

viewpoint. But there was also a return to the dogmatism and ambiguity of *Man, the Unknown*. He wrote that 'there are no sexual weaklings among heroes, the conquerors, the truly great leaders of nations ... Inspiration may come from repression of sexual appetite'. The second article took a holistic approach to health and had sensible advice on diet and healthy living. With the *Digest* fees and continuing royalties from sales of *Man, the Unknown*, in 1939 alone, Carrel received $16,697. Nevertheless, Carrel may not have been particularly well-off, and the bank statements surviving in his archives show a modest balance in spite of a good salary and considerable earnings from his writing.[49] These statements show regular transfer of money to France, and his letters mention his need to provide for his wife and others, as if Mme Carrel, after all, was not wealthy and had needs, and he was supporting some less well-off relatives in Lyon.[50]

The *Digest* articles brought in a new wave of letters from the public. Carrel was pleased to be reaching out to an even larger audience than before as if he had found his *métier*. He wrote to Wallace that 'the powerful voice of the *Reader's Digest* is heard everywhere. And it renders alive ideas, which expressed otherwise would remain dead'.[51] Carrel's secretary deplored the usual rewriting of his prose by the magazine which removed his characteristically empathic style. Nor did she approve of the risqué topics he chose.

Dispersal

Carrel's staff steadily moved elsewhere. Lillian Baker transferred to another group in the Institute, and then she became a teacher. Raymond Parker took the talented Miss Hollender, his 'best ever technician', with him to a research position, first with E.R. Sqibb in New Brunswick, and

---

[49] His estate after his death in 1944 was not great — see Chapter 19.
[50] The mystery deepens since, prior to her departure from New York in May 1938, Mme Carrel sold two gold bars held in France for $27,120, transferring the money to America.
[51] Carrel to Wallace, box 38 folder 59, GULBFC (note 19).

then moved to the Connaught Laboratory in Canada, poignantly dropping the viral culture work. There he became well known for producing Medium 199, the first synthetic medium to support tissue culture without the mysterious need to add serum or tissue extracts. Miss McFaul went to medical school and, as noted earlier, she assisted Dr. Leon Chesley in Jersey City with his organ pump work. With Carrel's unit reduced to the new post-retirement allowance, only Ebeling, two technicians and his secretary were still in place.

Carrel sailed as usual for his French island in July 1939 and would shortly be caught up in the War. After he left, his secretary was concerned to hear that Carrel, never popular at the Institute, was under renewed criticism, and there were murmurings about his use of the *Digest*. She was inclined to agree and confided in Lindbergh, now living nearby, that 'a great deal of harm would come to Dr. Carrel's reputation'.[52] She asked Lindbergh to call in and give her advice about handling the matter.

Other Retirees

The senior retirees at the Institute had all reached amicable agreements with Gasser. Landsteiner, Levene and Osterhout all chose to stay on and took up the offered post-retirement laboratory space and support. Only Florence Sabin left the Institute and, moving to Colorado, became a prominent public health activist. And the post-retirement scheme proved surprisingly productive at the Institute. Far from being a gentle let down for these distinguished senior scientists, their return to small-scale personal studies proved to be an invigorating change. Phoebus Levene's post-retirement work on the nucleotides of DNA soon led to the crucial demonstration at the Institute by Avery that DNA could transfer genetic information, and the final proof from Avery came in 1944, one year after he also had retired and continued under the new scheme. Karl Landsteiner carried on with his research, and in 1942, age 74, added to his fame when

---

[52] Crutcher to Lindbergh, 28 July 1939, Lindbergh Papers, box 025 folder 0752, MS 325, YULMA (note 15).

he published, with Merrill Chase, their classic paper on the transfer of immunological memory by lymphocytes, a finding now taken as the start point of modern cellular immunology.[53] This late burst of activity by the retired group greatly revived the reputation of the Institute and prevented what would otherwise have been a rather negative historical verdict on its work during the 1930s.

---

[53] K. Landsteiner and M.W. Chase (1942) 'Experiments on transfer of cutaneous sensitivity to simple compounds' *Proceedings of the Society for Experimental Biology and Medicine* 49: 688–90. They did not quote Murphy in this classic paper, but Chase liked to think that they soon after realised and acknowledged Murphy's earlier work; see Merrill W. Chase (1985) 'Immunology and experimental dermatology' *Annual Review of Immunology* 3: 1–19.

CHAPTER SEVENTEEN

To France and Back

Carrel, now retired, settled into his island home in France in July 1939. Two months after he arrived, Germany invaded Poland, and on 3 September, Britain and France, with no options left, declared war. No military action by the relatively weak Allies could be contemplated as yet, and with no military engagement until the following spring, Europe settled to a period of 'phoney war'.

Lindbergh's Moves

Lindbergh still hoped that Germany would not move against France and would instead threaten Russia, and that war between them would weaken both nations. If America stayed out of the European conflict, he considered, it might help direct Germany towards Russia. Lindbergh started his campaign to keep America out of the war, and to feel free to speak out, he resigned his reserve Air Force commission as a colonel. But the Roosevelt administration was increasingly inclined to assist Europe, and started to send supplies and armaments. Lindbergh was given a chance by the three major radio networks to speak on 15 September, and he again suggested that Germany should be allowed to expand its territory. Although American public opinion was strongly behind Lindbergh, the administration made fresh personal attacks on him, predictably bringing up Lindbergh's earlier visit to Germany and the acceptance of a Nazi medal. Lindbergh, in favour with the public, was also in favour with the owner of *Reader's Digest*, and wrote on 'Aviation, Geography and Race' in the November 1939 issue, taking the view that 'our civilisation depends upon peace among Western nations'. Lindbergh's isolationist stance caused problems for Carrel in France, and he asked Lindbergh to offer military support for France, which Lindbergh declined to do.

In France, Carrel's views were sought by the media and, taking a patriotically anti-German stance in a radio broadcast, he talked of 'the wonderful human strain which inhabits France'. He then called for a national effort to win the imminent war:

> You know what awaits us if we do not: forced labour for life for our workers and peasants, deportation to Africa for large masses of the population in our richest provinces and mass executions. ... Our sole hope at this moment is America. I believe we are capable of resisting the Boche.[1]

This view anticipated many later events, but in private he was more ambiguous and less patriotic. Writing to his nephew, he explained that he had to take this stance 'because the Jews control the French radio'.[2]

Carrel's War Work

In France, Carrel was not of an age to serve in the army, but was keen to help France in some way. He was taken on first as an advisor to the Secrétariat d'état de la famille et de la santé and then he moved to Raoul Dautry's Ministre de l'Armement. There he was a 'haut conseiller', and his remit was to promote surgical technology and also, mysteriously, 'social biology'. Dautry was Carrel's kind of person. He was a 'technocrat' who had been in charge of the French national railway system from 1928 and was brought in as a minister in the new French government of September 1939. Dautry understood Carrel and

---

[1] 'Dr. Carrel Warns French of Plight if They Lose' *NYT*, 7 December 1939.
[2] Carrel to Gigou, 4 January 1940, box 40 folder 3, Georgetown University Library Booth Family Center for Special Collections (GULBFC) and Malinin Collection of the Papers of Alexis Carrel and Charles Lindbergh, box 5 folder 28, FA 208 Rockefeller University Archives, Rockefeller Archives Centre (RUA RAC). See also Philip Nord, *France's New Deal: From the Thirties to the Postwar Era* (Princeton: Princeton University Press, 2010): 61.

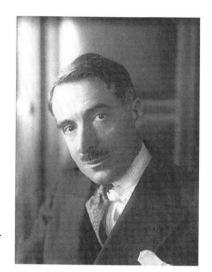

In 1939, Raoul Dautry in Paris enrolled Carrel in his wartime Ministry of Armaments. (*Wikipedia*)

knew of his book and hence gave him this vague extra remit. To be ready for the defence of France, there was much activity, and a revival of interest in military medicine. The French military hopes were that any war with Germany would be stalemated along the impressive French defences of the Maginot Line now in place along France's border with Germany, but Carrel, influenced by Lindbergh's view that aerial power would be crucial, foresaw a less static war and that planning for mobile hospitals was required. Carrel was pleased that many other pet projects, left unfinished at the end of World War I, were now back on the agenda.

New Projects

Carrel wished to take up studies of wound healing again, and also wanted to look at the effects of poison gases. Studies on shock had largely ceased after World War I, and although blood transfusion was now in civilian use, it still came by direct transfer from donors, and the arrangement for blood storage which had emerged in the last months of World War I had, perhaps surprisingly, not emerged in civilian life. The news from the Spanish Civil War was that during the bombing of Barcelona in the previous summer of 1938, blood banking had been extensively used by the Republican army medical staff. Carrel knew that these blood preservation methods used the Peyton Rous citrate-glucose storage technique devised at the Rockefeller Institute during World War I. Carrel wrote back from France to the Institute for details, and Rous was delighted at the news that blood storage was at last being revived. He replied that 'you have a great opportunity ... our work seems to have been forgotten'.[3]

Carrel was less pleased to hear that the Spanish military surgeons, notably Josep Trueta, treated their war wounds, not with Carrel's antiseptic irrigation method, but instead used a variant on Winnett Orr's radically different method — débridement first then a simple dressing applied to the open wound with the area covered by an unchanged plaster cast. Carrel was not pleased and complained to his surgical friend and supporter William Sherman that 'the modern surgeons are as ignorant as their predecessors 25 years ago ... such ignorance is bound to cause the loss of innumerable lives and limbs'.[4]

By January 1940, Carrel had a promise of research support in Paris and Dautry allocated funds for a personal unit, designed by Le Corbusier, at Garches on land owned by the Pasteur Institute. Carrel brought in his old friend Lecomte du Noüy from the Pasteur Institute to start blood transfusion studies, although du Noüy soon concluded that the Spanish surgeons were wrong to claim that red cells survived well in storage. The two couples renewed their earlier friendship. Mme Carrel joined a Red Cross voluntary nursing organisation which organised soldier's hostels placed close to the Belgian border. One of her staff was well-known as having had worked with Edith Cavell, the nursing heroine of World War I, but Carrel was unimpressed — 'a mere school teacher, an unrestrained liar, avid for publicity'.

---

[3] Crutcher to Carrel, 23 October 1939, Malinin Collection, box 4 folder 39, RUA RAC (note 2).

[4] Carrel to Sherman, 24 March 1939, box 42 file 'GULBFC (note 2). Trueta's method was much admired thereafter, but was forgotten when the advent of antibiotics radically changed wound management.

Dr. Carrel's Immortal Chicken Heart

Present, Authentic Facts about This
Oft-Falsified Scientific "Celebrity"

ALBERT H. EBELING, M.D.
Lederle Laboratories, Inc.

A TINY fragment, removed in 1912 from the heart of an unhatched chick embryo by the eminent Dr. Alexis Carrel, began then the most extraordinary career ever enjoyed by a chick or a part of a chick. It has attained potential immortality. The present descendants of the cells in this fragment, now spoken of as Carrel's immortal chicken tissue, or the "old strain," are in their 30th year of independent life in the wholly artificial environment of laboratory glassware. Their growth is independent of time. Under the established conditions, the cells do not grow old, and now, after practically three times the lifetime of a normal chicken, they are as young and healthy as

is closely bound up with the progressive development of tissue culture technique as carried out in Dr. Carrel's laboratory. The procedures are used in the cultivation of numerous pure strains of cell types other than the original "immortal chicken tissue" of Carrel, such as, for example, various types of epithelial cells, cartilage, thyroid, liver, certain cell types from the blood as well as various strains of malignant cells (sarcoma and

prolifer
and th
known
pedigre
tion ac
nearly
the bes
ing the
of subs
mercial
them n
the acti
of the
living t
vide a
antisept
compou
tic, a su
to bact

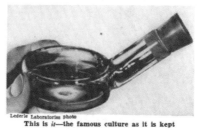

Lederle Laboratories photo
This is *it*—**the famous culture as it is kept**

After Carrel's retirement, Albert Ebeling took the 'immoral cells' to the Lederle laboratories, and wrote about them in the *Scientific American* of January 1942.

Changes at the Institute

When it was likely that Carrel would remain in France, Albert Ebeling felt there was no future for him at the Institute, and he left to take up a post with Wyckoff at the Lederle company. Only Miss Crutcher, Carrel's secretary, now remained from the large department, but she was kept busy with his articles and correspondence, and she would nobly support him in the difficult times to come.

Ebeling took with him two of Carrel's technicians from the Institute and also the 'eternal' chicken heart fibroblast cell line.[5] On 17 January 1940, New York's *World-Telegram*, wishing as always to mark the birthday

---

[5] Albert Ebeling 'Dr. Carrel's immortal chicken heart' *Scientific American* January 1942, 22–4.

of the cells, made its usual enquiry to the Institute. A manager seemed vague about the whereabouts of the cells. 'Listen,' he said to the attentive journalist, 'the Institute didn't encourage this business about the birthday of the chicken heart'. The newspaper, sensing a story, announced with mock solemnity that there had been a 'natural and painless' death of the much-loved cell line. Realising that the Institute had handled the matter badly, Gasser sought some damage limitation and told the press next day that the strain was in fact safe, in another laboratory, and that previous statements to the contrary were influenced by 'reasons of confidentiality'. Later, the cell line was discontinued without fuss when Ebeling retired in 1946.

Carrel's Return

By early 1940, Carrel was restive in Paris and, as ever, grumbled about France and the French, now complaining about delays in setting up his promised personal unit. Although the laboratories did appear shortly afterwards, Carrel returned to New York in May 1940, after only a nine-month stay, leaving Mme Carrel behind and in danger, still involved in her nursing projects. Carrel had no major reason for his return, but did bring French government instructions to seek the support of the American Volunteer Ambulance Corps, the formidable organisation which in World War I had provided about 300 ambulances and 600 drivers to support the Allied armies. In New York, Carrel contacted the Corps director James J. Johnson and they agreed on a design for a new 100-bed hospital which used 25 trucks and 16 large tents and which had impressive surgical and X-ray facilities. Charles Butler, an old friend of Carrel from the Demonstration Hospital days, was again involved in the design; it was quite like old times. With Carrel back, there were new suggestions for research support and laboratory space for him, and an offer came from John H. Kellogg at Miami Springs in Florida. Raymond Parker said Carrel could have a place in his new laboratory as did Wyckoff again at the Lederle laboratories.

His supporters also rallied round to resurrect Carrel's idea of an Institute to 'study man'. But the mood was not right. America might be going to war and the need was for the nation to feel virile and confident.

Carrel's view that the nations were decadent and needed rescue had no support among politicians and even Carrel's *Reader's Digest* fans may now have disagreed. With the European situation discouraging any further moves in this direction in America, Carrel was increasingly confident that instead in demoralised France he might now be listened to and that support for his ideas might emerge there. Carrel's relations with Lindbergh now cooled, since Carrel still favoured American intervention in Europe.

French Defeat

The expected German attack on France had come on 10 May 1940, just after Carrel left. Germany's new mobile armoured units, backed by overwhelming air support, moved unexpectedly through the wooded Ardennes into France and, overrunning Belgium to the north, also skirted round the French Maginot Line defences and moved towards Paris. The French government fell and France capitulated on 22 June. Thereafter, the Germans fully occupied the northern part of France and the rest of the nation to the south was put under a new German-supervised, demilitarised French government. Based at Vichy, it was headed by France's World War I military hero Marshal Philippe Pétain, one of Carrel's favourite Frenchmen. The new government did not have a democratic structure, and all forms of election were replaced by nomination. With this collaborationist arrangement, Germany was relieved of much of the civil administration, and it allowed Hitler to contemplate military aggression elsewhere, notably to draw up a plan for an invasion of Britain.

America pragmatically accepted the situation in France and recognised the new government by sending an ambassador to Vichy. A few French military men and politicians rejected the Vichy settlement and Charles de Gaulle, an Army officer, departed to London where he set up a government in exile, working with the British government towards defeating Germany. Resistance within France to the German occupation started immediately in a small way and only later grew in strength.

After the German invasion, communication with France from America was difficult. However, Mme Carrel was reported to be safe at their island home, now in the sensitive maritime military area — the 'zone interdite' — facing Britain across the English Channel. The Germans had taken the Carrel's motor boat and their two cars, and the Lindbergh's house had been steadily looted.

Carrel and Vichy

Carrel, back in New York, spent his first summer in the city for about 30 years, and watched the situation in France closely. By autumn 1940 he made a decision. For Carrel, France had been defeated and was at peace in a strange way. His world view, before the War, was that the West, and France in particular, was decadent and that this decay had invited unrest, war and military defeat. Carrel now considered that the France of old was no longer worth saving by a British or American military rescue. It was best that France be left alone to work something out and in particular to deal with the pre-war degeneration which he had detected. Though he had earlier called for American involvement in Europe, Carrel felt that this was no longer required.[6]

He was still ambivalent about Hitler, and Hitler had triumphed:

We do not know whether Hitler is going to found a new Islam. He is already on the way; he is like Mohammed. The emotion in Germany is warlike and Islamic. ... That can be the historic future.[7]

Carrel considered that a 'Pax Teutonica' might have arrived, giving Hitler's planned 'New Order' in a pacified Europe under German control. For Carrel, the new situation was not unattractive. In France, there was a stability of sorts. Moreover the news was that in Paris, something like normal life had resumed. Those who fled had returned, and the fabric of the city was intact. Certainly, there were curfews, Nazi flags, rationing

---

[6] The discussions between Lindbergh and Carrel on the European war are given in James D. Newton, *Uncommon Friends: Life With Thomas Edison, Henry Ford, Harvey Firestone, Alexis Carrel and Charles Lindbergh* (New York: Harvest Books, 1989): 175–99.

[7] 'Essay on Hitler', box 9 folder 29 and box 81 folder 26, GULBFC (note 2).

and bilingual road signs, but the German troops were strictly disciplined and behaved well, even apologetically, on the streets. For Carrel there was perhaps an opening for him, now that his old friend Pétain had considerable power within the limits allowed by the Germans. Vichy policy was carried out with little direction or oversight by the German victors, and in the now-technocratic state, experts rather than politicians were brought in to run the ministries.[8] Many pressed forward to assist Pétain at Vichy. The writer Georges Bernanos recalled how he and others rejoiced at the French defeat and the opportunity it gave:

> All that is called the Right … spontaneously united and cohered round the disaster of my country like a swarm of bees around their queen. I am not saying that they deliberately wished the disaster. They were waiting for it.[9]

Others said that 'the possibility of doing something new, thrills men of every walk of life', and that the emergence of Pétain was 'a divine surprise'. Former internal critics of pre-war France were now listened to, and among them, some old acquaintances of Carrel were drawn into Vichy politics. Jean Coutrot (of the Pontigny conferences and the CEPH) was offered a role by the Vichy regime, but died in 1941.

Carrel judged that the Vichy government would be sympathetic to his ideas and would listen to his long-trailed pre-war plans for improving the human race. He and Marshal Pétain had much in common, and they were known to each other before the war through contacts in French organisations. Pétain had announced that national reconstruction was now required and that a new French nation would emerge from the defeat.

Around the summer of 1940, Carrel decided that he should go back and get involved.

---

[8] These 'technocrats' included CEPH members and the related Group X-Crise of the 1930s.

[9] Francine Muel-Dreyfus, *Vichy and the Eternal Feminine* (Durham, Duke University Press, 2001): 16.

Vichy Contacts

Carrel's archives show that he made international phone calls from the Century Association to Vichy twice in September and again on 25 November 1940. At this early stage, he was perhaps sounding out the Vichy government, or at least seeking the difficult travel documents for a visit. There may have been a number of opportunities opening up for him at Vichy. Pierre Laval at this time was the all-powerful minister of state under Pétain, and American security reports later said Carrel's name was put forward to Laval as a possible Vichy ambassador to the United States. But Laval turned it down, saying: 'I don't want any bug hunters'. Instead, in late 1940, Laval appointed Gaston Henry-Haye, the mayor of Versailles.[10]

Vichy was regarded with suspicion in America and opinion was turning against Petain's regime. Carrel kept information about his Vichy contacts to himself; there were few in whom Carrel could confide, and Fred Coudert, his closest friend, was one. Coudert was a Vichy supporter and Vichy was using Coudert's legal services in America in the purchase of their new legation in New York. Coudert disliked the word 'collaboration', and instead he sought to depict the new Vichy regime as a 'shield for France' against Germany. He claimed improbably that during the invasion 'the French gave in only inch by inch', and that in defeat 'the French will do all that human beings can be expected to do to impede and delay the ruthless invader...'[11]

France Calls

In late 1940 Carrel started moves to get back to France. He steadily disengaged in New York, which was easily done, since he was completely out of experimental research and now had only some minor speaking engagements. He declined a request to write an article on tissue culture

---

[10] U.S. National Archives, OSS intelligence report, Heinzen to Allen Dulles: 'The Carrel affair' Record Group 226, box 122 folder 13.
[11] Letter from Coudert, *New York Herald Tribune*, 24 May 1941.

and passed it on instead to Ebeling at Lederle to write it, and had a surprising response. Ebeling wrote back that

> I should perhaps consider myself highly flattered, in view of the fact that, after all these years you should consider me capable of writing an article on tissue culture. You will recall, no doubt, through all the years of my association with you, that I never wrote any article acceptable to you. You were always extremely critical, unhelpful and at times unjust from my point of view.[12]

Carrel was, for once, ruffled and wrote back in pained tones, and Ebeling retracted much of his complaint. Carrel's last public appearance was in December 1940 at the New York State Health and Physical Education convention, where he proposed that exercises should be used to counter national degeneration and called for 'the development of men of greater physical and spiritual value than have lived at any other time'.[13] He saw less of Lindbergh, though both now were isolationists — Lindbergh wished to keep America out of the European war, as Carrel now did.

'America First Committee'

During 1940, Lindbergh had an increasingly high public profile. His support for an American isolationist policy on Europe made him the star speaker at the rallies organised by those wishing to keep out of the European war, who soon took the name 'America First'. Suggestions that Lindbergh had pro-German leanings were revived again when, in late 1940, his wife Anne produced a slim pamphlet titled *The Wave of the Future*. In it she concluded that the democracies suffered from 'blindness, lethargy, selfishness, smugness, weakness and moral decay', and this had led to the world crisis.[14]

---

[12] David Le Vay, *Alexis Carrel: The Perfectibility of Man* (Rockville: Kabel Publishing, 1996): 198. Ebeling's outburst is odd, since he did write a number of articles without Carrel's name, but a sense of grievance is clear.

[13] 'Dr. Carrel Urges High Defense Aims' *NYT*, 27 December 1940.

[14] Anne Morrow Lindbergh, *The Wave of the Future* (New York: Harcourt, Brace, 1940); see also Joyce Milton, *Loss of Eden: A Biography of Charles and Anne Lindbergh* (New York: HarperCollins, 1993): 392.

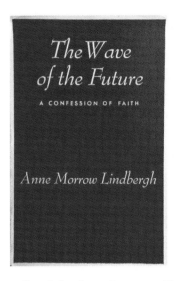

Anne Lindberg's book on European Fascism.

To this she added that a failure to 'absorb and use our scientific accumulations and discoveries' had contributed.

This analysis came straight from Carrel's table-talk at Saint-Gildas, which she had heard so often. A possible direct reference to Carrel was her praise for 'those far-sighted in Europe who wanted reform, but are now overrun. That the effort of these pioneers should apparently be wasted is one of the great calamites of our age'. Recalling her European travels with Charles, she concluded that what they had seen in Germany was 'the wave of the future', and that Germany had taken the actions which all nations would need to face up to eventually. She extended the metaphor by saying that powerful waves could have some scum on top, and she conceded that the European fascist leaderships had some faults. The pamphlet was initially well received and sold well, and was supported by condensation in *Reader's Digest*. But the Roosevelt administration, now leaning strongly towards intervening in Europe, had to neutralise these politically unwelcome views of this daughter of a former ambassador to Mexico, and they turned against her. A senior politician labelled her essay as 'the Bible of every American Nazi, Fascist, Bundist and

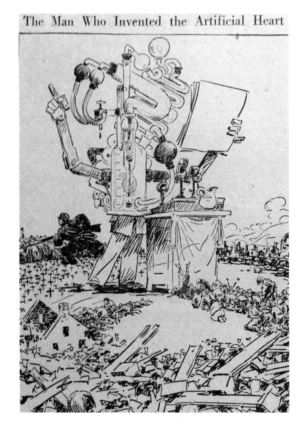

The Man Who Invented the Artificial Heart

With support for war growing, Lindbergh was depicted as heartless and insensitive to Europe's sufferings. (From the *New York Herald Tribune*, 9 October 1941.)

appeaser'.[15] The book was soon widely deplored by commentators, and for a while it meant social isolation for her.

Carrel's Plan

Carrel soon announced that he was proposing to go to France to do 'a survey of the conditions among the population of the occupied region, especially the children, from the point of view of malnutrition and infectious disease'. Strangely, a Rockefeller Foundation team was already

---

[15] A. Scott Berg, *Lindbergh* (New York: G.P. Putnam's Sons, 1998): 406–7.

in France doing such a nutritional survey, but Carrel had no part in it. His other agenda was his grand, long-standing aspiration to save France. To say he was planning this nutritional survey perhaps diverted probing questions about his travels. But others were clear why he was going. In a long article in the Paris journal *Esprit* in December 1940, Pierre Delore, a friend of Carrel, enthused about Carrel's plans to 'remake man' in France.[16] When Coudert wrote to Carrel wishing him bon voyage, he said that Carrel would 'begin the rebirth of the ancient races that built our civilisation'.[17] Lindbergh by now also knew something of Carrel's intentions. He handed Carrel a long friendly letter to take to Mme Carrel in France, avoiding the censors, and in it he spoke with feeling about their friendship in the past. In the letter, Lindbergh also wrote about Carrel's journey and seemed to know that Carrel would be in negotiations with the government. He said that

> the Vichy government must be reminded that [Carrel] foresaw exactly what was happening in France many years ago. He told people what it was leading to, but they would not listen. Now he has been demonstrated right, and now is the time to make use of his services in the constructing the nation along sound and enduring lines.[18]

There was no mention of a nutritional survey. But Lindbergh shrewdly saw problems ahead. He noted in his diaries that Carrel's notorious tactlessness might ruin his chances in Vichy and waste 'the powers he could otherwise contribute to the reconstruction of France'.[19]

Carrel had a last-minute flurry of letter–writing and visits, and he obtained the re-entry visa he required as a French citizen to return to

---

[16] Pierre Delore 'La médecine et la science de l'homme' *Esprit,* December 1940, 43–59. Delore and the Lyon connection are described by Weisz in Christopher Lawrence and George Weisz (eds.), *Greater Than the Parts: Holism in Biomedicine, 1920–1950,* (Oxford: Oxford University Press, 1998), 68–93 and 257–79.

[17] Robert Soupault, *Alexis Carrel* (Paris: Libraire Plon, 1952): 213.

[18] Letter to Mme Carrel, Lindbergh Papers, box 037 files 1131 and 1151, Yale University Library Manuscripts and Archives.

[19] Charles A. Lindbergh, *The Wartime Journals of Charles A. Lindbergh* (New York: Harcourt Brace Jovanovich, 1970): 444.

Dr. Carrell Sails for Survey in Europe;
Will Study Effects of Cold and Malnutrition

Dr. Alexis Carrel, French scientist and author, sailed yesterday for Europe on the American Export liner Siboney to study the effects of malnutrition and cold on the undernourished populations of war-ravished nations. He traveled on a French passport and plans to visit Spain first after landing at Lisbon, then will go wherever his studies best can be furthered.

"This is a one-man expedition which I started years ago," he said. "It is purely a medical study of the effects of starvation and cold and the spreading of disease as a result. It has no connection with the Rockefeller Institute. I am going for as short a time as possible."

Dr. Carrel explained that his trip will carry him to small towns and villages off the beaten path.

Dr. Carrel's most recent achievement was the designing of a mobile tent hospital to be used to fight post-war epidemics in the field. At the time of its announcement the scientist said he hoped "to be with the hospital now and then in France, or wherever else it may go."

Another passenger on the Siboney was James W. Johnson, president of the American Volunteer Ambulance Corps, which had 125 drivers and 110 ambulances in France.

Three Wright Field Army men from Dayton, Ohio, also sailed. One was Major Charles H. Cummings. to be assistant military at-

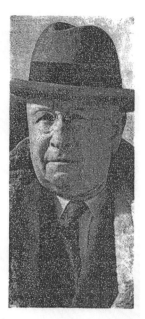

Dr. Alexis Carrel as he left yesterday on the liner Siboney.
Times Wide World

Carrel's press conference described in the *New York Times* 2 February 1941.

America. This would expire in three months' time. Carrel took this care to make plans to return to America, in case he was stranded unwillingly in France without a visa. He told *Reader's Digest* he would continue to write for them on his return, and three days before leaving, Carrel wrote to his old friend Karl Beck in Washington saying that he would do the Introduction to the surgeon's autobiography on his return. He declined to speak on a radio programme entitled *I'm an American*, saying delphically: 'I am an American only at heart. I have for important reasons, remained a citizen of France'. With only days to go, he had an urgent meeting in Washington with the Vichy ambassador Henry-Haye, to arrange contact soon with Maréchal Pétain and other ministers in Vichy. When thanking the ambassador, he added his sympathy for Henry-Haye's difficult role in Vichy's 'grand task'. While in Washington, and after obtaining documents to travel through Spain, Carrel lunched with Franco's ambassador and on return to New York wrote back praising 'the intelligence, beauty and saintliness of the Latin races', thanking the ambassador for helping the 'new growth of an old plan'.

The Journey

In this venture into Europe, Carrel conveniently joined up with the philanthropist James Wood Johnson, related to the Johnson and Johnson family's medical supplies company, who had organised charitable emergency supplies for Europe. Johnson wished to make the difficult journey to France taking vitamins, medications and powdered milk to help deal with the food shortages in France. Getting into France was difficult, and the route was a tortuous one via non-aligned Portugal, then into Spain, and then north over the border into France. At the New York docks on 1 February 1941, Carrel spoke to the press and there was a photo opportunity.[20] Charles Lindbergh and Jim Newton waved the two travellers off as they sailed on the freighter *Siboney* to Lisbon. Both were booked on a flight back to the U.S. three months later, on the transatlantic seaplane 'clipper' flight from Lisbon. Johnson returned to Lisbon to take the flight; Carrel did not, and was to stay in France until his death.

---

[20] 'Dr. Carrel Sails for Survey in Europe *NYT*, 2 February 1941.

CHAPTER EIGHTEEN

Back to France

Heading for Europe, and ostensibly planning to do a survey of the nutritional problems in France, Carrel had his extra, more ambitious agenda. He planned to make personal contact at a high level with the new German-installed collaborationist Vichy government, and to reacquaint himself with its leader, 85-year old Maréchal Philippe Pétain. Carrel also wished to reach his French island home and to be reunited with his wife. He planned to return to America in mid-April and had booked a return flight on the 'Clipper' from Lisbon.[1]

His companion James Wood Johnson's declared aim was to deliver Red Cross humanitarian aid to France, including vitamins, the only goods allowed through the British blockade of Atlantic trade which prevented supplies useful to Germany getting through. Johnson may have had undeclared reasons for this extended sojourn. European sales by the two family companies Johnson and Johnson and Mead Johnson Nutrition had declined as a result of the British naval blockade, and he may have hoped to study the political and military developments. Like Carrel, Johnson had managed to get a French visa, and he was expected in Vichy, possibly helped by General Robert C. Davis, head of the New York Chapter of the American Red Cross. Davis was also chairman of the

---

[1] Inaugurated on 28 June 1939, this Pan Am flying boat service, stopping at Horta in the Azores, took 29 hours, thus speeding up transatlantic travel, but at a price. The luxurious Boeing B-314 carried 74 passengers and mail; the return fare was $675. With Europe in crisis and Portugal alone open, the flight was much used by diplomats and the military.

Transradio Consortium, which owned the Vichy radio company Compagnie Generale.

Whatever their reasons, both were keen to get into France, and decided to travel together, taking the gift of vitamins with them. Carrel had, in addition, brought extra medical supplies which he had ordered from the Rockefeller Hospital's pharmacy. They left New York and headed by sea for a land-fall at Lisbon, planning then to get into France via Spain.

In Lisbon and Spain

Sailing on 1 February, with their two trunks of medical aid following on another ship, the travellers stopped first in Bermuda for the necessary clearance by the British authorities. For Carrel, a Frenchman, this involved questions on his attitude to the participants in the war. Sailing again, they arrived in Lisbon on 11 February. Lisbon was the only portal of entry into Europe and, as it was an open city, the hotels were full of refugees, military staff and diplomats, and it was also a centre for European intrigue. The two travellers noticed the effects of the nearby recently-ended Spanish civil war and heard of the exodus into Portugal of Spanish and French refugees, including many Jews. Moving inland over the border into Spain, they reached Madrid and saw more of the legacy of the war, won by Franco's fascist regime. The two visitors were regarded with suspicion, and a Madrid pro-German paper newspaper *Informaciones* made the unlikely accusation that

> Johnson in company of a famous scientist is an American who under the guise of charity is actively engaged in Red propaganda. He distributes money only to the Reds, giving them at the same time political tracts.[2]

The paper added that the money came from the exiled left-wing former premier Juan Negrín.

---

[2] Johnson wrote up his experiences later as 'We saw Spain starving' *Saturday Evening Post*, 28 June and 5 July 1941.

Another sceptic was an American intelligence source who said sarcastically that Carrel's Spanish 'survey' thus far 'consisted of a call at poor families, asking if they had enough to eat and leaving a donation of $10–$15'.[3]

But Johnson's vitamin shipment was seriously delayed and was eventually left behind and handed over to a Madrid hospital. In spite of the loss of their charitable aid, they pressed on and, reaching the French border to the north on about 15 March, both were successful in entering into France and travelling on to Vichy. On arrival, Carrel was met by a reporter and photographer from the government-controlled newspaper and, as ever, gave an interview. He diplomatically said that he found the situation in France was better than was perceived in America. This assessment was relayed back to America and was not well received, since the privations in defeated France were well known. It led to the first suggestions, which were to increase, that Carrel had pro-German sympathies.

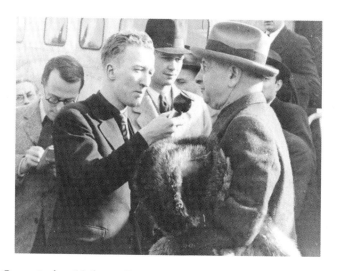

On arrival at Vichy in France, Carrel gave a press conference.

---

[3] 'Conditions in France', box 34 folder 7860, RG 0226, Office of Strategic Services, U.S. National Archives and Records (NAR). This was a summary made by the British censors in Bermuda of information gathered from personal letters sent home by the Rockefeller Foundation staff doing the nutritional survey and based then in Marseilles.

America had decided to maintain diplomatic relations with France and Admiral William D. Leahy was appointed ambassador in 1941. But the Vichy government was annoyed at America's increasing sympathy and support for Britain, and used the Paris newspapers to denounce Leahy as 'a freemason, a representative of Jewish bankers and a British agent'.[4] While Carrel was in Vichy, the American intelligence agencies used local contacts to take an interest in him. If Carrel had been seriously suggested as American ambassador, he was lucky to have avoided the post. The hapless Gaston Henry-Haye was soon ridiculed by the Washington diplomatic world and ostracised as a German stooge. Further black propaganda coming from British intelligence within America led to his internment in November 1942.

Pétain Contact

Carrel had the first of two meetings with Pétain on 16 March, and they would recall their pre-war contacts and discuss the new situation. In Vichy, there were opportunities for Carrel, and a discussion on Carrel's ideas was probably planned even before Carrel left America. Pétain would be a ready listener, and had heard Carrel's view on these subjects before the War. At his meeting with Pétain, Carrel could point to the success of *Man, the Unknown* as evidence of popular acceptability of his views, and the need for an institute to work on his agenda for improving the French nation. Pétain's chief civil servant recalled the meeting and that Carrel

> received some encouragement and threw himself into the creation of the Human Institute. Carrel fascinated us by his penetrating glance, his exceptional culture and the almost challenging ease of his answers. Was he, as he claimed, an admirer of the Axe (German-Italian-Japanese Alliance)?[5]

---

[4] For American relations with Vichy, see ambassador William D. Leahy's *I was There* (New York: Whittlesay House, 1950). After Leahy left, S. Pinkney Tuck served as interim chargé d'affaires until France severed diplomatic relations with the U.S. on 8 November 1942, at the time of the Allied invasion of North Africa.
[5] Henri du Moulin de Labarthète, *Le temps des illusions* (Geneva: Editions du Cheval Ailé, 1946): 252.

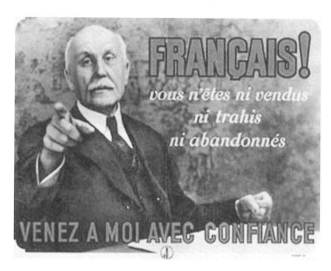

Marshal Petain, after France's defeat by Germany in 1940, headed the French collaborationist Vichy government and called for national renewal.

COMMENTS ON DR. ALEXIS CARRELL, French scientist who is ostensibly studying nutrition conditions in Europe:-
Written by Schwentker:- "Saw Alexis Carrell at dinner. Still the smooth diplomat but still very much out for old A.C. (Alexis Carrell) He has been making a private survey of the nutritional state of the children of France, knowing nothing about children and less about nutrition. But the French newspapers think he is wonderful. His publicity dwarfs ours."
Written by Youmans:- "If I felt more like writing, I'd write more about A. Carrell. He is a great nuisance. Comes over with a big fanfare and announces he will make the most important study of nutrition ever made. In the next breath says he will stay 40 days!! Knows nothing of nutrition of course, but fools a great many people. His inopportune arrival probably explains why he did not get the 'laissez passer' I spoke of in connection with my visit to Paris. He was here in Marseille a day or two - I didn't care to meet him but Strode and Wright did. He has a sort of body guard and is with a Johnson, of "Johnson & Johnson" Surgical Supplies. The French Health people are leery of him and the Rockefeller Foundation people disgusted. He made a big investigation of nutrition in Spain too; though investigation consisted of a call at poor families, asking if they had enough to eat and leaving a donation of $10 - $15."

American intelligence obtained intercepts of letters from Rockefeller Foundation nutritional scientists in France, mentioning contact with Carrel. (*Courtesy of the U.S. National Archives and Records: from Reference 3.*)

After spending some time in Vichy, Carrel and Johnson obtained a car and toured in the south of France from Roanne down to Marseilles, but there is no evidence that Carrel was doing a serious nutritional survey. He had no staff, nor an office or a base. Moreover, the Rockefeller Foundation already had a team of 11 staff and a secretary in Marseilles doing exactly that, although this Rockefeller's Institut des Recherches d'Hygiene lasted only for the first six months of 1941 after which, concerned at the events, they left France.[6] Carrel called in to see them. The Rockefeller Foundation nutritionists knew him well and were not impressed:

> Saw Alexis Carrell [sic] at dinner. Still the smooth diplomat but still very much out for old A.C. (Alexis Carrel). He has been making a private survey of the nutritional state of the children of France, knowing nothing about children and less about nutrition. But the French newspapers think he is wonderful. His publicity dwarfs ours. ... Knows nothing of nutrition of course, but fools a great many people. He has a sort of bodyguard and is with a Johnson of "Johnson and Johnson" Surgical Supplies.[7]

When they returned to Vichy, Johnson wished to travel north with Carrel into the Occupied Zone and towards Carrel's island home, but he did not get the necessary permit, and they parted company. To reach his island, Carrel did have permission to travel into the Occupied Zone, and would be warned that once he was in, it might be difficult to get out, particularly as all Americans were now prevented from leaving. There were further difficulties in reaching his island, since it was in the coastal militarised 'Atlantic Wall' facing Britain. But the island was also a farm, which simplified access, and at last he reached home on 18 April. From there, his contacts with Vichy continued and a plan began to mature. Mme Carrel meanwhile took a post as a social worker at the town of Penvenan on the coast nearby.

This region of France had its own niche pro-German politics. Before the declaration of war, the Breton National Party had contacted the Germans seeking independence from France, and this movement increased in strength after the German invasion. A supportive German military governor was put in place who encouraged the separatists.

---

[6] The Foundation's brief, forgotten venture in France is described in detail by William E. Schneider (2003) 'War, philanthropy, and the National Institute of Hygiene in France' *Minerva* 41: 1–23.

[7] 'Conditions in France' NAR (note 3).

Johnson instead travelled south to the Pyrenees to visit the refugee camps on the northern French side which held mostly German Jews but also republican Spanish refugees driven out by the civil war and who had braved the difficult mountain crossing to reach safety. All these refugees were unwelcome in France and were badly treated, notably at the internment camp at the town of Gurs. Impoverished France hoped to obtain outside humanitarian aid, and Johnson's mysterious mission may have involved these negotiations. When he returned to Lisbon there was a cable from Carrel stating 'Impossible vous rejoindre'; Carrel now no longer wished to take his return flight. Johnson left for home, as planned, by the clipper and reached America on 15 May. He telephoned Miss Crutcher at the Institute and reported to her on their travels, adding that he thought Carrel had now exceeded the time allowed on his re-entry visa to America.

New York Watching

At the Rockefeller Institute, there was understandable interest in Carrel's movements and activities, but communications between France and the outside world were increasingly difficult. Even within France, the postal services were tightly controlled. A few letters from Carrel sent via his

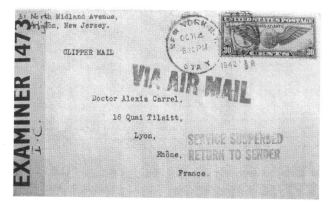

Carrel's secretary attempted to contact Carrel via his brother's address in Lyon, but her letters were returned by the British censors in Bermuda. (*Courtesy of the Georgetown University Library Booth Family Center for Special Collections.*)

brother Joseph in Lyon did get to America but, because of censorship, Carrel was careful not to say too much. He did report that the food was 'not good and in too small quantity', and that travelling was extremely difficult. Carrel's devoted secretary was increasingly concerned, and although she wrote regularly, many letters failed to reach him, and some were returned by censors, since all post from America to France was intercepted and read in British Bermuda.[8]

Because Carrel had not returned as planned, speculation in America about his activities increased in 1941. A suggestion appeared in the newspapers that he was being held against his will, but a press release from Vichy on 16 May said he was 'not detained, but working on a report on malnutrition'. This press release added the interesting information, which could only have come from Carrel, that he was seeking election to the Académie français as one of their elite 40 'Immortels'. For Carrel, this was a long-standing ambition, and for him to announce this goal suggests a confident mindset at the time. He would have the support of Pétain, now a powerful member of the Académie.[9]

Vichy Rule

Germany's unexpectedly sudden military success in subduing France had given Hitler encouragement to plan an invasion of Britain, and this looked set to follow in autumn of 1940. But after heavy German losses in the aerial Battle of Britain, Hitler's ambition turned east instead towards Russia. This left France demilitarised, defeated and initially pacified. 'Collaboration not subordination' was a reasonable face-saving mantra used by the German-installed French government. After introspection on the defeat, the official analysis was that France had not suffered a purely military disaster, but that defects in the nation were responsible, defects which dated back to the 1930s. Carrel and other declinists now seemed vindicated.

---

[8] See Lawrence Sherman 'United States mail to France in World War Two' *American Philatelist* January 2013: 42–51 and 126–36.

[9] The Académie still gives this, France's highest honour, to intellectuals, and has a role in zealously guarding the purity of the French language. Carrel was already an 'associate' member.

Pétain soon announced a national reconstruction plan. In his 'Révolution nationale', he changed the famous French motto from 'Liberté, égalité, fraternité' to 'Travail, famille, patrie' (work, family, fatherland). The list of pre-war problems now identified included the alleged defects of democracy, and a 'technocratic' government was in place instead. Carrel had always agreed with this strategy. Vital in the reconstruction was to achieve an increase in the size of the French population. Pétain, within days of the defeat, blamed 'too few babies, too few weapons, and too few allies' in his assessment.[10] In the Vichy 'pronatalist' policy there was a drive for more children, and Vichy urged that women should return to traditional domestic roles. This was always Carrel's view and would soon be noticed:

> Carrel, cited by everyone and everywhere, placed all his scientific authority into imposing the idea of an 'eternal feminine' founded this time on biological and physiological determinism.[11]

In October 1940 new legislation excluded women from the civil service and professions, and Mother's Day was re-established and emphasised from May 1941, highlighting a new, heroic but limited role for women in the home. Maternity was all-important, and in returning to an enclosed domestic sphere, as man's help-mate, women would be educated for this role. Women were also blamed for the defeat. Some strident French verdicts concluded that

> intoxicated with herself, in love with direct action, personal ambition [to be a] lawyer, doctor, business "man" — woman has little by little turned away from her eternal role. ... the French woman of today carries her share, a heavy share, of the responsibility for the defeat of France. The new men have understood this.[12]

Carrel was one of the 'new men'.

---

[10] Francine Muel-Dreyfus, *Vichy et l'éternel feminin* (Paris: Editions du Seuil, 1996), translated as *Vichy and the Eternal Feminine* (Durham, Duke University Press, 2001): 70.
[11] Muel-Dreyfus, *Vichy* (note 10): 286.
[12] Muel-Dreyfus, *Vichy* (note 10): 38.

Island Negotiations

Carrel, settled back at his island, was in touch with Vichy. Soon after he arrived, he had a visit in April 1941 from Félix-André Missenard. Carrel had written prefaces in the late 1930s for both of Missenard's books, and Missenard, as described earlier, had acted in pre-war France as Carrel's go-between in promoting Carrel's plans for a French 'Institute of Man'. Missenard was now involved with the Vichy administration as a member of the Conseil supérieur de la recherché scientifique. He arrived at the island bearing some details of Pétain's government's thoughts on support for an institute along Carrelian lines. In this, Missenard was soon joined on the island by the physicians André Gros and Jaques Ménétrier, who also had ties with Vichy ministers, and together they had authority to negotiate with Carrel. Some accounts say that Carrel was reluctant to proceed, but since the idea had been in the forefront of his mind for six years or more, and he now had powerful support, it is unlikely that he needed much encouragement, although the times were not particularly favourable. Carrel also involved his wife and local clerical friend Dom Alexis Presse in the discussion, and between them, the group doubtless added practical detail to Carrel's grand, long-held but rather nebulous ideas for the future of man.[13] Soon, a story reached the American newspapers in June 1941 that Carrel would head a new government department in Vichy, but Carrel got word out via Vichy denying it, saying that he had simply advocated an organisation of this type. In New York, Miss Crutcher was confused by the news:

> Having thought that I knew his attitude about ever working in France again, especially under German domination, I am at a loss to under-stand this report, if it is true.[14]

---

[13] For the group discussion, see André Missenard 'Sombre souvenirs: La vérité sur le séjour d'Alexis Carrel en France de 1941 à 1944' *Journal de médecine de Lyon*, June 1980, 397–411. Carrel's deepening friendship with Dom Alexis and other clerics is described in Daniel Lindenberg, *Les années souterraines* (Paris, La Découverte, 1990): 182–3.

[14] Crutcher memorandum, Malinin Collection of the Papers of Alexis Carrel and Charles Lindbergh, box 5 folder 1, FA 208, Rockefeller University Archives, Rockefeller Archives Centre (RUA RAC).

Discussion and negotiations were indeed going on with Vichy and extended over many months. Carrel and his advisors may have held out for some time, and when the institute was set up, it was lavishly funded.

Carrel's 'Fondation'

After these negotiations, on 1 November 1941, the Vichy government finally announced the establishment of the Fondation française pour l'étude des problèmes humains — the French Foundation for the Study of Human Problems. Its name and even its aspirations were close to that of Coutrot's defunct CEPH (Centre d'études des problèmes humains), with which Carrel had been associated, but Coutrot had died that year. Carrel was to be in charge as 'Regent' of the new institute and, often called the 'Fondation Carrel', it was to be based in German-occupied Paris, not in Vichy. It had unique ambitions, and its large budget, obtained at this time of economic difficulty, suggested that Carrel and his supporters had successfully made a strong case in Vichy. A remarkable budget of 40 million French francs was allocated to Carrel's venture in the first year, and this increased in the second. In comparison with other government departments, only the long-established Centre national de la recherche scientifique had a larger allocation. Carrel's Fondation was unusual in other ways. It had not emerged from any existing French government department, nor did it resemble conventional government departments, or institutions in other countries. It was fairly independent of government and was not linked to the prestigious Pasteur Institute nor to the universities of Paris.[15]

His appointment and the new institution were welcomed by the tightly controlled pro-German local Paris press.[16] In a government press release announcing the establishment of the Institute, Carrel let it be known that France was 'in good shape'.

---

[15] For a detailed account, see Alain Drouard, *Une inconnue des sciences sociales: la Fondation Alexis Carrel 1941–1945* (Paris: Editions de la Maison des sciences de l'homme, 1992): 286–7, and the shorter account in Andrés H. Reggiani, *God's Eugenicist: Alexis Carrel and the Sociobiology of Decline* (New York: Berghahn Books, 2007).

[16] See Reggiani, *God's Eugenicist* (note 15): 127–57.

The Fondation's Plan

The aims of Carrel's new institute were set out in its charter:

1. To study all possible means of safeguarding, improving and developing the French population.
2. To synthesise efforts undertaken by its own members or by others and to develop the science of man.

This was a broad remit clearly based on Carrel's long-held hopes for national revival via the 'bio-power' of scientific study; he was now usefully assisted by the absence of politicians and a population which was more regulated and directed by government than usual and was available for wartime study:

> France became an immense human laboratory in which medical and psychological experts manufactured massive amounts of sociobiological data and devised "scientific" responses ...[17]

In one of the few articles written by Carrel during the Occupation, he called his approach 'anthropotechnics', aiming for 'the systematic construction of civilised man in the totality of his corporeal, spiritual, social and racial activities', hoping to 'develop to the greatest extent the hereditary qualities which are still untouched, though dormant, in its population'.[18]

Carrel wished to look at all aspects of human activity, and he planned that experts would gather data relevant to public health, nutrition, the family, child care, education, housing, architecture, sociology, industrial productivity, economics and social insurance; after 'synthesis' of the findings in each area, the whole being considered to be greater than the parts, a plan would be put towards national improvement. His plans also included some favourite fringe projects of his own, notably on psychophysiology, hypnosis,

---

[17] Reggiani, *God's Eugenicist* (note 15): 127.
[18] Alexis Carrel 'La science de l'homme' in Sequana Broché (ed) *La France de l'esprit 1940–1943* p. 112, and Muel-Dreyfus, *Vichy* (note 10): 399.

telepathy and extrasensory perception. He favoured bringing in biotypology, as in Italy, to classify children and predict their aptitudes and
performance.

Accommodation Sought

His new large Fondation required a home, and Carrel moved quickly to
find space. First, he tried to move some of his new staff into the Pasteur
Institute, now depleted of personnel through loss to the French army and
captivity. A move by Carrel into the Institute required German approval,
and this Carrel obtained. But the Institute staff, largely unsympathetic to
the Vichy regime, objected, and they played a trump card. They told
Carrel that his actions were ill-timed, because he was being considered
for election as an 'Immortel' to l'Académie française. The death of
Marcel Prevost, the novelist, had given a vacant chair among the 40 elite.
Though Carrel backed off from his plans, an Académie election never
transpired. No elections could be made during the Occupation because
many members were interned and a quorum could not be obtained.
When Alan Gregg, director at the Rockefeller Foundation headquarters
in New York heard of Carrel's attempted 'storming of the glacis
[fortifications] of the Pasteur Institute', he seemed amused and commented
that 'Carrel has no horse sense'.[19] Carrel's action to gain space in the
Pasteur Institute produced lasting tensions. Pasteur Vallery-Radot, the
Institute's director, had been on Carrel's Christmas card list, and was later
active in the Resistance, and Carrel could no longer expect any favours
or co-operation from him. As Lindbergh had predicted before Carrel left
America, he was steadily alienating old friends and colleagues, and
gaining new critics.

Carrel's next target was the Institute for Physico-Biology (the
'Rothschild Institute') founded in 1927, an impressive Jewish-run physics
research organisation which had attracted Rockefeller Foundation
funding. Although the Germans had acted against most Jewish institutions

---

[19] Rockefeller Foundation, 1.1 Projects Series 500, France 500D, Rothschild Institute,
folder 127 box 12, RUA RAC (note 14).

in Paris, the Rothschild Institute had been spared initially, although many of the staff thought it prudent to leave. Carrel was granted permission by Pétain to take it over, and the director and the remaining staff were told by Carrel to move out immediately. The staff resisted these attempts, and Carrel said he would only desist if the Académie requested that the Institute be spared. The Académie did so, and Carrel had again to look elsewhere for space.[20]

Carrel then got permission from the German occupiers to take over the Rockefeller Foundation's Paris headquarters on the Rue de la Baume, left empty when the staff doing the nutritional survey wisely decided when internment was likely to leave for Marseilles. This building now became the Fondation's administrative centre. The Rockefeller Foundation headquarters in New York had little say in the matter and heard about Carrel's occupation after the event, and were not pleased. Carrel found other space in the deserted Carnegie Endowment for International Peace on the Boulevard Saint-Germain, and he used it to house the unit for mother and child, and biology of inheritance studies. Some facilities for laboratory work, including 'psychophysiology', were set up later in the suburbs at Vulaines-sur-Seine. Eventually, as staff built up, three more smaller satellite locations where established.

Administration

Carrel's lavish funding allowed his Fondation to build up, reaching 230 full-time staff by January 1943; there were others working part-time and many outside advisors. Missenard and Gros were rewarded for their early support by appointment to senior posts as vice-regents. Jacques Ménétrier (1908–1986), his other supporter, was the Fondation's first general secretary, but he was soon replaced by François Perroux (1903–1987), a distinguished academic and economist who was also an advisor

---

[20] The Rothschild incident is mentioned in the OSS intelligence report (note 38); other accounts say that the Rothschild staff successfully appealed to Pétain. See also Leon Sokoloff (1995) 'Alexis Carrel and the Jews at the Rockefeller Institute' *Korot* 11: 66–81.

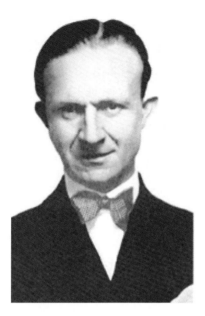

François Perroux, the distinguished Paris economist, was Carrel's senior administrator at the Fondation, but relations soon soured. (*Wikipedia*)

to Pétain at Vichy and an admirer of the Portuguese dictator António Salazar. Carrel had experience in setting up new organisations, and he had no problem with recruiting staff, since wartime work was scarce. To add to his staff, he usually appointed young, otherwise unknown, doctors, social scientists, economists, architects, chemists and engineers, often coming fresh to this work. Carrel, hostile as always to universities, looked outside academia for most of these appointments, complaining that he did not require 'ineffectual, tuberculous intellectuals'.[21] By avoiding links with the staff of the universities of Paris and the Pasteur Institute, who were both short of money at the time, and encouraging the view that his Fondation was a new kind of institution apart from all others, Carrel was steadily adding to his alienation from French scientific and academic circles.

---

[21] Reggiani, *God's Eugenicist* (note 15): 142.

The Structure

Carrel chaired a Board of Directors linked to associated supervisory and technical committees, and he had a secretary-general as his administrator. Below this complex structure, the Fondation had 10 departments, called *équipes* (teams), each also overseen by large committees which included advisers brought in from academia, medicine, public health and industry. Carrel came from a world of undirected research, and from the start he favoured freedom of action within these departments, with each making their own agenda within his broad directives. This also suited his dislike of meetings and routine committee work. The three larger *équipes* looked at demography (under Robert Gessain), nutrition (headed by Jean Sutter), and housing (under Jean Merlet). Any particular project was approached in a multidisciplinary way with the desired 'synthesis' of the input to follow later. The Fondation had a statistical department and used pioneering opinion polls conducted by Jean Stoetzel (1910–1987) who, when studying in America, had met George Gallup. This was the first such polling carried out by any national government.

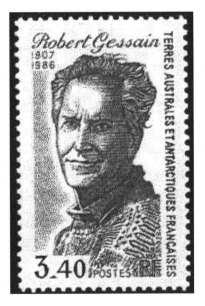

Robert Gessain, the French anthropologist, headed one of the many departments in Carrel's Fondation.

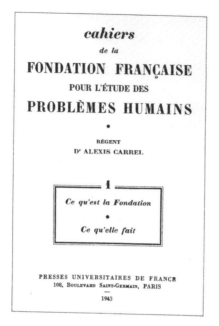

cahiers
de la

FONDATION FRANÇAISE
POUR L'ÉTUDE DES
PROBLÈMES HUMAINS
•
RÉGENT
D' ALEXIS CARREL.

— 1 —

Ce qu'est la Fondation
•
Ce qu'elle fait

PRESSES UNIVERSITAIRES DE FRANCE
108, BOULEVARD SAINT-GERMAIN, PARIS
—
1943

The Fondation's slow start meant publications appeared much later, close to the time of the Liberation.

Carrel's Fondation staff did not start to grow until mid-1942, and as a result the Fondation was fully functional for only about two years before the Allied invasion of 1944. With so many new inexperienced staff, it took time for substantial research publications to appear. Many of Carrel's more controversial beliefs and personal projects are not prominent in the reports, and his grand social engineering plan for mankind perhaps had to wait because there were other priorities at first; the early work of Fondation occupied fairly conventional areas.

The first of its major public publications (its *Cahiers*) came out in 1942, and after extensive quotation of Carrel's early writings, it outlined a much needed public health programme.[22] It dealt with the pressing problem of the war-time nutritional deprivation resulting from the combination of food shortages, severe rationing and the particularly hard winters. Epidemic diseases, like diphtheria, were increasing, and cases of tuberculosis were rising. The Fondation devised schemes to maximise

---

[22] *Cahiers de la Fondation française pour l'étude des problèmes humains*, No. 1 (1942).

agricultural food output and obtain high nutritional value from neglected and ersatz sources. Jean Sutter, later a respected figure in post-war technocratic French government, worked on advice for affordable meals, and he arranged that the nutritious 'Oslo breakfast' — milk, rye bread, margarine and goat cheese — would be available in all schools, together with advice on nutrition. To improve child health, 'puericulture' was a theme, seeking care of the child from conception onwards, through infancy and into school years. The Fondation broke new ground when it announced the first systematic national child health survey, and the government supported it by introducing a new health and dental record for each child, called the *carnet de santé*, completed steadily from birth onwards.

Pronatalism Drive

To deal with the declining population of France, Pétain had immediately brought in pronatalist policies. With a target for each family of three children, Fondation studies confirmed that family size was related to the family economy, and that lower-income families needed family allowances and 'birth bonuses' to contemplate having further children. 'Social security' was a new phrase now used at the Fondation. The Fondation's opinion polls also found that the public was sympathetic to measures to help single mothers and their children, Added to this, pioneer clinical studies on infertility were supported by the Fondation, together with efforts to discourage abortion.

In education, plans were made for girls and boys to have different school curricula to fit new national policy which saw women primarily as home-makers and mothers. Perhaps surprisingly, given Carrel's support for 'survival of the fittest', French special schooling for the handicapped school children was expanded. The French leaning towards Lamarckian genetics meant the belief that after proper nurture to overcome the defects of nature, any improvement in these children would be a permanent genetic gain.[23]

---

[23] For the French fondness for Lamarckian genetics, see William H. Schneider, *Quality and Quantity: The Quest for Biological Regeneration in Twentieth-Century France* (Cambridge: Cambridge University Press, 1990): 70, 86–8, 283–4.

Biotypes Sought

Plans at the Fondation proposed wider use of 'biotypes'. This meant study of the body using physical and psychological measurements, starting with height, weight and body shape and then adding tests of physical skill and intellectual ability. These, it was believed, would predict much about the person's capabilities in life. This approach was already favoured in Italy by Nicola Pende, the high-profile Italian demographer who Carrel had met and praised in the 1930s. Pende also hoped that a person's biotype could be modified leading towards a 'total and harmonic man' after cultivation and orientation by educators with new skills.[24] In the Childhood Development *équipe*, biotype collection commenced. The plan was for a further biotype examination on leaving school which, linked up with the *carnet*, would give advice on aptitude for types of work and even the type of sport to be favoured. This long-term plan would have intruded into life choices, with personal choice yielding to this 'science of man', but these aspirations did not emerge during the short life of the Fondation.

Race and Immigration

In the Fondation's 'science of man', biotypes were also thought to be linked to race, and the biotypes of ethnic groups in two areas in Paris were studied by the Fondation. The conclusion was that a biotype could predict failure to be assimilated. National biotypes were identified, and the Poles were said to have least favourable measurements. Robert Gessain at his *équipe* of the Biology of Hereditary, outspoken on bio-politics, claimed that

> many hundreds of thousands of racially unassimilable immigrants, I mean, for example due to Mongolised or Negrified or Judaicised racial elements, profoundly modify the hereditary heritage of the nation.[25]

---

[24] Pende's career is described in Francesco Cassata, *Building a New Man: Racial Studies in Twentieth Century Italy* (Budapest: Central European University Press, 2011). Biotypology had hints of the ancient physiognomy of the Italian Giambattista Della Porta (1535–1615) and Johann Lavater (1741–1801), and also fitted Carrel's belief in physiognomy.

[25] Drouard, *Une inconnue* (note 15): 231.

Immigrants with these biotypes were therefore seen as a genetic danger to the nation and could be identified at border immigration test stations — *centres de triage* — but firm plans for this action did not emerge during the lifetime of the Fondation.

Environment and Health

The health and environment of the workforce was a particularly French preoccupation in pre-war days, with hopes of improving industrial output and optimising performance. The Fondation continued these studies of conditions in the workplace, including the effects of temperature, light and noise, and these were to be adjusted to fit human capabilities. Health in the workforce would involve medical examinations, and occupational health schemes were introduced for all companies employing over 50 workers. There was concern about conditions of work and their effect on women's fertility. Care of disabled workers was also planned, starting with support of an industrial rehabilitation unit in the now-depleted American Hospital in Paris. After the war, these innovations were accepted internationally and were widely acknowledged by historians of occupational health as an early French initiative:

> The presiding genius behind these changes [occupational health] has been France where, starting already during the German occupation (for reasons which I still do not fully understand) a comprehensive occupational health service has been developed for industry, mines and transport. ... This French initiative has had wide outside repercussions.[26]

Better housing for moderate income families was an aspiration, and the work of the Fondation brought in architects, psychologists, physicians and sociologists to pool their understandings toward an agreed synthesis. The influential architect Le Corbusier was approached to join the planning for 'houses for living', although the Vichy government eventually turned down his designs.

---

[26] R. Murray (1963) 'Occupational health in other countries' *Transactions of the Association of Industrial Medical Officers* 13: 89–92.

Some of Carrel's personal thinking is seen in a Fondation study of *isolats*, the remote village communities admired by Carrel in *Man, the Unknown*. The findings in the report discouraged this idea of a 'noble peasant', one who had an elevated spiritual life and who retained the genetic material of an earlier, superior French race. It found instead that the inhabitants of these areas were often in poor physical and mental health, had poor hygiene and were prone to alcoholism.[27]

Eugenics Studied

Eugenic thinking and proposals for action at the Fondation were cautious. Though some French activists had earlier made strident calls for eugenics measures, the response in France was mild when compared with the events elsewhere.[28] None of the pre-war French eugenicists had any links with the Fondation. Also, in France's pro-natal drive, an increased 'quantity' of births in France was a priority, rather than seeking only 'quality' in the new French population. However, the Fondation still wished to encourage 'superior' parents to have large families, and Missenard at the Biology of Lineage *équipe* sought to locate and encourage families of 'good genetic constitution'. There was Fondation discussion on attempting to reduce the birth of those 'unfit' and withhold family allowances from the 'poorer stock'. The writings of Jean-Jacques Gillon at the Child and Adolescence *équipe* show admiration for the works of the American white racist Lothrop Stoddard, but otherwise these vague, positive and negative eugenic ideas seldom reached practical implementation via Vichy legislation.

Missenard supported discussion on sterilisation of those having and carrying hereditary disease, but the Fondation was cautious on the matter. The Catholic Church was steadfastly opposed to compulsory sterilisation,

---

[27] Reggiani, *God's Eugenicist* (note 15): 136, 144.

[28] However, the Nobel Prize-winning immunologist Charles Richet (1850–1935) rivalled the worst of eugenic thinking outside France, and favoured banishing those with tuberculosis, syphilis or alcoholism to distant French colonial islands, also proposing that the *anormoux* — newly-born defective children — be left to die; see Schneider, *Quality and Quantity* (note 23): 110.

and while other nations had gone ahead, there was no comparable action in pre-war France. The Fondation's only action in this area was to recommend a study of the sterilisation measures already in place in America, Germany and Scandinavia. Carrel's extreme views in his *Man, the Unknown*, notably suggesting use of gas chambers for the criminally insane, cannot be detected in the publications of the Fondation.

One French negative eugenic measure brought in was to prevent marriage among those with hereditary disease. A compulsory prenuptial examination was supported by the Fondation and was put in place in France by the Vichy marriage law of 16 December 1942. Germany had led the way in this in 1935, and although the eugenicist's long and seriously flawed list of supposedly genetically-controlled diseases had by now shrunk considerably, there was still a list of afflictions said to be preventable in the population by marriage control. Carrel's *L'Homme cet inconnu*, widely available in France the 1940s, still warned the young not to risk genetic danger by marrying into families with syphilis, cancer, tuberculosis, nervousness or 'weakness of mind'. This was as bad, Carrel added gratuitously, as marrying into 'les familles pauvre'.

The *Bulletin*

The Fondation's monthly *Bulletin bibliographique* was for internal use, and had a role in the Fondation's stated policy of seeking 'synthesis' of all relevant knowledge. This publication aimed at identifying contemporary published work of importance to the Fondation, and although it was international in outlook, some of the items and authors quoted highlight the chilling prejudices emerging in Vichy France.[29] The *Bulletin* included the work of racists like René Martial, who was hostile to immigration, mixed marriages and the Jews, believing that 'half-Jews are more dangerous than pure Jews'. Martial had a grant for his work from the Fondation in 1942. The *Bulletin* also noted George Montandon's antisemitic books and the articles he published in the magazine *L'Ethnicity Française*, funded by Paris's German Institute. Montandon,

---

[29] This comes from Muel-Dreyfus' account of the *Bulletin's* contents (note 10).

later murdered by the Resistance, from 1941 was head of Vichy's notorious state-supported antisemitic L'Institut d'études des questions juives et ethnoraciales.[30]

What If?

The Fondation had less than two years of full activity until it stalled after the liberation of Paris. If instead Germany had established a stable military conquest of Europe, Nazification of the entire continent under Hitler's 'Pax Teutonica' would have followed. In this united Europe, Fondation policy might then have shifted to take it along some of the paths already favoured in Germany. Carrel's second annual report hinted at such future trends and states circumspectly that 'the implementation of eugenic concepts is not for the moment in the domain of the more or less near future. Scientific research must still progress …'[31] In Germany, handicapped children had already been identified and removed from their families, and in France, the Fondation's national survey and listing of handicapped children was available.[32] Even the Fondation's population and demographic studies had potential for grim consequences. Their official data-gathering included racial classifications, and Nicola Pende and other institutes in Italy offered data on 'mixed marriages' and minorities, including Jews. This was passed to Mussolini, at his request, enabling him to use 'dictatorial demography' to act with precision against the Italian Jews.

German Contacts

The Fondation was largely ignored by the occupiers. The German presence in Paris at this time was not large, since Vichy was so cooperative that little German oversight was needed, other than by a

---

[30] Other extremist French authors featuring in the *Bulletin* included Georges Mauco, Xavier Vallat and Darquier de Pellepoix.
[31] See Schneider, *Quality and Quantity* (note 23): 279.
[32] See Suzanne E. Evans, *Hitler's Forgotten Victims: The Holocaust and the Disabled* (Stroud: Tempus, 2007).

few Gestapo agents assisted by the complicit Paris police. There were occasional visits to Paris by German academics, and in December 1941 the Nazi sympathiser Eugen Fischer, director of the Kaiser-Wilhelm-Institut of Berlin, lectured in Paris at the Maison de la Chime, an organisation sympathetic to the Nazis. In his lecture, Fischer blamed 'blacks and Jews' for the world's problems and praised the French nation as being of 'Nordic' origin. The Institut Allemand, the German propaganda organisation in Paris, hosted a lecture by Otmar von Verschuer after he succeeded Fischer. Carrel is said by some to have visited the Deutsche Institut, the German cultural centre favoured by local Paris Nazi sympathisers like Robert Brasillach, Ernest Fourneau and Jean Cocteau.

Otherwise, Carrel had little formal contact with the Germans. He had met them earlier when looking for a home for the Fondation, and later he met the local German administration to discuss the rationing policy as it impinged on the Fondation studies of nutrition. All European countries, including Germany, had rationing, but the allowances imposed on France were particularly severe, and it is said that Carrel did make a protest at a meeting with the Germans.[33] Another contact with occupiers was when Carrel appealed, with success, to obtain the release of Dr. Morris Sanders, an interned American anaesthetist, to allow him to work at the industrial injuries unit of the American Hospital. Carrel also approached the Germans in April 1944 on behalf of his lawyer friend Frederic Coudert to seek German permission for Coudert's long-established law firm to continue to operate openly in Paris. Before America declared war, Coudert's firm's letters to and from his Paris office were transmitted in the diplomatic pouch via the Paris embassy, but with America now at war with Germany, Carrel's request was refused. However, a staff member, Mr. Robinson, did keep the Coudert office functioning independently in a small way in Paris during the war.[34]

---

[33] Louis Winter (1987) 'Souvenirs de la Fondation' *Bulletin de l'Association des amis du docteur Alexis Carrel*, No. 20, 5–7.

[34] A letter from Miss Crutcher to Carrel's brother in Lyon, opened by British censors and passed to the FBI, showed that Coudert was keen to re-establish contact with

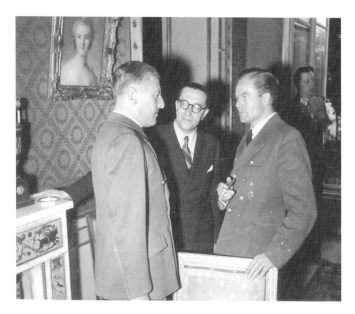

Otto Abetz (left), the Francophile German ambassador to France, entertained local intellectuals in Paris. (*Jan Doets/www.thestorycurator.net.*)

One incident played up by Carrel's detractors later was that he and Mme Carrel had attended a reception in his honour at the German Embassy. Carrel's friends later explained that he called in to the Embassy earlier on an administrative matter, but was told to come back in a few days at a specified time, and when he arrived they found that Otto Abetz, the German ambassador, had arranged a reception in his honour.[35] This was part of Abetz's drive to win over French intellectuals to the German cause, and to assist this, he had set up a collaborationist Comité France-Allemagne.[36] Carrel did not join this group, but his portrait did appear

their Mr. Robinson in their Paris office: Department of State, RG 59, box 5192, NAR (note 3).

[35] Report to European Desk SIS [Britain's intelligence gathering MI6], 11 October 1942, FBI folder 62-HQ-43687, NAR (note 3).

[36] For Abetz, see Barbara Lambauer, *Otto Abetz et les Français ou l'envers de la Collaboration* (Paris: Fayard, 2001).

in an issue of the Comité's journal *Cahiers franco-allemands* devoted to scientists. Not all of those featuring in the articles in that issue were sympathetic to the German cause.[37]

Agency Interest

Information about Carrel in France reached intelligence organisations in America. The OSS (Office of Strategic Services, later renamed the Central Intelligence Agency) was based in unaligned Switzerland, where they could watch European events. In 1942, the OSS obtained news of Carrel from 'a reliable source', namely Ralph E. Heinzen, head of the United Press agency in Vichy. He briefed Allen Dulles of the OSS that

> responsible persons in Paris scientific circles report that Doctor Alexis Carrel has become 100% Nazified in his political outlook and affirms his conviction that the United States and Great Britain were whipped from the start and that politically they are on the wrong track anyway… . His Parisian scientific fellows have no liking for him, because when he had money and power in the Rockefeller Institute, he was very crusty towards anything French … [he] is also suffering from a highly exaggerated idea of his own importance.[38]

A second American informed on Carrel in early 1942. Therese Bonney, the American photographer, who worked with the Red Cross in France, reported that

> friends of mine who have just come out of Paris say Dr. Carrel is most chummy with the Germans and reigns supreme in the former Rockefeller Foundation headquarters in Paris. The Germans are soft-soaping him it seems a great deal and he, being I fear a bit "seniley" vain, falls.[39]

---

[37] *Cahiers franco-allemands* No. 2, February 1942.

[38] OSS intelligence report, Heinzen to Allen Dulles: 'The Carrel affair' Record Group 226, box 122 folder 13, NAR (note 3); it has some factual errors.

[39] Bonney to Ruth Shipley, Head of Passports: 'Alleged German subversive activities of Dr. Alexis Carrel', Department of State, RG 59, box 5500, case number 862.20200, Carrel, Alexis, NAR (note 3).

This letter was to Mrs. Ruth Shipley, Chief of Passports at the State Department, who was making a name for herself by denying entry visas rather capriciously to large numbers of applicants when there was any suspicion that they might be a threat to America. Edgar Hoover at the FBI was also keeping a watch on his old friend Carrel, now deeming him 'of interest'. The FBI obtained news from a 'reliable confidential source', namely the Duchesse de Chaules, née Théodore Shonts, the Paris socialite. She reported that

> Doctor Carrel is considered in France to be entirely pro-German. And that the older scientists are very much against him on this account … that naturally left only the young men to be associated with him … Dr. C expressed distinctly pro-fascist ideas and spoke of Mme Carrel's interest in such ideologies, especially in de la Roque's.[40]

The U.S. Immigration Department was told to notify Hoover if Carrel arrived.[41] Another FBI contact was with Pierre du Noüy of the Pasteur Institute. When he managed to reach America in safety, as noted below, he again said that Carrel was entirely pro-German and had lost the support of the older Paris scientists.[42] However, these apparently independent assessments have close similarities, and it is possible that there was only one hostile source or perhaps collusion in France to discredit Carrel.

Later, the American agencies decided to leak the adverse intelligence to the American press and briefed against Carrel. In February 1944 Fulton Oursler, speaking on radio WOR, an outlet often used by Hoover for planted stories, said that 'unbelievable as it sounds, officials of the French Press and Information Service have assured me that Dr. Carrel has

---

[40] François de La Roque headed the right-wing semi-fascist Crois de Feu organisation until its dissolution in 1936, and then led the more moderate Parti Social Français. Mme Carrel's links with these organisation were noted in Chapter 15. The Duchesse de Chaulnes was known to Carrel in New York and Paris, and also to the FBI's J. Edgar Hoover.
[41] Hoover to Donovan 'The Carrel Affair' (note 38).
[42] Crutcher to Coudert, 6 October 1942, RU 650-5 Malinin Collection, box 3 folder 17, RUA RAC (note 14).

become an ardent pro-Nazi'.[43] Carrel was in some danger. He was still a French citizen, and his two-month re-entry visa had expired. If he wished to return, the American immigration authorities could have made things difficult for him.

Americans in Paris

Many Americans had left in good time before America declared war, but a few stayed on and were interned or had to report to the police and Gestapo weekly. These measures did not affect Carrel as a French citizen.[44] The American Library in Paris kept going bravely, overseen by the wealthy Ohio-born Comtesse de Chambrun, protected through her son's marriage to a daughter of Pierre Laval, Vichy's prime minister. The American Hospital also survived and continued its role in giving free care to Americans. Carrel, never gregarious, did not join up with any of the remaining Americans. His old friend du Noüy was still working as a scientist in Paris, but as a Jew, he was in danger and asked Carrel for help in obtaining a post in America. Carrel declined to assist, and cut off contact with the couple.[45] The du Noüys, aided by false medical documents, managed to get to Vichy, then obtained American visas, and escaped.

The Carrels had a new Paris apartment at 56 Avenue de Bretteville, passed to Mme Carrel from a relative. Paris life had largely resumed. The buildings were unaffected, but Nazi symbols, flags and drapes were everywhere, and the streets were empty of cars since petrol was scarce. There was an evening curfew. The German army was well-behaved in public, but the Gestapo was ever-present. The Carrel's had a garden and a greenhouse, and Mme Carrel still produced her herbs and herbal medicines. As the war continued, there were food shortages, particularly in the cities, but the Carrels may have had an extra supply from their garden and their island farm, which still sold its produce. The black

---

[43] 'Gone to Devil' remark was broadcast by Fulton Oursler in his '*The People's Reporter*' 24 February 1944.

[44] See David Pryce-Jones, *Paris in the Third Reich* (London: Collins, 1981).

[45] Mary Lecomte du Noüy, *The Road to "Human Destiny": A Life of Pierre Lecomte du Noüy* (New York: Longmans, Green and Co., 1955): 252–8.

market could supply many things, but coal was in short supply, being diverted to Germany; Carrel's supporters later said that he was offered extra fuel by Germans, but declined.[46] They attended séances together, and Carrel still grudgingly approved of Mlle Laplace, the clairvoyant friend of his wife. Later, she rightly predicted that the Germans would lose the battle at Stalingrad but spoiled her record by confidently asserting that an Allied invasion and attempt to liberate France would be repulsed by the Germans.

As ever, Carrel had no time for his fellow citizens. He wrote to his nephew that 'the great mass of government officials is composed of cowards, liars, thieves, imbeciles and villains'. He took a sour view of the French youth, 'the young Frenchman of the defeat; rude, slovenly, slouching about.' This misanthropy was extended ungallantly to the local Paris girls: 'The young women are surprising by their ugliness, the idiotic expression on their faces and their vulgarity.'[47]

The Resistance

Carrel took no part in the Resistance. Others in Paris did so, including some staff at the Fondation. One American who assisted was Sumner Jackson, the surgeon at the American Hospital, who gave false certificates of illness to Jews and sheltered shot-down Allied airmen as patients. When they recovered, he encouraged them to slip away undetected in civilian clothes to reach the escape routes to Spain. Braver still were those in France who guided British Special Operations Executive (SOE) agents in and out of France to organise sabotage. Carrel's former colleague du Noüy and his wife had occasionally assisted in this way and passed on useful information.[48]

---

[46] SIS Report (note 35).

[47] Carrel to Gigou, Malinin Collection of the Papers of Alexis Carrel and Charles Lindbergh, box 14 folder 10, FA 208, RUA RAC.

[48] Du Noüy gave information to the French entomologist Alfred Balachowsky, who assisted the British SOE spy network called Prosper (later called 'Physician' in his honour). Balachowsky was betrayed, arrested and moved to Buchenwald, but survived.

The strength of Carrel's sympathies with Germany may be unclear, but what is clear is that he did not assist the Allies in any way, even on the eve of the Liberation. In particular, he disapproved of the exiled de Gaulle's plans to rescue France.

Carrel's Attitude

Carrel's situation was a strange one. But he stuck to his new post at the Fondation, though, as ever, grumbling in his family letters about France and French politicians, but not about the Germans. Vichy seemed pleased with his contributions. It is said Carrel was approached about taking other posts, but declined to be minister of public health or head of the French Red Cross. He made no moves to return to live in America, and never wavered in his view that France should be left alone and not rescued. A friend recalled Carrel's thinking in the early stage of the Occupation. Carrel told him that:

> Travel would soon be quite free again, as the fall of Britain would shortly end the war. Apparently convinced that America was on the verge of revolution and would remain neutral, he [Carrel] argued that the only possible course was to accept the inevitable and work with the Germans for the benefit of France.[49]

Even in late 1943, he wrote to his nephew that 'only the Germans were capable of imposing order in Europe and particularly in France'.[50] Carrel concluded at this time that Europe was now unified and the widespread defects of the West could be dealt with since

> times have changed. ... It is no longer a question of debating or fighting against people belonged to the same culture. It is the entire Western civilisation that is involved and not only the interest of such and such a nation.[51]

---

[49] Du Noüy, *Road* (note 45): 253.
[50] Carrel to Gigou, 14 September 1943, Malinin Collection, box 14 folder 9, RUA RAC (note 14).
[51] Carrel to Gigou, 7 May 1943, Malinin Collection, box 14 folder 9, RUA RAC (note 14).

Carrel, fond of seeking the moral high ground, might at least have deplored the intolerance and fanaticism around him but he did not. In November 1941, five French left-wing scientists were arrested, then questioned, and two were given prison sentences. Antisemitism pervaded the newspapers and radio. Vichy needed little encouragement from the Germans, and often went willingly well beyond the occupier's wishes in their own actions against the Jews. In Paris, Jews were identified with a badge and were banned from public places, restaurants and cinemas. One effect obvious to Carrel was the virtual exclusion of Jews from medical practice and scientific work.[52] In particular, Carrel knew through his Lyon family links of the details of the arrest and deportation of the city's Jews. In Paris from summer 1941, Jews from France and Poland were held at the Drancy internment camp in the northeast suburbs before transportation to their death in Germany. A few escaped, and some who were ill were released and told Paris about the camp's role. In July 1942 the Paris police rounded up 12,884 Parisian Jews and held them in the Vél d'Hiv sports ground, close to Carrel's Fondation headquarters, before moving them later to Drancy and Auschwitz. This complex operation lasting five days could not be concealed, and crowds gathered outside the stadium — all Paris knew of this outrage.

Paris Writings

His *L'Homme cet inconnu* still sold well during the Occupation at about 35,000 copies annually. Even so, Carrel wanted to make it more widely available, since he felt the book explained the Vichy philosophy. He wrote to his publisher:

> I had foreseen and indicated the path to follow. It is indispensable that my book be accessible to all those who in France are capable of understanding, reflecting and acting.[53]

---

[52] Application of Vichy's antisemitic laws to the doctors was accepted by Carrel's old friend René Leriche, who was from 1940–1942 president of the Conseil supérieur de l'orde national des médecins, the doctor's representative body.
[53] The full letter is in Drouard, *Une inconnue* (note 15).

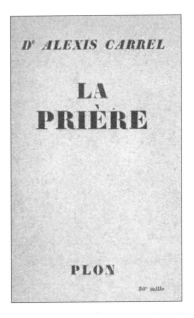

Carrel's book *La Prière* was published during the German Occupation.

Vichy put his book on the nation's list of required reading. In this convergence of the views of Carrel and Pétain, it was said that Carrel was 'the scientific double of Pétain'.[54]

To add to this, *La prière*, a book on prayer, based on his *Reader's Digest* article, was published in May 1944 and sold out quickly. In it he urged that special areas for prayer — 'islands of peace' — be set aside at work. As ever, he attributed cures at Lourdes to prayer and concluded that the decline in miracles at the shrine as the century progressed was because prayer was not as common as before, and that the pilgrims were now 'merely tourists' and did not pray correctly. Still in *Readers' Digest* inspirational mode he advised that:

> Prayer lets man reach God, restores mental equilibrium, patience, assists sleep and man begins to change from selfishness, pride, greed, and intemperance and gives up golf on Saturdays and Sundays and gives time to the family.

---

[54] See Lindenberg, *Les années* (note 13): 177–94.

Carrel continued work on his *Réflexions sur la conduit de la vie*, a sequel to *Man, the Unknown*, although it did not appear until much later. Fond of lecturing the world on how to behave, yet ignoring the wickedness on his doorstep in Paris, he could, without any insight, write:

> Most people do not distinguish clearly between good and evil. ... Just as the tradesman keeps his account books and the scientist his experimental notebook, so every single individual ought to register every day the good and evil for which he has been responsible. ... Christian morality is incomparably more powerful than lay morality ... tolerance of evil is a dangerous error. ... any act or thought which tends to diminish, disintegrate or destroy life is a sin.[55]

In Paris, he had to curb his usual attachment to publicity, and as a government employee in an occupied country he lacked the usual freedoms. In France, newspapers were few and were necessarily pro-German, with closely controlled content. He knew the editor of *Le Matin*, later imprisoned after the Liberation. A rare interview with Carrel did appear in the notably anti-American weekly journal *Gringoire*, in which he criticised American public health policy; this disloyalty was promptly relayed to American intelligence sources. An Argentinean fascist journal *La Fronda* carried an article by Carrel in 1943 — possibly an old reworked one, and this was again dutifully reported to J. Edgar Hoover at the FBI.[56]

Another frustration was that Carrel had no facilities for experimental work, and as a result had no 'show and tell' exhibits for visitors. Perhaps missing this traditional work, in March 1943, he used the property at Vulaines-sur-Seine near Fontainebleau for a new project 'to raise dogs and do experiments on fertilisers ... Elizabeth de la Motte [a cousin of Mme

---

[55] Alexis Carrel, *Réflexions sur la conduit de la vie* (Paris: Ploné, 1950), translated as *Reflections on Life* (London: Hamish Hamilton, 1952): passim. The book remained unpublished until his wife arranged for it to appear posthumously in 1950.

[56] Carrel also contributed a short orthodox article on 'Le rôle future de la médecine' in *Médecine officielle et médecines hérétiques*, a multi-author book devoted to holistic medicine eventually published in 1945.

Carrel] is superintendent'.[57] This was a revival of his old interest in the in-breeding of dogs, doubtless again hoping to find Mousery-type links between nutrition, physique and intelligence. By 1944 there were Fondation moves towards conventional biochemistry and biophysics studies, with lavish expenditure on purchase of two ultracentrifuges and an electron microscope to be used at the Fondation's property in the Avenue des Villars.

There were annual reports, but the first bulky *Cahier* with its report on public health had been slow to appear, and the next two emerged only after the Liberation — No. 2 in October 1944, No. 3 in March 1945 and No. 4 in November 1945.

New York

Carrel's office at the Institute in New York, though empty, was initially preserved, but with his prolonged absence and lack of contact, his equipment was taken away by others, and eventually a Dr. Horsfall took over his office in late 1942. After a decent interval, in Carrel's continued absence, Miss Crutcher, his secretary was moved to work in another unit, but she wrote that 'I've not been so bored in 24 years'. In a rare letter from Carrel that did get through to her, he asked Herbert Gasser, the director, to send him some recent articles on nutrition. But Gasser declined to do so, much to Miss Crutcher's annoyance, on the grounds that America was now at war with Germany. One other letter did say that he 'hoped to be in New York in May 1942 to attend 4th Race Betterment Conference of Dr. Davenport'. But the conference organised by this prominent eugenicist was never held, since growing anti-German sentiment in America and a new awareness of Nazi racial policy meant that the American eugenicists, though not completely discredited, were now silent.

Miss Crutcher nobly continued to look after Carrel's interests. She dealt with difficulties at his bank, since, as a Frenchman, his assets were

---

[57] Alexis Carrel Papers, box 38 folder 46, Georgetown University Library, Booth Family Center for Special Collections, Washington DC (GULBFC).

frozen. His penthouse flat at 56 East 89th was sublet, and she arranged for the cleaner to be paid. His clothes had to be preserved from deterioration, and she insured his car, paid his bills and kept up his regular subscriptions. Considerable royalties continued to come in from his writings, as did his generous pension, and she drew up his tax return. She kept up links with Lindbergh, Newton and Coudert, and at all times hoped he would return.

Charles Lindbergh's star had faded. At a rally at Des Moines in September 1941, he again said that dark forces were behind American support for war against Germany, and listed them as 'the Roosevelt administration, the British, the Jews, capitalists, anglophiles and intellectuals'. But he particularly emphasised the Jews, saying that 'the greatest danger to this country lies in their [Jewish] large ownership and influence in our motion pictures, our press, our radio, and our government'.[58] Religious leaders, newspapers and the administration demanded retractions. And as he was now a liability to the America First movement, they hesitated to use his further support. But shortly after, on 7 December 1941, the unexpected Pearl Harbor attack by the Japanese meant that American opposition to joining the War vanished. Lindbergh asked to rejoin the military, but was snubbed and, only slowly forgiven, was later allowed to restart in a lowly military capacity in the Pacific campaign.

Coudert and Vichy

In New York, Carrel's lawyer friend Frederic Coudert was still keen to have news from France. A letter from Carrel did get through to Coudert, written during a visit to Vichy in July 1942, and in the necessarily bland

---

[58] Jewish ownership was prominent only in the American motion picture business, but as their pre-war profits came largely from Europe, including Germany and Italy, these owners carefully kept out of European politics. Lindbergh was correct in his allegation that there was a British covert operation to bring America into the war, as was revealed much later; see Nicholas Cull, *Selling War: The British Propaganda Campaign Against American Neutrality in World War II* (Oxford: Oxford University Press, 1995).

account of his activities he said that he was trying to get on with his new book, but was having difficulty. He added that he missed Coudert's friendship, and that 'their conversations are necessary to elaborate these ideas'. Coudert's international law firm, with its long-standing links with France, obtained international legal work in these fraught times, obtaining briefs from the French munitions company Schneider et Cie based near Vichy, now making armaments for the Germans. He was now also acting for the Vichy government by helping with the purchase of their New York consulate, and when he acted for them in a major dispute, his name would be forever linked with the Vichy era. Before the German invasion, Belgium had shifted their gold reserves to apparent safety in France, but after the Occupation, this Belgian gold was now in the hands of Vichy and the Nazis. The Belgian government in exile in London sued the Bank of France in a New York court for the return of their $228 million bullion, but Coudert, retained by the Vichy government, argued successfully that Vichy need not hand it back to the Free Belgians.[59]

Coudert wrote letters to the New York press asking for an 'understanding' not only of Vichy but also of the Franco regime in Spain. A cartoon in the American socialist magazine *The New Masses* in September 1942 showed Coudert in bed with Pétain, surrounded by Nazi symbols.[60] Coudert's pro-Vichy stance also gave him a local problem when running for re-election in October 1942 as a Republican senator in the New York state legislature. His Democrat opponent smeared him as a fascist, but Coudert survived, with a reduced majority.[61] Coudert was increasingly prominent in local New York politics and co-chaired New York's notorious Joint Legislative Committee to Investigate the Educational System, which

---

[59] Coudert had been an attorney for the Russian Tzar, and also acted for exiled Tzarist clients. The Coudert firm used the services of Boris Brasol, the Tzarist supporter who claimed to have translated the anti-Semitic forgeries *The Protocols of the Learned Elders of Zion*. Brasol sold them to Henry Ford, who notoriously published them in his *Dearborn Independent* newspaper.

[60] Barbara Giles, 'Coudert — Vichy lawyer' *The New Masses*, September 1, 1942: 13–15.

[61] *NYT,* 29 September, October 20, 21, 24, 30 and November 2 1942.

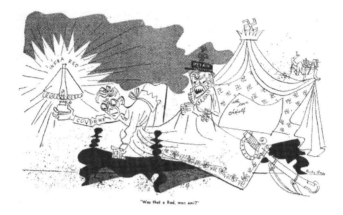

In New York, the leftist magazine *New Masses* satirised Frederic Coudert for his pro-Vichy sympathies.

sought out alleged communist sympathisers, hearings later regarded as a 'dress rehearsal for McCarthyism'.[62]

Tide Turns

The first opposition to the Vichy government came from small left-wing or communist groups. But the French citizens soon started withdrawing support, since Pétain's national revolution had not been delivered and instead there was rationing, lack of fuel and shortages added to poverty, disease and lawlessness. Vichy policy was seriously discredited when in February 1943 they agreed to move young Frenchmen to work in Germany, and the Resistance started to grow in strength and confidence. In Paris, Pasteur Valléry-Radot, head of the Pasteur Institute, and the paediatrician Robert Debré, the sole Jewish staff member remaining at Paris's Rothschild Hospital, gave their support to the Resistance and set up the Comité médical de la Résistance in Paris, and the Groupe médical de secours, which later joined the military arm of the Resistance.[63] Debré

---

[62] For rather bland biographies of Coudert, see Paula Murray Coudert, Paul B. Jones and Lawrence Klepp, *Frederic R. Coudert Jr: A Biography* (1985) and Virginia K. Veenswijk, *Coudert Brothers: A Legacy in Law* (New York: Truman Tally Books, 1994).
[63] F. Goursolas (2005) 'Le «Groupe Médical de Secours» de Pierre Deniker' *Histoire des sciences médicals* 39: 373–84.

and Vallery-Radot were denounced but, going underground, eluded arrest and survived, and were honoured later for their actions.[64] The French citizens now increasingly looked towards Britain and America for assistance, and the first bombing of Paris in March 1942, denounced by Pétain, gave hope to the city.

His Illness

Carrel had a heart attack in August 1943 and was off work for some months. There had been tensions at the Fondation after Carrel had fallen out with his chief administrator François Perroux, who criticised Carrel's loose and devolved administrative approach, which gave rather vague general remits to the departments. In Carrel's absence while ill, Perroux was in charge and complained to Vichy about the 'anarchic and incoherent' studies of the Fondation and the failure of the much-heralded 'synthesis'. He added that there had been waste of money. Perroux took his chance and appointed some talented academics; he also tried to remove Carrel's wife as a manager of the Fondation's out-station at Vulaines-sur-Seine. When Carrel returned to work in December 1943, restored to health, he managed to move Perroux out, and undid the changes. Perroux obtained a university appointment and responded with an attack on Carrel and his book *L'Homme cet inconnu*, criticising its 'massive and unproven assertions made in the name of science'. Some staff resigned in sympathy with Perroux, but Carrel had survived and was pleased at the 'cleansing'.

Liberation Nears

By the spring of 1943, the Allied armies had success against the Germans in North Africa and were poised to enter Europe. The Allies started daylight raids on Paris factories (which also destroyed much of the

---

[64] Vallery-Radot and Debré were denounced along with Frédéric Joliot-Curie and his wife Irène, joint recipients of the Nobel Prize for Chemistry in 1935. Joliot-Curie evaded the Gestapo and, living in Paris under a false name, organised the production and storage of explosives at his laboratory at the Collège de France.

Fondation's archives). The population welcomed these signs that France might be liberated, but Carrel was not pleased. What did please him was that during a visit by Pétain in April 1944, he was well treated by the Paris crowds. Carrel commented: 'What an unexpected blow to de Gaulle and the traitor Giraud.'[65] Giraud was then the co-president with de Gaulle as leaders of the Free French outside France.[66] At a lunch about this time he spoke out against de Gaulle, and his lunch companions advised him to be more diplomatic, since de Gaulle might soon be in charge.[67]

Carrel gave no hint that he had realised the personal danger he was in. He was a prominent appointee of the increasingly shaky Vichy government, and he had made enemies in Parisian academic and scientific circles, some of whom were now prominent in the Resistance. If France was liberated, Carrel's position was untenable. If he wished to leave, difficulties in getting back to America were likely, since he was regarded there with suspicion. Carrel's letters to his nephew had an increasingly resigned tone. On 19 April 1944 he wrote 'we await at Paris whatever is fated to come. We scarcely 'see' the future. The future will be what it will be ... people are leaving Paris as quickly as possible'. He had a second heart attack in August, five days before the liberation of Paris.

The Liberation

As Allied troops neared Paris, Frederic Coudert in New York knew that Carrel's position in Paris was perilous and made attempts to have him rescued and protected by the agents who would arrive with Eisenhower's troops. Coudert's plea was made to Adolf A Berle, Assistant Secretary of State, a confidante of Roosevelt. But Coudert had no response — Berle would have seen all the FBI and OSS reports.

Prior to the arrival of the liberating troops in Paris, from 15 August the city was first deliberately paralysed by strikes organised by the

---

[65] Carrel to Gigou, April 1944, Malinin Collection, FA 208, box 14 folder 6, RUA RAC (note 14).

[66] Because Giraud had served at Vichy for a while, then changed sides, Giraud, in Carrel's view, was a traitor.

[67] Missenard, *La vérité* (note 13): 404.

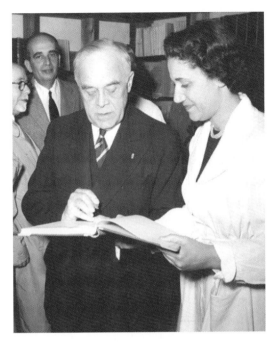

After the Liberation of Paris in 1944, the new minister of health, the physician Pasteur Vallery-Radot, dismissed Carrel from his post at the Fondation. (*Courtesy of the Helenic Pasteur Institute.*)

Resistance and then the citizens rose up against the Germans. On 23 August, two days before the triumphal arrival of French troops in Paris, the Resistance made appointments to a Provisional French Government. Pasteur Vallery-Radot of the Pasteur Institute was appointed as head of Public Health, and Vallery-Radot's first action in office was to take action against Carrel, suspending him and announcing that the new ministry 'would modify deeply' the work of the Fondation, which was 'notorious for its actions detrimental to the nation'. Old scores were being settled.

Two days later, on 25 August, de Gaulle arrived in triumph and 13 days later, Vallery-Radot was confirmed in his government post under de Gaulle's new administration. United Press Agency staff also got through and, settling in Paris, their office gave out the first non-censored news from the city since 1939. They carried a story that Carrel had been arrested and a rumour that he was on the Resistance list for a death sentence. A better authenticated story later was that he had been blacklisted by the French National Committee of Writers as one of 'those whose attitude or writings under the Occupation brought moral or material help to the oppressors'.[68] In America, Coudert sought news of Carrel from the Free French representatives in Washington, who confirmed that Carrel was 'possibly under some form of arrest' but assured Coudert that they would urge de Gaulle to ensure Carrel's safety.[69] In the chaotic period which followed, Vallery-Radot let it be known that there was evidence against Carrel as a collaborator.[70] Carrel, although not well, managed to get a defiant response back to the press:

> I was living in tranquillity in the United States when I decided that France needed me. I came and founded my institute for the children of my country and put my theories into practice. I had one aim and I reached it. I am convinced I did nothing against France.

The first of the most notorious collaborators had already been executed, and this gave further concern among Carrel's friends. Some contacted the Rockefeller Institute in New York and made offers of help to Miss Crutcher. Simon Flexner wrote to Henry Stimson, secretary for war, a member of the Century Association, about fellow member Carrel's plight. Flexner also offered to remonstrate with Vallery-Radot, but nothing came of it.

Meanwhile, Vallery-Radot's ministry said of Carrel that it had discovered 'important new evidence against him'. This may have been a further complaint to the government from François Perroux, still smarting and hostile after his removal from the Fondation, saying that little of value had come from the Fondation and there had been financial irregularities. Perroux also improbably accused Carrel and his deputies of being part of the shadowy rightist Synarchy conspiracy preparing for a

---

[68] *New York Herald Tribune*, 5 November 1944.
[69] Shay to Coudert, Malinin Collection FA 208, box 5 folder1, RUA RAC (note 14).
[70] 'French Health Chief Dismisses Dr Carrel' *NYT*, 29 August and 1 September 1944.

coup.[71] There was further discomfiture for Carrel next month when Vallery-Radot, now a French hero, was elected on 12 October as one of the 'Immortels' of the French Academy, the very honour Carrel had always desired.[72] In the continuing turmoil, little more emerged, but Carrel was still unwell and at home. On 5 November 1944 a radio broadcast said he had fled from Paris and was being searched for by the police as a collaborator.

This claim was quickly withdrawn by the station: Carrel had died that day.

---

[71] Drouard, *Une inconnue* (note 15): 219. Historians have doubted that the Synarchy group existed, classing it with other conspiracy theories.

[72] Three appointments were the first since 1940, and Louis de Broglie, André Siegfried and Vallery-Radot were honoured at this séance of the Academy.

CHAPTER NINETEEN

Aftermath

There was a short burial service in Paris, to which the British government sent a representative, but there was none from France or America. Carrel's body was later re-buried on his island home in Brittany. Back in New York, the anaesthetist Paluel Flagg held a memorial mass for Carrel on 11 November 1944 at his own chapel. Two days after Carrel's death, the French government told the Marquis Guy de St. Perier, as Carrel's 'Chef du Cabinet' and his chief administrator, to make a report on Carrel's wartime activity to assist with the investigation of the accusations of collaboration. Perier's two-page report listed only four contacts with the Germans, beyond those necessary in his work. These were the incident when Carrel had attended a reception in his honour at the German embassy; when he asked for the release of Morris Sanders the American anaesthetist; when he sought permission for his friend Coudert's legal firm to operate in Paris; that he had contacted the Germans to seek mercy for Yves Tolédano, the son of a Fondation staff member, convicted of working for the Resistance.[1] Shortly after the Liberation, Charles Lindbergh, sent to assess the state of German aviation and rocketry, arrived in Paris with the incoming American army. Keen to get information on Carrel's work in Paris, with the help of the lawyer Robinson, Coudert's man in Paris, Lindbergh was shown Perier's list of the complaints against Carrel. He noted that they seemed 'trivial'. An FBI agent also quickly obtained a copy of this report and it was passed on to J. Edgar Hoover in Washington.

---

[1] Tolédano's own famous account of his escape does not mention assistance by Carrel; see Marc Tolédano, *The Franciscan of Bourges* (London: George G. Harrap, 1970).

Hoover soon made the favourable assessment that Carrel was not involved in political matters and that German propaganda was instead behind the stories hostile to his reputation. Hoover reported his conclusions to the State Department.

Another American arriving in Paris was 'Tibby' Mott, a retired American military man, who had managed to visit Carrel earlier that year, and he wrote to Coudert on 10 December:

> I was deeply affected by the details of Carrel's death. He died really of a broken heart; he could not stand the accusations made against him and his sensitive soul broke under them. Alas, these purifiers have done to him what some others did to Einstein and to Mann. But he saved for us the home of the Rockefeller and Carnegie Institutes here and his work *must* go on.[2]

Mott also urged the American government not to support de Gaulle, but instead to reinvigorate Vichy rule.

Obituaries

Normally, reflective obituaries suitable for a Nobel Prize-winning scientist would have appeared, but the times were not normal. Carrel's move to Paris and his work in Occupied France had changed everything, and his reputation was clouded by the taint of collaboration. Assessing his career at this time was a sensitive and difficult matter and the few notices of his death were cautious. The *New York Times*, which had followed his career so closely, had only a short obituary, and the *Journal of the American Medical Association* and the *British Medical Journal* carried guarded accounts of his career.

---

[2] Mott to Coudert, 23 May 1944, FA 208, Malinin Collection of the Papers of Alexis Carrel and Charles Lindbergh, box 5 folder 17, Rockefeller University Archives, Rockefeller Archives Centre. Mott (1865–1952), a retired military man, married a Frenchwoman after WWI, and they settled in Biarritz from where he ran the American Fund for the French Wounded, and later the American Battle Monuments Commission. In WWII he was interned, but released, and was one of Carrel's rare visitors in early 1944.

There had however been some interesting comment on his career in America just after his dismissal and shortly before his death. The *Washington Post* offered a perceptive assessment. It asked for

judgment to be reserved until less feverish times. Dr. Carrel's politics have very little to do with his scientific attainments, and we should be careful not to confuse one with the other. Some of his colleagues, no doubt, considered him more imaginative than a scientist ought to be. ... The reputation he had gained before and during the war of 1914–18 gave him almost the status of a minor divinity in the eyes of those for whom science, and particularly medical science, had become a substitute for religion. Thus his frequent and oracular pronouncements on such questions of philosophy, politics, love, and what-not were now listened to with as much reverence as his views on surgery, medicine or biology. And when, about a decade ago, he proposed, as a cure for the social evils of the time and as a shortcut to Utopia, a benevolent dictatorship of surgeons and medicos, his book was received here with a serious enthusiasm.

As we can now perceive, the fact that Dr. Carrel was a great scientist did not prevent him from being pretty muddle-headed on matters of history and politics. This truth, however, also works in reverse and it would be stupid to suppose that because Dr. Carrel was politically myopic, he was never a really great scientist.[3]

The *Post's* journalist clearly had insider help, possibly from the distinguished tissue culture scientists at Baltimore nearby, who had watched Carrel's unusual career from the earliest days. Another thoughtful and charitable verdict came 10 days after his death:

The scientific borderland where Carrel toiled is a happy hunting ground for certain types of ideological schemers. The effects of such association appears to have left him in an exposed and somewhat politically helpless condition at the liberation of France.[4]

---

[3] *The Washington Post*, 14 September 1944.
[4] John La Farge in *America*, 18 November 1944.

Collaboration Allegations

In the disorderly times shortly after the Liberation, the first purge — the *épuration sauvage* — featured revenge, rough justice and summary executions. For those escaping the vengeance of the mob, 86,000 were interned, some for their own safety, and many were released later to await trial. 125,000 cases of collaboration were considered in the courts and tribunals in the next year, and 6,700 death sentences were passed.

The label 'collaboration' which Carrel attracted, then and since, has to be looked at carefully, since allegations of collaboration covered a range of activities. The worst French offenders were those who carried out repugnant acts against their own countrymen, with little prompting by the German occupying power. At the other end of the spectrum were those who accepted senior government roles under the Vichy rule, but simply did their job. Carrel's possible offences were somewhere between these extremes. There were also other niche categories of collaboration, and one of these was the actions of academics that had 'disgraced the French intelligence'. Another category included those whose writings or broadcasts assisted the Nazis, and when the more orderly *épuration légale* started in October, those on trial included two writers: Albert Lejeune, the publisher, and journalist Robert Brasillach were quickly found guilty and executed. Others facing less serious charges included André Missenard, one of Carrel's vice-regents at the Fondation, but he was cleared by a tribunal.

No immediate moves were made to review Carrel's Paris activities. There was a story that a list of charges had been drawn up, but no details have survived; his friends said later that these allegations were withdrawn. If there was a case against him, it would not be a priority. The courts and tribunals were busy: moreover, Carrel was dead.

His Actions

Reviewing his possible collaborationist activity, Carrel was certainly prominent in heading a large government department in Paris under the Vichy government. But there was no obvious German input to policy, and he had no regular day-to-day contact with the Germans; any meetings were infrequent and seem only of administrative necessity. He had to ask the local German-controlled administration for permission to take over the various Paris buildings for his Fondation, and he had other meetings with the Germans to discuss rationing. Carrel did attend, perhaps unwittingly, a reception at the German embassy in his honour, arranged by an ambassador who was courting support from French intellectuals. But these contacts seem minimal, and in the fraught environment in which Carrel functioned, allegations of significant, culpable, regular collaboration with the Germans occupiers are not proven. Nor was it Carrel's style — he had never sought close political or organisational allegiances, believing at all times in his own agenda.

Many reminisced after the War about the activities of the Fondation and many commented on Carrel's role. But no one made detailed accusations of collaboration. Instead, the verdict of those who knew him, including some who were in the Resistance, was that there was political naiveté. Those who earlier had portrayed him to American intelligence as a Nazi did not repeat it, and were silent after the War. One of the most impressive witnesses is Morris Sanders, the Red Cross Hospital anaesthetist liberated from internment by Carrel, who also had part-time work at the Fondation. After Carrel's death, in a long letter to his sister, Sanders lists Carrel's faults, mentioning his dogmatic indiscretions and fascist-like manner, but he clears Carrel of collaboration, pointing out that if he had collaborated, he would have received favours, and the Germans would have promptly and enthusiastically used Carrel's name.[5]

Nor is there evidence in the work of his Fondation of any significant influence from Germany's increasingly Nazified academic world. Carrel had not damaged France in any obvious way, other than by Vallery-Radot's initial accusation that Carrel had failed to support the other French institutions, notably the universities and the Pasteur Institute.

---

[5] Morris letter to 'Sis', James D. and Eleanor F. Newton Papers, box 6 'Letters' folder, MS 1592, Yale University Library Manuscripts and Archives (YULMA).

What If?

If Carrel had survived, without legal action taken against him, his new personal problems would have been acute. He was disliked by the French academic world and his chances of election to the Académie were now gone. The new 'immortels' soon elected to the Académie included Vallery-Radot and two others who had been in the Resistance, and they took decisive action against the members deemed to have collaborated during the war. Pétain, later sentenced to death, but reprieved, an Académie member since 1929, was expelled together with three others.[6] If Carrel had survived and decided to return to America, judging that the new environment was hostile, he might have encountered difficulties. Although his old admirer Hoover now felt that Carrel was of 'no interest' to the FBI, the other agencies had reasonably doubted his patriotism and obtaining his usual re-entry visa for a return might have been a problem.

Carrel's Estate

After his death, Mme Carrel immediately travelled to New York. Frederic Coudert, Carrel's friend and lawyer, dealt with his estate and, in his will in America, he left $76,974. Although this seems a substantial sum, it is hardly more than the royalties which had mounted up in New York during the War, plus his unused Institute pension of $10,000 per annum. It is likely that he had moved funds to Mme Carrel in France, and doubtless Coudert had advised him well on his finances. His French estate amounted to 2.5 million francs, including a 2 million valuation of his island.[7]

In dealing with Carrel's death and estate, Mme Carrel also had then, and for years after, the devoted assistance of Charles Lindbergh. He helped her by clearing the New York apartment, and characteristically

---

[6]The expelled Académie members included Abel Bonnard, poet, novelist and Vichy minister of education, who fled to Spain, gaining political asylum from Franco, but was condemned to death in absentia. Also expelled were Abel Hermant, who contributed to the pro-Nazi daily *Les Nouveaux Temps*, and Charles Maurras of the fascist party Action Française.

[7]Carrel's two estates would have been worth about $1 million in 2016.

made a careful inventory of its contents, including a catalogue of Carrel's books. Carrel's friends discussed his life and works regularly and they kept in touch with Miss Crutcher. Coudert, Bakhmeteff and Lindbergh agreed to start raising a fund for a memorial — 'The Alexis Carrel Foundation Inc.' — to support study of his ideas. Fund-raising proved to be slow and instead the money was eventually handed over to assist with creating a memorial on his island, a project organised by his former Fondation administrator Marquis Guy de St. Perier, Mme Carrel's nephew. He had hoped that Mme Carrel would gift her husband's continuing royalties to the project, but she did not and the project evolved later into the 'Fondation Alexis Carrel (Saint-Gildas)', which only lasted until 1956.

Carrel's personal papers at the Rockefeller Institute were removed by Lindbergh, and Mme Carrel, seeking a home for the substantial archive, decided that the papers should go to a Jesuit organisation, because of Carrel's long association with that religious order. She and Lindbergh contacted Georgetown University in Washington, and although this Jesuit university did not have a formal archive at that time, it accepted this gift. This collection has survived administrative and storage crises, and with the repeated reappraisals of Carrel's career, this important holding has been much studied.

Mme Carrel soon returned to France, and lived in France for five more years. The houses on both islands were reasonably preserved during the Occupation. Mme Carrel assisted with setting up a religious community near her island, and in the next few years, she successfully arranged for the appearance of Carrel's unpublished works. The first was *Le voyage de Lourdes* of 1949, a novel written much earlier, possibly in his Lyon days, based on his experience at Lourdes. Lindbergh loyally wrote an Introduction, and it sold well. Carrel's *Réflexions sur la conduit de la vie*, the delayed sequel to *Man, the Unknown*, followed in 1950, and Mme Carrel added an Introduction. It sold well in France, but was not a success elsewhere.[8] Publication of his introspective diaries *Jour après jour: journal, 1893–1944* came later, in 1956.

---

[8] Carrel's book *Réflexions sur la conduite de la vie* (Paris: Librarire Plon, 1950) was reprinted six times in France up to 1991, occasionally combined with *La Prière*. The

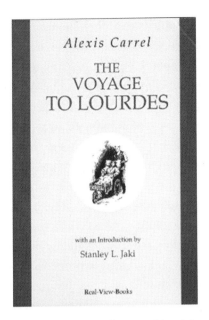

Carrel's novel was published posthumously in 1950, with an Introduction by the prominent Catholic academic Father Stanley Jaki.

In the early 1950s, Mme Carrel moved to Argentina, where much earlier her son had settled to join his father-in-law's cattle ranch. There, she took a low-key role in right-wing politics and worked to establish Carrel's reputation, emphasising his role as a Catholic thinker.[9]

Immediate Reputation

After his death, although Carrel had escaped formal allegations of collaboration, his name came up at the Nazi War Crimes Trials in 1946. One of Hitler's doctors, Karl Brandt, who headed the Nazi euthanasia program from 1939 onwards and was involved in the crude, culpable human medical experiments on prisoners, appeared at the Nuremberg

English translation *Reflections on Life* (London: Hamish Hamilton, 1952) may not have sold well.
[9] Andrés H. Reggiani, *God's Eugenicist: Alexis Carrel and the Sociobiology of Decline* (New York: Berghahn Books, 2007): 169.

'Doctors Trial' session. His lawyer, attempting a defence, pointed out that from the 1920s the United States had supported compulsory sterilisation, and the lawyer quoted Carrel's suggestion in *Man, the Unknown* for use of gas chambers to dispose of the criminally insane. This pleading was to no avail — Brandt was found guilty and executed in June 1948.

Man, the Unknown was, perhaps surprisingly, reprinted by a London publisher in 1948, unaltered and with no explanatory introduction, and in Paris, Plon also issued a new French reprint. These editions still had the passage on the use of gas chambers and praise of Mussolini. Bentley Glass, a distinguished geneticist and editor of *The Quarterly Review of Biology*, was shocked when he read it:

> Penguin Books have reprinted many worthwhile books, but this is not among them. That a noted scientist [Carrel] could hold such unsound biological ideas and turns them to such pernicious ends is truly ground for consternation. The book is seeded with the virus of racial superiority. The chief value of this book is that it will reveal to the reader why Carrel was a Nazi sympathiser and from what source Lindbergh became infected.

Even the reviewer in the libertarian conservative journal *The Freeman* was unimpressed, and noted that Carrel's views were 'sharply offensive'.[10] In America, Carrel's *Reflections on Life* also had bad reviews, and the *New York Times* science correspondent Waldemar Kaempffert, still writing at age 76, who had followed and praised Carrel's every contribution before the War, now deserted his hero and wrote that 'this is a bitter book. It brings to mind the fulminations of the ancient prophets'.

The Fondation's Fate

As Paris returned slowly to peacetime activities, Carrel's Fondation survived intact for a while. The new communist minister of health in the de Gaulle government pondered the Fondation's fate for a year. Then,

---

[10] James Burnham in *The Freeman*, 16 November 1953.

urged to retain the institute in a modified form by Alfred Sauvy, the minister of family and population, and by Robert Debré, the Jewish paediatrician hero of the Resistance, the minister decided to keep on almost half of the staff, renaming it as the Institut national d'études dèmographiques. It had a role in the technocratic post-war French government, though missing from the Institut's agenda was any grand 'reconstruction of man'. Those retained in the new organisation, soon headed by Sauvy, included Jean Sutter, André Gros and the psephologist Jean Stoetzel. Sauvy remained in charge until 1962 and gained an international reputation as a demographer and as a liberal social scientist. The new Institut was soon admired for its work, and in calmer times later, some looked back and acknowledged that Carrel's Fondation had laid useful groundwork and had achieved some wartime successes.[11]

Geopolitical Landscape

Had Carrel lived and survived the turmoil he would have found himself in a strange new environment. Carrel had been in a frontline position in the bio-politics of the 1930s. Many had listened to him and agreed with his assumption that something had to be done about the human race. But in the aftermath of World War II, attitudes in the Western world were transformed, and many of the major pre-war debates in which Carrel was involved had simply disappeared. The alleged decline of the human race was no longer accepted as a given, and claims of terminal moral failure now came only from preachers and evangelists. The widespread inter-war view that democracy had failed, and that non-elected technocrats should be in charge, another of Carrel's standpoints, had vanished. In pre-war Europe, fascist leaders had emerged in Germany, Italy, Spain and Portugal, and to Carrel and others, this seemed the new normal. But the Axis dictators eventually took their nations over the cliff, and with the Allies triumphant in their victory over fascism, communism was now the enemy. The West's tradition of democracy was seen as a good thing after all, and democracy returned steadily to France and to Germany, and eventually to all the European nations, with Spain and Portugal being last to change.

---

[11] See Philip Nord, *France's New Deal* (Princeton: Princeton University Press, 2010).

Many of the biological ideas favoured by Carrel had also gone. His shaky understanding of genetics included the view that diseases like cancer, tuberculosis and epilepsy were hereditary and that acquired changes in life could be passed on, and these concepts were now shunned in embarrassment. His use of physiognomy and the support of biotypes, particularly in social policy, were ridiculed and forgotten. Carrel's belief in intuition as a reliable and useful mechanism in research no longer had serious supporters. Scientific support for the existence of telepathy and clairvoyance had shrunk, and the academic department of parapsychology at Duke University, which Carrel had admired, was actively closed down.[12]

To add to this, all forms of eugenic discourse were studiously avoided. With the post-war discovery of the horrors of the Nazi's systematic extermination policies, not only of Jews, but also others considered 'unfit', even thoughtful positive eugenicists kept their thoughts to themselves. The new tolerance also meant a retreat from ideas of 'race'. The earlier unchallenged view that there were various races of man, and that some were more valuable than others, was dumped and criticised. A defining moment was the confident statement in 1950 by UNESCO (the United Nations Educational, Scientific and Cultural Organisation), which signalled an end to scientific racism:

> The myth of race has created an enormous amount of human and social damage. In recent years it has taken a heavy toll in human lives and caused untold suffering.

There was, UNESCO stated, only one human race, within which they suggested, seeking a neologism, there were 'ethnic groups'. The alleged horrors of miscegenation (marriage between 'races') were now conceded to have no biological basis.[13]

---

[12] See Seymour H. Mauskopf and Michael R. McVaugh, *The Elusive Science: Origins of Experimental Psychical Research* (Baltimore: Johns Hopkins University Press, 1980).

[13] *The UNESCO Statement by Experts on Race Problems* (New York: UNESCO, 1950). Comments on this radical document were then sought from others and analysed in *The Race Question in Modern Science: The Results of an Inquiry* (Paris: UNESCO, 1952). Julian Huxley was head of the UNESCO at this time. Outright rejection of the UNESCO consensus in Britain came from Sir Ronald Fisher and Cyril D. Darlington,

Blacks, yellows and browns were slowly accepted as equal partners in the human world and steadily gained political rights and access to scientific, sporting and artistic fame. The Jews were given a homeland. The 'unfit', who had been targeted internationally, were not only safe from hostile government action, but the disadvantaged and disabled were shown a new tolerance, and affirmative action added some privileges. The mentally ill, seen as a burden by Carrel, were shown new compassion. An old word 'autonomy' — the freedom of individuals to determine their own destiny — soon gained new currency in public and academic discourse, and steadily rose to be a cardinal ethical principle, soon regarded as timeless and self-evident. Support for autonomy had, however, been widely absent in pre-war discourse, notably in Carrel's clerical-fascist mantra urging that 'we are not free to live according to our fancies'.

Carrel's major proposal that technocrats and scientists should routinely be in charge of the affairs of the nations was also now regarded with suspicion. Any moves towards Huxley's *Brave New World*, a world created by biocrats, was now watched with concern, particularly as nuclear scientists had delivered the new atomic weapons, but had been slow to show awareness or responsibility for the serious consequences. Carrel's technocratic bio-political regime, which would have told the citizens who they should marry, if they were allowed to marry at all, was off the agenda.

Also gently marginalised from post-war public discourse were the generalist intellectuals who had status in public discourse in the inter-war years. Carrel's role as a scientific guru, someone who knew all the answers and was worth listening to, would have gone.

The New France

Post-war France now showed considerable vitality, just the revival Carrel had hoped to engineer under Vichy. The pre-war cultural despair was no

---

who both asserted that 'races differ in their innate capacity for intellectual and emotional development'; see also Gavin Schaffer (2005) "Like a baby with a box of matches': British scientists and the concept of race in the interwar period' *British Journal of the History of Science* 38: 307–24.

longer around. French science, literature, and philosophy blossomed, and the French style of living was widely admired, particularly by Americans. France became a tolerant haven for artists and writers, and the French films of the 'New Wave' broke new ground. In particular, French biological sciences entered an innovative golden era in which French talent emerged in strength. Jacques Monod, André Lwoff and François Jacob, all active in the Resistance earlier, were awarded their Nobel Prize in 1965 for their post-war cell biology work.

The ultimate irony was that in this confident post-WWII era, France took an international lead in Carrel's main interest — blood vessel surgery and organ grafting. Fear of infection, which had discouraged attempts at such human surgery, was lifted by the arrival in the 1940s of antibiotics, and added to this, new X-ray methods could localise areas suitable for surgery in blood vessels.[14] It was Jacques Oudot (1913–1953) and Charles Dubost (1914–1991) in Paris who carried out the first regular replacement of human blood vessels along Carrelian lines when they used cadaveric human artery grafts to replace diseased segments of the aorta.[15] From 1948, Jean Kunlin in Paris was first to use human vein grafts in dealing with disease in smaller vessels.[16] Soon after, cold preserved vessels were also shown to be as effective as fresh grafts, just as Carrel had shown decades before.[17]

Surgical ambition increased dramatically at this time in Paris and it was the French surgeons who were first to embark on human kidney

---

[14] During WWII, injuries to the blood vessels of the limbs were dealt with by simply tying off the main vessel above — a surprisingly successful emergency procedure in young men.

[15] Jean Natali (1992) 'Jacques Oudot and his contribution to surgery of the aortic bifurcation' *Annals of Vascular Surgery* 6: 185–92. Oudot was medical officer on the famous French Himalayan Annapurna expedition.

[16] J.O. Menzoian, A.L. Kosher and N. Rodrigues (2011) 'Alexis Carrel, Rene Leriche, Jean Kunlin, and the history of bypass surgery' *Journal of Vascular Surgery* 54: 571–4.

[17] R.E. Gross, A.H. Bill and E. Converse Peirce (1949) 'Methods of preservation and transplantation of arterial grafts' *Surgery, Gynecology and Obstetrics* 88: 689–701. They were commendably aware of Carrel's earlier work but, surprisingly, thought that the cells of the cold preserved homografts had survived. They were unaware that Carrel had shown that these preserved grafts were successful merely as inert tubes.

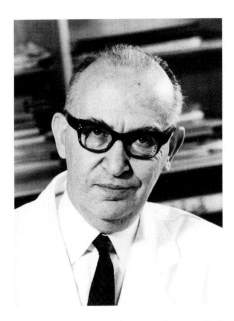

Jean Hamburger revived Carrel's transplant studies, and the pioneering French human kidney transplants followed.

transplantation. Vallery-Radot, the medical hero of the Resistance, and Carrel's accuser, headed a post-war Paris university medical department. In 1947, one of his staff, the physician Jean Hamburger, carried out dog kidney transplant experiments, exactly in the manner of Carrel.[18] Hamburger's published paper, perhaps deliberately, did not acknowledge Carrel's dog kidney work of almost 40 years earlier. Human attempts followed in Paris in January 1951, when two teams of surgeons carried out the first series of human kidney transplants, initiating the modern era of organ transplantation. Hamburger was involved, as were the surgeons Oudot and Dubost, adding their vascular experience. In Boston, attempts at kidney transplantation followed on quickly.[19] Carrel's earlier

---

[18] At this time, Vallery-Radot published a volume on WWII French medical research carried out during these 'les années d'oppression', and Carrel's Fondation work does not feature.

[19] These human kidney grafts were carried out without using significant immunosuppression. In the early 1950s, the British surgeon James Dempster was one of the first to try the Carrel–Murphy suggestion of radiation for experimental immunosuppression, but poignantly, radiation is ineffective in dogs. After Dempster's seven years of fruitless

lead was sometimes acknowledged by these surgeons, sometimes not. French authority in the science of tissue transplantation continued, and France gained a Nobel Prize when Jean Dausset (1916–2009), a wartime member of the Free French Army, from 1958 opened up the first understanding of tissue typing and organ matching. Not until the early 1960s was Carrel's suggestion of immunosuppression by radiation or marrow-depressing chemicals used regularly with success, at last.

France and Carrel

In the immediate post-war years, France had been understandably cool towards Carrel, who had ended up on the wrong side of history. But with the new awareness, particularly in the surgical community, of his remarkable early contributions, by the early 1950s a public rehabilitation in France could commence. With the detailed memories of Vichy repressed, the new generation was reassured by the French leadership that the wartime events were the result of patriotism and that the Vichy government was a 'wartime shield' for France. The now-prosperous and confident French nation moved on, encouraged by de Gaulle's wish for reconciliation and unity. An amnesty for all but the most serious wartime actions was announced in 1951, attempting to draw a line under the Vichy events.

It was time for a reconsideration of Carrel. With the success of the biological sciences in this new *belle époque* and the vitality of French surgery building on Carrel's work, it was felt, after all, that Nobel Prize-winner Carrel could be added to the French pantheon. His rehabilitation commenced slowly, reaching saintly status on occasions.

Carrel Biographies

It was now safe to attempt a biography, and the first of many in the exemplary genre appeared in 1952 written by Paris surgeon Robert

---

attempts with radiation in dog kidney transplants, Roy Calne, in 1959, in the same lab, turned to the successful chemical immunosuppression using 6-mercaptopurine thus starting the modern era of organ transplantation.

Soupault.[20] He was a Petainist in the Vichy era and had been accused of collaboration, but although he was cleared by a tribunal, he lost his hospital post and moved to America. He returned in more tolerant times, and he was keen to show that Carrel was a genius who had first been forgotten and then judged unfairly in recent times. Soupault had excellent material to use from Carrel's scientific work, but other matters were problematic. There were the embarrassing passages in *Man, the Unknown*, but Soupault could point to the huge sales of *Man, the Unknown* as evidence that the book was a treatise of major importance, and hence Carrel was not only a scientist but also a philosopher, mystic and religious thinker, as well as an ascetic, saintly figure. In dealing with the more recent possibility of collaboration, Carrel had apparently been cleared of any blame, and there were his useful pre-war anti-German quotes to neutralise any suggestion that he supported fascism. Another difficulty for his supportive biographer was Carrel's regular denigration of France and the French. Soupault dealt with this by blaming petty Lyon provincialism for Carrel's move to America, and he used the scattered patriotic statements also to be found in Carrel's writings.

A remarkable number of short, admiring, popular French biographies followed, all based on Soupault's larger work.[21] French medical journals regularly praised him and his work in short historical articles.[22] France had now taken serious responsibility for their hero, and Carrel's fame

---

[20] Soupault's biography had help from many who knew Carrel, including interviews in America, and Mme Carrel had a powerful influence on the narrative and opinions offered. Soupault attached a thorough bibliography of Carrel's many publications, drawn up by Jean Sutter, formerly on his Fondation staff. Soupault's hard-to-find travelogue *Une ère chirurgicale nouvelle* was published in Argentina in 1946.

[21] The biographies which followed are H. Delaye-Didier-Delorme, *Alexis Carrel, humaniste chrétien, Prix Nobel 1912* (Paris: Apostolat des editions, 1963), J. Descotes, *Alexis Carrel 1973–1944* (Lyon: Simep-Editions, 1966), Jean-Jaques Antier, *Alexis Carrel* (Paris: Wesmael-Charlier, 1970) followed by his *Carrel cet inconnu* (Paris: Éditions S.O.S., 1974). There is a collection of supportive essays in Yves Christen (ed.), *Alexis Carrel: L'ouverture de l'homme* (Paris: Editions Féline, 1986).

[22] J.J. Gillon, who assisted in 1935 with Plon's French translation of *Man, the Unknown*, wrote 18 supportive articles between 1954 and 1989 dealing with Carrel or Carrelian policy; these are listed in Drouard's *La fondation Carrel* (note 67): 533–4.

again rose to rival that of Einstein in France.[23] On the centenary of his birth in 1973, there were many tributes in the journals. In Britain and America, Carrel's *Man, the Unknown* was ignored and forgotten, but it still had cult status in France, without the contents being studied closely, and the Paris publisher Plon continued to reprint the book. There were steady sales elsewhere. In Argentina there was a final printing in 1957 and the last edition outside Europe was in Mexico in 1982. The last edition in Spain was in 1970 and the final Italian edition of *L'uomo, questo sconosciuto* came in 2006, introduced by the publisher as a 'lucid analysis of modern society'.

Further Honours

To acknowledge Carrel's new status as a scientist and thinker, in the 1960s French cities started to re-name streets in his honour, as did municipal authorities in South America and francophone Canada. The University of

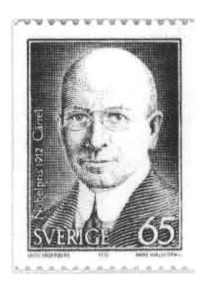

With Carrel's post-war reputational recovery, his surgical contributions and his Nobel Prize were increasingly recognised.

---

[23] Public fame can be judged by Google Books 'Ngram reader' data, which counts entries in printed books.

Lyon now sought to honour him and used his name to re-christen one of the faculties of the medical school. A Carrel fan club emerged in Nantes, with Lindbergh's help, called 'Les Amis du Docteur Carrel', and for a while they issued the *Bulletin de l'association française des amis de Carrel* and also their *Journées Carrel*. In Nantes, the group raised a subscription to put up a statue in 1970; another appeared at Carrel's birthplace. In 1972, Sweden issued a Carrel postal stamp, as did Micronesia, and in 1979, astronomers gave Carrel's name to a lunar crater. In France in 1971 André Gros founded the Centre international de réflexion prospective based on Carrel's teachings. Eponymous institutions emerged, like the Instituto Alexis Carrel in Cordoba, Argentina, with 300 students, and there was a similar college in Cuba. A Psycho-Somatic Clinique honouring his name opened in Mallorca. In Milan, schools were often named after scientists including Volta, Einstein and Marconi, and they now attached Carrel's name.[24]

Catholic Links

Supporting this rehabilitation, Carrel's status as a mystic and Christian was revived. Post-war Catholicism had a problem, since having earlier opposed the theory of evolution, and now changing stance, the Church sought to catch up and seek a reconciliation with the world of science. In particular, the Church looked for scientist-believers who were practising Catholics. Carrel's writings were studied with interest and his books, including *Voyage to Lourdes* and *Prayer*, showed him to be a supporter of spiritual values, and even of miraculous healing. His works and beliefs therefore had merit.

One of the first post-war Catholic commentators to notice Carrel was Liam Brophy, who said that Carrel had set out with 'passionless detachment' the case against 'modern man's utter lack of the religious sense and the terrible effects of secularism'.[25] Other Catholic writers soon

---

[24] Reggiani, *God's Eugenicist* (note 9) lists other celebratory institutional use of his name.
[25] Liam Brophy (1946) 'Hermann Keyserling, Knight of the Holy Ghost' *The Irish Monthly* 74: 376–83.

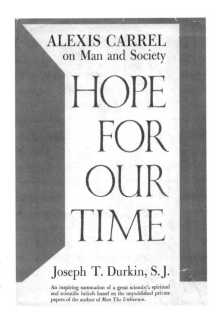

In 1965, Father Durkin, the Jesuit Georgetown University historian, gave a sympathetic account of Carrel's beliefs.

wrote in approval of Carrel, and John O'Brien and Albert Bessières found Carrel useful in their books on scientists who had religious faith.[26] The Catholic *Life Annual* of 1957 carried a condensed version of Soupault's biography. The staff at the Jesuit Georgetown University, now holding Carrel's archive, also showed an interest. Considering Carrel to be 'one of us', Father Joseph T. Durkin, Georgetown's professor of history, set to work on exploring Carrel's beliefs, starting with *Man, the Unknown*, and assisted by the huge archive, thus far little consulted. Durkin, as a historian, had to face up to the unattractive side of Carrel, and he privately noted that some findings were 'ticklish items'. Avoiding these, he nevertheless found merit in some of scientist's religious beliefs, and these appeared in Durkin's book *Hope for Our Time* of 1965. In it, he concluded,

---

[26] John O'Brien, *Roads to Rome* (New York: Macmillan, 1954) and Albert Bessières, *La destinée humaine devant la science — Alexis Carrel, Lecomte du Noüy, Charles Nicolle* (Paris: Editions Spes, 1950). Charles-Jules-Henri Nicolle, of the Pasteur Institute in Tunis, was Nobel Prize winner in 1928 for his work on typhus, and published the popular work *La destinée humaine* of 1941; for du Noüy, see note 36.

as the title suggests, that Carrel's teachings did indeed offer hope for the spiritual life of mankind.[27] Durkin also wrote a short biography which was published only in France, and only after the author agreed to changes favourable to Carrel, notably regarding the World War II events.[28]

Catholic magazines continued to praise Carrel, not only for his support for the life of the spirit but also for his belief in unexplained Lourdes cures. These magazines and inspirational websites also carried extracts from his *Readers' Digest* articles and his wartime book on prayer *La prière*.[29] Father Stanley L. Jaki, the Catholic scientist, theologian and populariser, praised him and wrote a supportive Introduction to the last printing of *La prière* in 1994.[30]

Other Writers

With the steady rehabilitation of Carrel, other old supporters gained confidence, and André Missenard, his important pre-war admirer and deputy at the Fondation, felt it was time to produce his own book, *À la recherché de l'homme* (1954), translated as *In Search of Man* (1957).[31]

---

[27] Joseph T. Durkin, *Hope for Our Time: Alexis Carrel on Man and Society* (New York: Harper & Row, 1965).

[28] Joseph Durkin, *Alexis Carrel, savant mystique* (Paris: Fayard, 1969) had an Introduction by Charles Lindbergh. An unpublished English version is held at Alexis Carrel Papers, Georgetown University Library, Booth Family Center for Special Collections ACP-GULBFC.

[29] Alexis Carrel, *La Prière* (Paris: Plon, 1944) was reprinted four times, the last being in 1949, plus a special illustrated edition in 1978, and it was reissued, combined with *Réflexions*, from 1971 to 1991. An English translation was published by Hodder & Stoughton in 1947, and reprinted in 1948. *Reader's Digest* has reprinted extracts from *Prayer*, which is also still favoured by Christian websites.

[30] See the article by the prolific writer Father Stanley L. Jaki in *Catholic World Report*, November 1994.

[31] André Missenard, *In Search of Man* (New York: Hawthorn Books, 1957) was the translation of his *À la recherché de l'homme* (Paris-Strasbourg: Librairie Istra, 1954). Missenard also gave an account of Carrel's time at the Fondation in his 'Sombre souvenirs: La vérité sur le séjour d'Alexis Carrel en France de 1941 à 1944' *Journal de Médecine de Lyon*, June 1980, 397–411; Nord (note 11): 178 describes him as 'marginalised and embittered'.

It was largely a reprise of *Man, the Unknown*, and in his Introduction he dedicated it to:

> Alexis Carrel, teacher and friend, in an attempt to explain the scientific and humanitarian concern which brought him back to the humiliated and bleeding France of 1941.

Missenard, whose post-war career had not prospered, took up the cause where Carrel left off, and repeatedly echoed Carrel:

> Modern man is already an artificial creature, more and more disturbed and tormented as his life becomes more arbitrary. … The quest for means of procuring more and more superior men is a tragic necessity. The weak and defective are artificially kept alive. …[32]

Missenard copied Carrel's agenda on a long list of other minor matters, notably physiognomy, and praised the 'noble savages' in the isolated Lötschental Valley in Switzerland who 'live their lives in spiritual

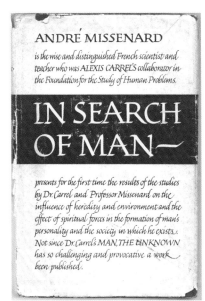

André Missenard's 1957 book attempted to revive his mentor Carrel's earlier teachings.

---

[32] Missenard, *Search* (note 31): 27.

harmony'. The Nordic races he considered to be naturally superior. Women should accept a return to motherhood and to the kitchen, and he tut-tuts about the trashy literature 'of the heart' for girls. Missenard openly hoped that the Lamarckian explanation of evolution would prove to be right and that characteristics acquired in life are passed on. Some of his educational proposals have Carrelian dogmatism: babies should not be fed on demand (it creates selfishness) and children should not be taught about Santa Claus, since 'it encourages other lies'.[33]

Missenard's book had little impact and the few reviews were hostile, noting Carrelian 'inexplicable disregard for statistics' and 'extravagant and unsupported views'.[34] Others thought it was 'vaguely cited ... simplistic ... elitist' and some noted 'an authoritarian thread'.[35]

Lecomte du Noüy, after his escape to America, where he found employment as an academic, also published after the War. Though estranged from Carrel, he agreed with many of his old mentor's views, and shared the Carrelian urge to speak to the public on man's future. To add to his book *La dignité humaine* of 1944, du Noüy produced his *L'Homme et sa destinée* in 1947.[36] But unlike the gloomy declinist assumptions of Carrel and Missenard, these were more optimistic works, and he believed, like the 'new mystics' led by Teilhard de Chardin, that man's physical and spiritual evolution was always upwards, directed by God. Du Noüy's book, aimed at a popular readership, sold well but received sceptical, even hostile, reviews in serious journals.[37] A reviewer, detecting the 1930s

---

[33] Missenard, *Search* (note 31): 240.
[34] John De Lucca (1959) 'In Search of Man' *Philosophy of Science* 26: 53–4.
[35] *American Anthropologist* 60 (1958): 1212–3.
[36] Lecomte du Noüy's *L'Homme et sa destinée* (Paris: La Colombe, 1947) was translated and issued as *Human Destiny* by Longmans, Green and Company from 1951, with a paperback edition following in 1963.
[37] Du Noüy's wife, in her biography, says there were editions in 12 languages and it was a non-fiction best-seller in 1947, helped by praise in *Reader's Digest*; see Mary Lecomte du Noüy, *The Road to "Human Destiny": A Life of Pierre Lecomte du Noüy* (New York: Longmans, Green and Co., 1955): 294–303.

thinking, classified it as 'clerical-fascism' and wrote that du Noüy was intent on the

> establishment of an ultra-conservative social order — an authoritarian, hierarchically-ordered society devoted to the leader-principle and dominated by an intellectual élite holding sway over an obedient, tractable, breeding mass of church-going inferiors.[38]

The Pierre Lecomte du Noüy American Foundation Award was set up in his name after his death, and it was awarded for the best book of the year reconciling science and religion. The last award was in 1973.

Further Surgical Fame

In the world of medicine and science, the new success with blood vessel surgery and kidney transplantation meant that Carrel's pioneering work was steadily acknowledged and honoured, to which was added some surprise and even embarrassment at the neglect of his surgical innovations. As Carrel's fame grew, surgical meetings and guest lectures named in his honour appeared. At Lyon, enthusiasts in the medical school organised a major symposium in 1966.[39] The speakers at this and similar events thereafter, found, to their surprise, the richness of Carrel's contributions. Added to this, it was easy to uncover new scientific findings in what was increasingly realised to be a pre-World War I 'lost era' of remarkably 'modern' transplantation studies.[40]

---

[38] Ferdinand Lundberg (1948) 'Human Destiny' *The Journal of Philosophy* 45: 152–61; for du Noüy's scientific status see Ralph Estling in *New Scientist*, 2 June 1983.

[39] Speakers at the Lyon meeting included René Leriche and Robert Soupault, joined by Jean-Michel Dubernard, one of the new generation of talented Lyon transplant surgeons. Also attending were André Gros, Theodore Malinin, Joseph Durkin and Charles Lindbergh; see J. Descotes (ed.), *Alexis Carrel 1873–1944: Pionnier de la chirurgie vasculaire et des transplantations d'organes* (Lyon: Simep editions, 1966).

[40] For this 'Lost Era' of organ transplantation, see David Hamilton, *A History of Organ Transplantation* (Pittsburgh: Pittsburgh University Press, 2012): 105–25.

In the mid-1960s, Dr. Theodore Malinin, director of the Miami Tissue bank, one of the new scientists working on tissue storage for transplant use, was particularly intrigued by Carrel's earlier organ perfusion experiments with Lindbergh. Yet again, it appeared that Carrel had been first in the field, this time with his organ pump 30 years earlier. Malinin also realised that Charles Lindbergh was still alive and active.[41] Malinin invited him to visit his laboratory and Lindbergh was pleased to co-operate, and they worked hard in constructing a similar but larger organ pump which could accommodate larger organs, such as monkey heart and kidneys. However the results with these organs were no better than in 1938.[42] In 1973, Malinin organised a Centennial Symposium at Georgetown celebrating Carrel's birth. The invited speakers gave celebratory papers on his life and work and Lindbergh, though seriously ill, managed to attend and speak.[43]

Two American biographies of Carrel appeared at this time, both by surgeons. The first, a short father-and-son work by Sterling and Peter Edwards was published in 1974,[44] and four years later, a longer account by Malinin followed, with an Introduction by Charles Lindbergh.[45] Both these biographies now had the fairly standard, but incomplete,

[41] Lindbergh and Ann Lindbergh were showing early environmental concern and her *Gift from the Sea* was a national bestseller in 1955. He published his wartime diaries with minimal changes.

[42] V.P. Perry, C.A. Lindbergh, T.I. Malinin and G.H. Mouer 'Pulsatile perfusion of whole mammalian organs' in Judah Folkman *et al.* (eds.), *Organ Perfusion and Preservation* (New York: Appleton-Century-Crofts, 1968): 203–16. There is further detail on their method, and poor results, in C.A. Lindbergh *et al.* (1966) 'An apparatus for the pulsating perfusion of whole organs' *Cryobiology* 3: 252–60 and T.I. Malinin and V.P. Perry (1968) 'Observations on contracting hearts maintained in vitro at hypothermic temperature' *Johns Hopkins Medical Journal* 122: 380–6.

[43] Joseph T. Durkin (ed.), *Papers of the Alexis Carrel Centennial Conference* (Georgetown University, 1973).

[44] W. Sterling Edwards and Peter D. Edwards, *Alexis Carrel: Visionary Surgeon* (Springfield: Charles C. Thomas, 1974).

[45] Theodore I. Malinin, *Surgery and Life: the Extraordinary Career of Alexis Carrel* (New York: Harcourt Brace Jovanovich, 1979).

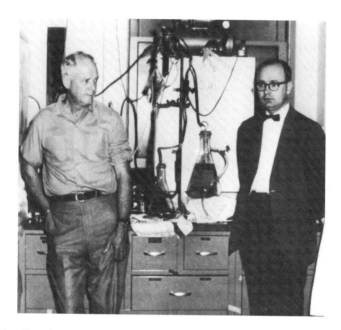

Charles Lindbergh at age 63 took up the invitation in 1965 to assist with new studies of organ perfusion in Miami. (*Courtesy of the Bureau of Medicine and Surgery, US Navy.*)

account of his life and described some of his surgical contributions, downplaying or ignoring Carrel's involvement in other matters. Thereafter, the secondary literature on Carrel blossomed, and these accounts, largely copied from these books, became simpler and more vivid over time. A series of surgical Carrel Symposia followed, starting in 1986 and ending with the eighth event in Sweden in 2001. In February 2002, as part of centenary celebrations of Charles Lindbergh's birth, the Medical University of South Carolina at Charleston established the Lindbergh–Carrel Prize for contributions to the 'development of perfusion and bioreactor technologies for organ preservation and growth'.[46]

---

[46] Michael DeBakey and nine other scientists received the quirky bronze statuette prize, created for the event by the Italian artist C. Zoli and named 'Elisabeth' after Elisabeth

Carrel's other work had revivals. As antibiotic resistance emerged and grew, recourse to chemical antisepsis was necessary again, and Dakin's solution re-emerged for use in various forms.[47] Even lavage of wounds with antiseptics had a return to favour.[48] Some suspected that there might be other important Carrel contributions which remained ignored or unpublished. Norman Orentreich, a dermatologist with an interest in ageing, noticed one of the lesser claims by Carrel that blood taken from younger animals would rejuvenate older ones. Orentreich was determined to find the details of the experiment, and he trawled through Carrel's papers at Georgetown University in vain trying to find details and data.

Tissue Culture

Carrel's prominence in the development of tissue culture was long recognised. Carrel's wider fame in this area was sustained because his immortal chicken heart cell line was established as a fundamental fact, featuring in all works on biology. This was in spite of the conspicuous failure of others to reproduce the findings, and that the cells were never successfully gifted to others. It had gained a lively place in imaginative writing and popular culture. In the novel *The Space Merchants* of 1952, a giant mass of cultured chicken cells is sliced regularly for food, as is a similar growing lump in the novel *Methuselah's Children* (1958). Comedian Bill Cosby in his stand-up comedy performances, and his 1966 album 'Wonderfulness', used the possibilities of an unfettered cellular growth which endangers the world. Carrel continued to have posthumous skill in catching the public imagination, and after his death schoolteachers and pupils still wrote to the Rockefeller Institute (by now

Morrow, sister of Lindbergh's wife Anne Morrow. Concern about Elizabeth's heart disease led to Lindbergh's links with Carrel.

[47] Jeffrey M. Levine (2013) 'Dakin's Solution: Past, present and future' *Advances in Skin & Wound Care* 26: 410–4.

[48] D.J. Keblish and Marlene DeMaio (1998) 'Early pulsatile lavage for the decontamination of combat wounds' *Military Medicine* 163: 844–6.

renamed as the Rockefeller University), for help with the chicken heart experiment as a laboratory project or to show it at the school Science Fair. The John Carroll High School in Birmingham, Alabama, even had an Alexis Carrel Club.

Tissue culture methods had slowly and steadily improved. The steady search for improved growth media gave new varieties of longer-lived (but not immortal) cell lines, with Raymond Parker from Carrel's lab having an important role. In the hunt for long-lasting cells, there was a denouement when George Gey found an immortal strain of malignant cells, the HeLa cell line, in 1951. He rapidly shared these robust 'eternal' cells with other labs.

Reputational Setbacks

Throughout his career, Carrel had regularly survived concerns about his scientific work and conduct. His early claim in 1911 for obtaining sustained culture of malignant cells was not confirmed, nor was he correct in reporting that his cultured cells grew into organs. In World War I his Carrel–Dakin system of wound care was clearly less successful than he claimed. His later announcement in the 1920s of success in transforming one cell into another or producing malignancy in tissue culture were quietly forgotten. His organ perfusion pump was a technical triumph, but the results with most organs were unconvincing. These flawed claims were decently ignored and were charitably balanced out by his undoubted innovations.

But in 1961 a serious new concern arose, this time over his 'immortal' cells.[49] In 1961 a new view of the lifespan of cells emerged. Leonard Hayflick (born 1928) showed that normal animal cells (unlike malignant cells) had a limited capacity for division, and that after about 50 divisions, they stop dividing. This new orthodoxy was the 'Hayflick Limit'.[50]

---

[49] John Paul in his standard work *Cell and Tissue Culture* of 1959 could loyally state that 'Carrel had demonstrated beyond all doubt that animal cells could be grown indefinitely in tissue culture'.

[50] Hayflick's first paper on his 'limit' was firmly turned down for publication in the Rockefeller's *Journal of Experimental Medicine* by Peyton Rous, Carrel's former colleague,

Attention returned to Carrel's famous cell line, since Carrel's claims now seemed improbable, as Hayflick pointed out. Detective work by Jan Witkowski, of the Carnegie Institution in Washington, concluded that the cell cultures in Carrel's lab were either inadvertently topped up with fresh cells, or this was done deliberately, to keep the boss happy.[51] Either way, the scientific community had been seriously misled. If fraud was involved then retrospectively this was a serious episode involving what was now called scientific misconduct, one of an increasing number of cases uncovered from the 1960s. Its implications were considerable because of the influence of these 'immortal' cells for decades on biological thinking. If cells are immortal, it followed that man's life span is constrained by other non-cellular factors. Now, new theories of aging were required — the gerontologists had been misled.

The Cells Persist

Although this reassessment affected Carrel's standing within the cell biology world in the 1970s, his public reputation largely survived. The 'eternal cells' had been accepted for so long, that it was remarkably difficult to correct Carrel's mistake. Even in serious reference works, the now-disputed cell line continued to have a useful extension of life, and continued to appear in Carrel's entry in scientific biographies.[52] Even serious medical journals continued to be unaware of the error, and Witkowski and Hayflick had to wearily correct the mistake in *The Journal of the American Medical Association* and the respected journal *Science*.[53]

---

then aged 82, with the agreement of three other editors. Leonard Hayflick also developed the first useable human diploid cell line WI-38 and made a large stock at the 8th passage. With his new view on gerontology, his sensible book *How and Why We Age* of 1994 sold well.

[51] J.A. Witkowski (1980) 'Dr. Carrel's immortal cells' *Medical History* 24: 129–42.
[52] Carrel's immortal cells are still described favourably in Carrel's entries in *Notable Twentieth Century Scientists* (1995), the *Encyclopaedia of World Scientists* (2000), *Doctors and Their Discoveries* (2002) and *The Complete Dictionary of Scientific Biography* (2008).
[53] Jan Witkowski had to correct the distinguished science writer Barbara Culliton when she praised Carrel's cells in her history of the Rockefeller University; see his 'Carrel's

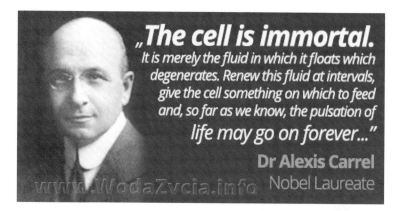

„*The cell is immortal.*
It is merely the fluid in which it floats which
degenerates. Renew this fluid at intervals,
give the cell something on which to feed
and, so far as we know, the pulsation of
life may go on forever..."
Dr Alexis Carrel
Nobel Laureate
www.WodaZycia.info

Carrel's faulty claims for cellular immortality are still used in justifying alterna-tive medicine strategies, notably supporting 'detoxification' regimens. (*www. WodaZycia.info*)

Adding to the confusion, some historians of tissue culture seemed reluctant to get involved.[54]

In the murkier depths of the Internet, the immortal cells are very much alive, and even beating. Since the immortal cells apparently needed regular 'washing' with new fluid, those who allege that toxin build-up causes human diseases still invoke Carrel's name when promoting detoxification regimens, like colonic lavage, extra daily water intake, alkaline diet, stimulation of lymphatic flow, and other strategies to remove 'badness' from the body.

---

cultures' *Science* 247 (1990): 1385–6. In 1983, *JAMA* reprinted a 'Landmark' paper by Carrel, and Dr. Hassan Najafi's added 'Perspective' had many inaccuracies. After Witkowski's criticism (*JAMA* 252: 44), the journal took the unusual step of retracting the article.

[54] Landecker does describe the affair briefly in her book *Culturing Life: How Cells Became Technologies* (Cambridge: Harvard University Press, 2010): 91 and 166. She diplomati-cally omits the controversy in her chapter on tissue culture in Darwin H. Stapleton (ed.), *Creating a Tradition of Biomedical Research: Contributions to the History of the Rockefeller University* (New York: The Rockefeller University Press, 2004): 151–74.

Guthrie Remembered

With the re-discovery of Carrel's major contributions to early transplantation and vascular surgery, more details emerged about his collaboration with Charles C. Guthrie in the period 1905–1906 in Chicago. Accounts of Carrel's early work traditionally described Guthrie as the junior partner in their early joint work. But with these concerns about Carrel's probity emerging, Guthrie's criticisms of Carrel, made 60 years earlier, were now noted with interest, particularly at Pittsburgh, where Guthrie had worked from 1909. The chairman of the Department of Surgery, Samuel P. Harbison, looked anew at the Carrel–Guthrie work and studied their correspondence preserved in Guthrie's archive. He now loyally proposed that Guthrie was instead the dominant partner and had contributed most of the ideas. He went further, and suggested that Guthrie should have shared Carrel's Nobel Prize, although the award could not be shared at that time.[55] Also taking a new look was J.B. deC.M. Saunders who, in his Introduction to a 1972 textbook on organ transplantation, also supported the view that Guthrie had been wronged when depicted as merely an assistant to Carrel.[56] Carrel loyalists were unimpressed with this revisionist verdict and spoke up, downplaying these new claims for Guthrie.[57] But Guthrie had been noticed, and in 1960, just after his 80th birthday, he was awarded a medal by the American Association of Plastic Surgeons, more than 50 years after his work with Carrel. The Association explained that the award gave

> belated but richly deserved recognition to the pioneer work of this great physiologist and vascular technician who established fundamental

---

[55] S.P. Harbison (1962) 'Origins of vascular surgery: The Carrel–Guthrie letters' *Surgery* 52: 406–18. In 1959, Harbison with Bernard Fisher edited, introduced and reprinted Guthrie's *Blood Vessel Surgery and its Applications* of 1912; see also Blair O. Rogers (1959) 'Charles Claude Guthrie M.D. PhD: a remarkable pioneer in tissue and organ transplantation' *Plastic and Reconstructive Surgery* 24: 380–3.
[56] J.B. deC.M. Saunders 'A conceptual history of transplantation' in J.S. Najarian and R.L. Simmonds (eds.), *Transplantation* (Philadelphia, Lea and Febiger: 1972): 3–25.
[57] For a rebuttal of Harbison's support for Guthrie's cause, see Serge J. Dos (1975) 'The Carrel–Guthrie controversy' *Surgery* 77: 330–2.

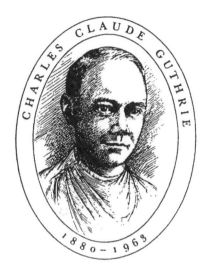

Interest revived in Guthrie's work with Carrel in 1905–06, and from 1980 he was honoured as patron of the Mid-Western Vascular Surgical Society.

principles and methods upon which many of our wonderful present day vascular operations are based.[58]

This effusive praise for Guthrie's vascular work, a tribute which seems to diminish Carrel's role, came from plastic surgeons and is perhaps a surprise. But these by-now senior surgeons had earlier been in the U.S. Army in World War II, and on return to America were the leaders in the post-war research in transplantation, only later handing over to the general surgeons. With their wartime involvement in Europe, they would know of, and disapprove of Carrel's Paris sojourn, and this perhaps explains their enthusiastic new assessment of Guthrie. Later, the Mid-Western Vascular Society also found they had a new hero and used Guthrie's likeness in their crest. In 2001 they brought out an elegant two-volume testimonial to his life and works.[59]

[58] Jerome P. Webster (1963) 'Dr. Charles Claude Guthrie, first recipient of Association Medal, dies' *Plastic and Reconstructive Surgery* 32: 482. Joseph Murray, the pioneer of American organ transplantation in the 1950s, emerged from this group of early transplant-orientated plastic surgeons.

[59] Hugh E. Stephenson, Robert S. Kimpton and G. Mallary Masters, *America's First Nobel Prize in Medicine or Physiology: the Story of Guthrie and Carrel* (Boston: Midwestern Vascular Surgery Society, 2001).

Public Setbacks

In France, the post-war attempts to forget Vichy had been largely successful for two decades, but interest in Vichy revived in the 1970s, and Carrel's involvement had further attention and renewed analysis. The reassessment started with the 1969 French semi-documentary film *Le chagrin et la pitié (The Sorrow and the Pity)*, which was followed in 1972 by Robert Paxton's influential revisionist book *Vichy France*. The debate continued, and former supporters of Vichy emerged again, joined by the far-Right politicians and writers. They took an interest in Carrel, and it was the praise from the Right that brought him, his book *L'Homme cet inconnu*, and his support for the Vichy government, to the front again in France.

In the late 1940s, after the defeat of fascism, writers and thinkers on Right were largely silent, but with new awareness of the Vichy era, a trickle of low-profile 'new Right' writing in France appeared, grouped together as the French movement *Nouvelle droite*.[60] Aware of the text of *L'Homme cet inconnu*, and that they had a French conservative thinker to honour, they started to use Carrel's name in some pronouncements. Alain de Benoist's manifesto *Vu de droite* of 1977, seen by some as a 'restatement of fascism', had a chapter devoted to Carrel, in particular supporting Carrel's claim that the white races were endangered. Benoist echoed Carrel's call for positive eugenics and rule by a hereditary elite. Benoist's journal *Nouvelle École* began to receive attention, and it influenced the righist politicians emerging as the Front national party in France, which gained significant support in the 1980s. Among those in this scattered group who invoked Carrel's name was Jacques de Mahieu (1915–1990), who had fled to Argentina after the Liberation and became one of the ideologues in the Peronist administration.

In 1991, Bruno Mégret, then the General Secretary of the Front national party headed by Jean-Marie Le Pen, made a prominent speech on the environment and used Carrel's name. Wishing to suggest that their

---

[60] Hardly noticed at the time, but admired later by neo-fascists, was the 1948 book *Imperium* by the American Francis Parker Yockey (1917–1960), a Spenglerian work favouring a united fascist Europe, similar to the Pax Teutonica likely under Hitler.

The Decay of Modern Society

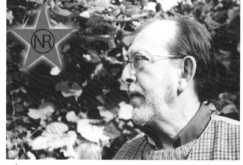

Alain De Benoist

Carrel's writings were revisited in the 1970s by the leaders of the French NR movement (Nouvelle Droite – New Right).

party cared about the environment, he claimed that Carrel was 'a man of the Right and founder of ecology'.[61] Carrel's thoughts on the environment in *Man, the Unknown* were largely limited to deploring city pollution, but Mégret was seeking to recruit Carrel to their broader cause. With his name revived by the far Right, critics of the Right looked again at *Man, the Unknown* and encountered not just a popular book on biology and the spiritual life, but one with attacks on democracy, praise for authoritarian government, hostility to women and unsophisticated support for eugenics. The forgotten passage advocating the use of gas chambers for the criminally insane was now found and widely quoted. Appearing that year was a slim, polemical work *L'Homme cet inconnu? Alexis Carrel, Jean Marie Le Pen et les chambres à gas*, which sought to link together Le Pen's party, Carrel and Nazi leanings.[62]

---

[61] Mark Wegierski (1993–4) 'The New-Right in Europe' *Telos:* 98–9, 55–74.
[62] Lucien Bonnafé and Patrick Tort, *L'Homme cet inconnu? Alexis Carrel, Jean–Marie Le Pen et les chambres à gaz* (Paris: Édition Syllepse, 1992). Bonnafé (1912–2003), a communist French psychiatrist, wrote in a polemical style.

The Lyon newspapers in particular took up the story and reminded readers that a faculty in the local Lyon medical school had been renamed in Carrel's honour.[63] Pressure grew on the University to reconsider and a commission of scholars was tasked with re-investigating Carrel's career. In their report, they separated Carrel's work as a scientist from his other views, and, supporting this partition, the University's governing body voted narrowly in December 1992 to retain his name in the medical school title.

More Pressure

Carrel's life and works were now part of a public debate in France, linked to the reassessment of the Vichy era and the rise of the Right in politics, and the matter would not settle. The febrile mood attracted some other more dubious accusations against Carrel, and a psychiatrist claimed that wartime directions from Carrel led to deliberate starvation of patients in psychiatric institutions. But no clear evidence to support this claim emerged.[64] More subtle was criticism in 1991 of Carrel from an advisor at the Institut national d'études démographiques (INED), the successor to Carrel's Fondation. He suggested that the INED, in their demographic studies, had inherited racist assumptions from the Fondation and that the INED's attitude to ethnic groups had encouraged the racist anti-immigration rhetoric of the Front national.[65]

The local debate in Lyon continued and was made more vivid by the trial in the city in 1994 of the fugitive Vichy collaborator Paul Touvier. He was brought to justice for his involvement in the wartime murder of Jews in Lyon and deportation of others to the German gas chambers. The Paris newspaper *Le monde* called their fate a '*mort toute*

[63] Bernard Fromentin 'De Pétain à Le Pen, en passant par Alexis Carrel' *Lyon Journal*, 21 November, 1991.
[64] Hervé Le Bras 'Logique biologique de la démographie: Alexis Carrel et l'élimination des 'déficients'' in M-C. Hook-Demarle and C. Liauzu, *Transmettre les passés: Nazisme, Vichy et conflits coloniaux* (Paris: Édition Syllepse, 2001): 21–37 and André Castelli and Armand Ajzenberg, *L'abandon à la mort* (Paris: l'Harmattan, 2012).
[65] Reggiani, *God's Eugenicist* (note 9): 6.

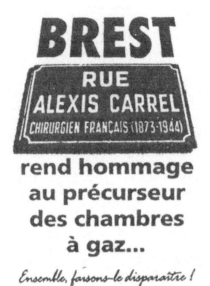

BREST

RUE
ALEXIS CARREL
CHIRURGIEN FRANÇAIS (1873-1944)

rend hommage
au précurseur
des chambres
à gaz...

Ensemble, faisons-le disparaître !

After Carrel was praised by the rightist National Front politicians in France, pressure grew to remove his name from street signs. (*Ras L'Front*)

'carrélienne'' and Plon, the publisher, temporarily withdrew stocks of *L'Homme cet inconnue*. This put further pressure on Lyon University, and in 1995 it again had to consider its use of Carrel's name. This time the governing body decided that Carrel's science and his attitudes should not be separated and voted decisively to rename the faculty. Instead they chose that of René Laënnec (1781–1826), the Parisian who had introduced the stethoscope into medical practice. Lyon's Contemporary Art Museum had a similar problem when an opportunity to honour local surgeons arose at this time. They chose to put up statues of Mathieu Jaboulay, Carrel's mentor, and René Leriche, Carrel's distinguished contemporary, but not one of Carrel.

The numerous city streets named after Carrel now attracted attention, and in Paris leftist politicians linked Carrel's name to Le Pen and his party. Pressure for *débaptisation*, i.e. renaming the streets, gathered force. Eventually 21 of the French cities using Carrel's name on public signs took this step, removing his name, with Paris being last to do so. Others were

556 The First Transplant Surgeon

less sensitive about links to Carrel. There was no change of the street name in Buenos Aires or Montreal, and the solitary eponymous road sign in São Paulo remained in place. Others unaware of the debate in France were some Scottish scientists. In Edinburgh in March 2000, five piglets were cloned by the new genetic engineering methods, and two of the young piglets were called 'Alexis' and 'Carrel'. The Scottish scientists, to their surprise, were criticised by the French media, who deemed the choices as unfortunate.[66]

A new assessment of Carrel was needed and it appeared in 1992 written by Alain Drouard, the historian who had been on the Lyon University investigative committee.[67] Drouard aimed to give a balanced account of the wartime events, and although he recognised the deficiencies in the earlier biographies, he took the view that Carrel and his writings were largely in tune with 1930s attitudes. Drouard was immediately assailed by Patrick Tort, a distinguished French biologist and left-leaning philosopher, who concluded that the new biography was 'an involuntary comedy which comes apart', and it was wrong to depict Carrel 'as a poignant victim of hindsight'.[68] Carrel's supporters in return showed loyalty, and Jean-Jaques Antier, a conservative Catholic playwright, returned to defend Carrel in his book *Alexis Carrel, la tentation de l'absolu* (1994).

Beyond France

Others beyond France who discovered and admired Carrel's writings included Kerry Bolton in New Zealand, who praised him in his book *Thinkers of the Right* (2003) and in it gave a long supportive critique of

---

[66]The other famous Edinburgh genetically-engineered piglets were Millie, Christa and Dotcom.

[67]Alain Drouard, *Alexis Carrel (1873–1944): de la mémoire à l'histoire* (Paris: Éditions L'Harmattan, 1995). He also published a detailed scholarly account of the Fondation in Vichy times; Alain Drouard, *Une inconnue des sciences sociales: la Fondation Alexis Carrel 1941–1945* (Paris: Editions de la Maison des Sciences de l'Homme, 1992).

[68]Patrick Tort in *L'Homme* 34 (1994): 162–4.

Man, the Unknown.[69] Bolton published with others in America using the journal *North American New Right*, a publication which admired the European New Right movement, and warned that

> our race [is] on the path to cultural decadence and demographic decline. If these trends are not reversed, whites will disappear as a distinct race. The incomparable light we bring to the world will be extinguished ...[70]

There was a balanced entry on Wikipedia on Carrel, but it was not safe and was 'attacked' by critics in 2006, giving a new unfavourable verdict. Supporters fought back, and there were unpleasant exchanges on Wikipedia's 'Talk' facility; Carrel's entry was 'frozen' to protect it.[71]

Islamic Interest

In the post-war period, a growing number of Muslim writers accused the West of exporting decadence and secularism to the East and claimed that it would undermine Islam and give a return to the barbarism (jahiliyyah) of pre-Muhammad times. When these writers came across Carrel's *Man, the Unknown*, they found, to their surprise, his prophet-like complaints about degeneration and lack of spirituality in the West and his call for a return to 'natural' laws. The first ideologues to note and praise Carrel's writings were Mehdi Bazargan, the French-educated Iranian prime minister, and Ali Shari'ati of the moderate 'median school of Islam'.[72] Writing the daily paper *Khorasan* of the city of Mashhad, Iran's second city and its cultural capital, Shari'ati supported Carrel's

---

[69] Bolton was associated with the New Zealand Fascist Union and was secretary of the New Zealand National Front from 2004.

[70] See the 2011 three-part essay 'Alexis Carrel: a Commemoration' at www.counter-currents.com.

[71] See Wikipedia Talk: 'Alexis Carrel' 2 January 2014.

[72] See Ali Rahnema, *An Islamic Utopian: a Political Biography of Ali Shari'ati* (London: I.B. Tauris, 1998).

predictions of a dismal future for the soul-less, materialist West.[73] He recommended Carrel's *Man, the Unknown* and his *Reflections on Life* as having 'illuminated the real value of Islam's noble tenets'. To add to this, Ali Shari'ati also translated and published Carrel's *Reader's Digest* article on 'Prayer'. Carrel was noticed next by the Lucknow Pakistani Islamist Abu al-Hasan 'Ali al-Nadawi, who had some links with the Muslim Brotherhood.[74]

Muslim Brotherhood

The most significant figure to invoke Carrel and recruit his writings to the Islamic cause was Sayyid Qutb (1906–1966). Born in Egypt, Qutb spent 1948–50 in America at a college in Colorado but was unhappy and unassimilated, and he viewed American culture with distaste. Returning to Egypt, Qutb became head of propaganda for the influential Muslim Brotherhood, now dedicated to removing British rule and replacing it with Islamic rule. Nasser broke Egypt's links with Britain but declined to set up an Islamic state. After the Brotherhood's 1954 assassination attempt, Qutb was imprisoned, and while in a Cairo jail he studied *Man, the Unknown*.[75]

Released but re-arrested, Qutb wrote his book *Milestones* in prison before he was executed in 1966.[76] Qutb advocated village utopianism, mysticism, fasting, intense prayer and a lowly place for women, and proposed that in the authoritarian Islamic state there would be a Carrel-like synthesis of education, ethics, economics and politics. Like Carrel, he urged a return to God-given 'natural laws'. Carrel's book was useful to Qutb in another way. The text of the Koran deals in generalities and lacks specifics — there is no clear itemised Islamic agenda which can be

---

[73] This difficult-to-find article is *Nashriyeh-e-Farhang-e-Khorshan* Yr 2 (1955) No. 6 Shahrivar (August–September): 1333–7.

[74] Ali al-Nadawi's writings, notably the many editions of *Madha Khasira al-'Alam bi-Ihitat al-Muslimin (What the world has Lost with the Decline of the Muslims)* were published widely in the Islamic nations from the 1960s.

[75] For general accounts, see Tariq Ali, *The Clash of Fundamentalisms: Crusades, Jihads and Modernity* (New York: Verso Books, 2002) and Ibrahim M. Abu-Rabi *Intellectual Origins of Islamic Resurgence* (New York: State University of New York Press, 1996).

[76] Sayyid Qutb, *Milestones* (Indianapolis: American Trust Publications, 2001).

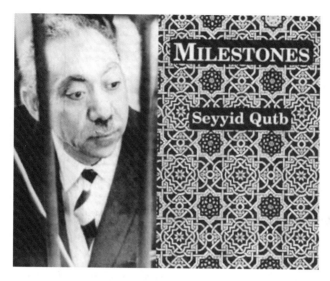

Militant Islamic ideologues admire Carrel's writings, and agree with his diagnosis of decadence in the Western world. (*Wikipedia*)

understood internationally. Qutb wished to use Western discourse, and Carrel's forceful writings in *Man, the Unknown* were valuable and his quotations from Carrel are only second in number to those from the Koran. He also adopted Carrelian language. Qutb wrote, echoing Carrel:

> Mankind today is on the brink of a precipice ... because humanity is devoid of those vital values which are necessary not only for its healthy development but also for its real progress. Even the Western world realises that Western civilisation is unable to present any healthy values for the guidance of mankind.[77]

Later, militants in the Algerian Front islamique du salut were guided by Qutb and Carrel's books when imprisoned in 1991 after election victories and an attempt to set up an Islamic state.

Carrel had warned that the white races were endangered by the expansion and confidence of others in the East and Orient. His remedies included rule by elites, and return to religion and prayer. At no point did

---

[77] Qutb, *Milestones* (note 76): 7.

Carrel realise how closely his agenda resembled the thinking and lifestyle in Islamic lands.[78]

Envoi

Carrel's remarkably durable legacy is still being tossed about inside and outside of science and medicine. In surgery and biology he has increasingly found his rightful historical place, although with some concerns. His other writings have been problematic but they endure because they touch on eternal political and personal issues. He is dismissed by many, but some regard him as an important thinker, and in the wider debate on mankind, he flits on and off the stage, with his life and works constantly revisited and used by advocates from remarkably different groupings. Carrel's persona changes with each analysis by supporters and critics, and his voice changes with each selective quotation from his writings. Carrel is long dead. His place in the history of medicine is unassailable, but beyond this, his life and works still attract an ever-changing verdict.

---

[78] In Carrel's time, there was minimal awareness of Islamic culture; his only possible sources were his neighbours in Brittany, the much-travelled brothers Jean and Jérôme Tharaud; see Mary du Noüy, *Human Destiny* (note 37): 128. In their writings about the Middle East, notably in their books *Fez* and *Alerte en Syrie*, they mostly described bourgeois Islamic culture. Importantly, Carrel does not quote Julius Evola (1898–1947), the Italian fascist writer who praised the East's 'spiritually superior earlier culture', but Carrel once did compare Hitler to Mohammed (Chapter 17, note 7).

Bibliography and Sources

There is a rich mother lode of primary sources available on Carrel's life and works. His personal papers survived well and passed to Georgetown University's Lauinger Library, where they are held in the Booth Family Center for Special Collections. His long career at the Rockefeller Institute has meant much information available at the Rockefeller University Archives, notably his scientific reports, and in the personal and administrative files. The Yale University Library Manuscripts and Archives have much on Carrel's joint work with Charles Lindbergh held in their Charles Augustus Lindbergh Papers, and Yale also has a small interesting cache of Carrel material in the James D. and Eleanor F. Newton Papers. Other essential primary sources are his books and his many general and scientific publications, some of which are listed below. Carrel's career was closely followed by the press, notably the *New York Times*, and these newspaper entries are increasingly available on the Net. Some of those who knew Carrel, notably the Lindberghs, left accounts of him, particularly in Charles's *The Wartime Diaries* (1970) and Ann's *The Flower and the Nettle* (1976), as did Mary Lecomte du Noüy in her *The Road to "Human Destiny": A Life of Pierre Lecomte du Noüy* (New York: Longmans, Green and Co., 1955).

The first Carrel biography came from Paris in 1952, and in Robert Soupault's *Alexis Carrel, 1873–1944*, like many others writing later on Carrel, he had an agenda, in this case aiming to restore Carrel's tarnished post-war reputation. Soupault's book has a commendable attempt at a full bibliography of his works. Thereafter, many other short French biographies added little to Soupault's work until Alain Drouard's *Alexis*

Carrel (1873–1944): de la mémoire à l'histoire (Paris: Éditions L'Harmattan, 1995), a more balanced and readable account.

The first English-language biographies were written in the 1970s by American surgeons who re-discovered Carrel's early perceptive surgical work. W. Sterling Edwards and Peter D. Edwards were first with their *Alexis Carrel: Visionary Surgeon* (Springfield: Charles C. Thomas, 1974), followed by Theodore I. Malinin's, *Surgery and Life: the Extraordinary Career of Alexis Carrel* (New York: Harcourt Brace Jovanovich, 1979). A later work by Angelo M. May and Alice G. May, *The Two Lions of Lyons: The Tale of Two Surgeons: Alexis Carrel and René Leriche* (Rockville: Kabel Publishing, 1994), linked Carrel with this other talented Lyon vascular surgeon. David Le Vay's difficult-to-find *Alexis Carrel: The Perfectibility of Man* (Rockville: Kabel Publishing, 1996) was more scholarly, but for a vivid tale of Carrel's work with Lindbergh, see David M. Friedman, *The Immortalists: Charles Lindbergh, Dr. Alexis Carrel and their Daring Quest to Live Forever* (New York: HarperCollins, 2007).

His spiritual beliefs were looked at tolerantly by a Jesuit historian in Joseph T. Durkin's *Hope for Our Time: Alexis Carrel on Man and Society* (New York: Harper and Row, 1965), but Durkin had difficulty with dealing with Carrel's darker side, unlike Andrés H. Reggiani's, *God's Eugenicist: Alexis Carrel and the Sociobiology of Decline* (New York: Berghahn Books, 2007), who emphasised Carrel's eugenics and his work in Vichy France.

For the background to tissue and organ transplantation at these times, see David Hamilton, *A History of Organ Transplantation* (Pittsburgh: Pittsburgh University Press, 2012), David Hamilton (1988) 'Alexis Carrel and the early days of tissue transplantation' *Transplantation Reviews* 2: 1–15, Susan E. Lederer, *Flesh and Blood: Organ Transplantation and Blood Transfusion in Twentieth-century America* (Oxford: Oxford University Press, 2008) and Thomas Schlich, *The Origins of Organ Transplantation: Surgery and Laboratory Science 1880–1930* (Rochester: University of Rochester Press, 2010). For the early development of vascular surgery, see Steven G. Friedman, *A History of Vascular Surgery* (Malden: Blackwell Futura, 2005). The best account of the early events is still by Stephen H. Watts (1907) 'The suture of blood vessels. Implantation and transplantation of vessels and organs. An historical and experimental study' *Bulletin of the Johns Hopkins Hospital* 18: 153–79. For the rise of laboratory medicine at this time, see Andrew Cunningham and Perry Williams, *The Laboratory Revolution in Medicine* (Cambridge: Cambridge University Press, 1992).

Carrel's Lyon Days

European medical schools at this time were surveyed in Abraham Flexner, *Medical Education in Europe* (Washington: Carnegie Foundation, 1912) and Thomas N. Bonner, *Becoming a Physician: Medical Education in Britain, France, Germany, and the United States 1830–1950* (New York: Oxford University Press, 1995).

Lyon's heritage in medicine is described in Alain Bouchet, *La Médecine à Lyon* (Paris: Éditions Hervas, 1987) and the city's strength in surgery, particularly vascular surgery, is reviewed in Fredric Jarrett (1979) 'René Leriche (1879–1955): father of vascular surgery' *Surgery* 86: 736–41, F. Collet (1960) 'Testut et Jaboulay' *Cahiers Lyonnais d'histoire de la médecine* 5: 3–10, and A. Bouchet (1994) 'Les pionniers Lyonnais de la chirurgie vasculaire: M. Jaboulay, A. Carrel, E. Villard et R. Leriche' *Histoire des Sciences Médicales* 28: 223–38. René Leriche's own memoires are *Souvenirs de ma vie mort* (Paris: Éditions du Seuil 1986). See also I.M. Rutkow, B.G. Rutkow and C.B. Ernst (1980) 'Letters of William Halsted and René Leriche: "Our friendship seems so deep"' *Surgery* 88: 806–25.

Lourdes 'miracle cures' at the time are described in Gustave Boissarie, *Heaven's Recent Wonders, or the Work of Lourdes* (New York: F. Pustet Co., 1909) and for a recent assessment see Ruth Harris, *Lourdes: Body and Spirit in the Secular Age* (London: Allen Lane, 1999).

Chicago Period

Carrel's early work in Chicago is described in William C. Beck 'Alexis Carrel and Carl Beck — a historical footnote' *Perspectives in Biology and Medicine* 30 (1986): 148–51, and William Baader and Lloyd M. Nyhus (1986) 'The life of Carl Beck and an important interval with Alexis Carrel'

Surgery, Gynecology & Obstetrics 163: 85–8. Carrel's pioneering work with
Charles C. Guthrie has been of enduring interest; see Hugh E. Stephenson
Jr. and Robert S. Kimpton, *America's First Nobel Prize in Medicine or
Physiology: The Story of Guthrie and Carrel* (Boston: Midwestern Vascular
Surgery Society, 2001), S.P. Harbison (1962) 'Origins of vascular surgery:
the Carrel–Guthrie letters' *Surgery* 52: 406–18, J.G. Walker Jr. (1974)
'The Carrel–Guthrie letters revisited' *Surgery* 76: 359–62 and Blair O.
Rogers (1959) 'Charles Claude Guthrie, M.D. PhD: a remarkable pioneer
in tissue and organ transplantation' *Plastic and Reconstructive Surgery* 24:
380–3. Guthrie's own book *Blood-Vessel Surgery and Its Applications*
(London: Edward Arnold, 1912) was reprinted in 1959.

Carrel's links with the Johns Hopkins surgeons are found in I.M.
Rutkow (1980) 'The letters of William Halsted and Alexis Carrel' *Surgery,
Gynecology & Obstetrics* 151: 676–88 and L.G. Walker Jr. (1988) 'The
letters and friendship of Carrel and Cushing' *Surgery Gynecology & Obstetrics*
167: 253–8. For the Hopkins surgical milieu, see Michael Bliss, *Harvey
Cushing: A Life in Surgery* (New York: Oxford University Press, 2005) and
Gerald Imber, *Genius on the Edge: The Bizarre Double Life of Dr. William
Stewart Halsted* (New York: Kaplan, 2011), and for Halsted's vascular
surgery, see Daniel B. Nunn (1995) 'Halsted and "The Vibrant Domain of
Surgery"' *American Journal of Surgery* 180: 356–65. The Hopkins Hunterian
Laboratory is described by Harvey Cushing in his 'Instruction in operative
medicine' *Bulletin of the Johns Hopkins Hospital* 17 (1906): 123–34.

Early Years at Rockefeller

General works on the Rockefeller Institute that contain assessments of
Carrel's scientific work are George W. Corner, *A History of the Rockefeller
Institute 1901–1953: Origins and Growth* (New York: Rockefeller Institute
Press, 1964) and the collected essays in Darwin H. Stapleton (ed.),
*Creating a Tradition of Biomedical Research: Contributions to the History of
The Rockefeller University* (New York: The Rockefeller University Press,
2004). Simon Flexner, the Director, lacks a biography, but there is a good
account in Peyton Rous 'Simon Flexner 1863–1946' *Obituary Notices of
Fellows of the Royal Society* 6 (1949): 409–45. For the origins of the

Rockefeller Institute, see Gerald Jonas, *The Circuit Riders: Rockefeller Money and the Rise of Modern Science* (New York: Horton, 1989) and E. Richard Brown, *Rockefeller Medicine Men: Medicine and Capitalism in America* (Los Angeles: University of California Press, 1979).

For antivivisection activity at the time, see James C. Turner, *Reckoning with the Beast* (Baltimore: Johns Hopkins University Press, 1980), Anita Guernini, *Experimenting with Humans and Animals: From Galen to Human Rights* (Baltimore: Johns Hopkins University Press, 2003), Susan Eyrich Lederer (1985) 'Hideyo Noguchi's luetin experiment and the antivivisectionists' *Isis* 76: 31–48 and also Bernard Unti 'The doctors are so sure that they only are right' in Stapleton, *Tradition* (above).

'Visible science' is dealt with in Bert Hansen, *Picturing Medical Progress from Pasteur to Polio* (New Brunswick: Rutgers University Press, 2009), and for Carrel's fellow Rockefeller celebrity scientist, see Paul Franklin Clark (1959) 'Hideyo Noguchi, 1876–1928' *Bulletin of the History of Medicine* 33: 1–20.

Vascular Surgery

For the background to Carrel's direct transfusion of a baby, see N. Nathoo (2009) 'The first direct blood transfusion: the forgotten legacy of George W. Crile' *Operative Neurosurgery* 64: 20–27. The creditable story of Mount Sinai Hospital's pioneers of blood transfusion is described in Richard Lewisohn (1943–44) 'The development of the technique of blood transfusion since 1907' *Journal of the Mount Sinai Hospital* 10: 605–22.

Tissue Culture

For a general history, see Hannah Landecker, *Culturing Life: How Cells Became Technologies* (Cambridge: Harvard University Press, 2010) and her description of Carrel's early work in 'Building "A new type of body in which to grow a cell": tissue culture at the Rockefeller Institute, 1910–1914' in Stapleton, *Tradition* (above): 151–74. For the controversy over Carrel's relations with Ross Harrison, see the lively account in 'Ross Granville Harrison' *Biographical Memoirs of Fellows of the Royal*

Society 7 (1961): 110–26. For Guthrie's complaint against Carrel, see C.C. Guthrie (1909) 'On misleading statements' *Science* 29: 29–31.

Other American tissue culture workers are described in A. McGehee Harvey (1975) 'Johns Hopkins — the birthplace of tissue culture: the story of Ross G. Harrison, Warren H. Lewis and George O. Gey' *The Johns Hopkins Medical Journal* 136: 142–49 and Frederick B. Bang (1977) 'History of tissue culture at Johns Hopkins' *Bulletin of the History of Medicine* 51: 516–37.

Cardiac Surgery

For the rival experimental and human anaesthetic respiratory ventilation methods at the time, see J.B. Brodsky and H.J.M. Lemmens (2007) 'The history of anaesthesia for thoracic surgery' *Minerva Anesthesiologica* 73: 513–24. Meltzer's work is described in A. Meltzer (1990) 'Dr. Samuel James Meltzer: physiologist of the Rockefeller Institute' *American Jewish Archives* 42: 49–56.

Carrel's shared projects with Tuffier are analysed in Saul Jarco (1975) 'Carrel and Tuffier (1914) on experimental surgery of the cardiac orifices' *The American Journal of Cardiology* 36: 954–6, and for the comparable attempts at Baltimore, see Saul Jarcho (1975) 'Experiments on heart valves (1908) by Harvey Cushing and J.R.B. Branch' *American Journal of Cardiology* 35: 506–8.

For Carrel's French surgical friends Theodore Tuffier and Samuel Pozzi, see Alexis Carrel (1932) 'Tuffier' *Revue de Paris* 39: 347–59, translated in Joseph T. Durkin, *Hope for Our Time: Alexis Carrel on Man and Society* (New York: Harper and Row, 1965): 102–10, and the biographies of Pozzi by Caroline de Costa and Francesca Miller, *The Diva and Doctor God* (XLibris, 2010) and Claude Vanderpooten, *Samuel Pozzi, chirurgien et ami des femmes* (Paris: V&O, 1992).

Transplantation

The European 'Lost Era' of transplantation is identified in David Hamilton, *A History of Organ Transplantation* (Pittsburgh: Pittsburgh University Press, 2012), and for Murphy's remarkable insights into immunosuppression at this time, see Arthur M. Silverstein (2001) 'The lymphocyte in immunology: from James B. Murphy to James Gowans' *Nature Immunology* 2: 569–71. Tissue typing is anticipated in R. Ingebrigtsen (1912) 'The influence of isoagglutinins on the final results of homoplastic transplantations of arteries' *JEM* 16: 169–77, and Carrel's visionary address to the International Surgical Association in 1914 is given in Alexis Carrel (1914) 'The transplantation of organs' *New York Medical Journal* 99: 839–40.

World War I

For a general description of military medicine, see Mark Harrison, *The Medical War: British Military Medicine in the First World War* (Oxford: Oxford University Press, 2010) and Ian R. Whitehead, *Doctors in the Great War* (London: Leo Cooper, 1999). For the changes in surgical policy, see Thomas S. Helling and Emmanuel Daon (1998) 'In Flanders fields: the Great War, Antoine Depage and the resurgence of débridement' *Annals of Surgery* 228: 173–81.

The American surgical presence in Paris is recalled in Eric I. Rutkow and Ira Rutkow (2004) 'George Crile, Harvey Cushing, and the Ambulance Américaine' *Archives of Surgery* 139: 678–85, and Crile's policy meeting is found in George Crile (1915) 'Symposium on military surgery at American Ambulance, Neuilly-sur-Seine, France' *Surgery, Gynecology & Obstetrics* 20: 708–16.

Carrel's hospital has been much described — see Georgette Mottier, *L'ambulance du Dr. Alexis Carrel 1914–1919* (Lausanne: Éditions la Source, 1977), and L.G. Walker (2002) 'Carrel's war research hospital at Compiegne: Prototype of a research facility at the front' *Journal of the American College of Surgeons* 195: 870–7. For Dakin's career, see *Obituary Notices of Fellows of the Royal Society* 8 (1952): 128–48 and his interesting review H.D. Dakin 'Biochemistry and war problems' *BMJ*, June 23 1917, 833–7.

Carrel's approach is assessed in Perrin Selcer (2008) 'Standardizing wounds: Alexis Carrel and the scientific management of life in the First World War' *British Journal for the History of Science* 41: 73–107. For Almroth Wright and his involvement in WWI, see Michael Dunnill, *The*

Plato of Praed Street: The Life and Times of Almroth Wright (London: Royal Society of Medicine Press, 2000). The controversy on antiseptics involving Wright started with W.W. Cheyne's 'On the treatment of wounds of war' *British Journal of Surgery* 3 (1915–16): 427–50 and finished with Wright's polemic in *The Lancet*, 16 September 1916, 503–13.

For new WWI military surgery ideas, see Peter C. English, *Shock, Physiological Surgery, and George Washington Crile* (Westport, Conn: Greenwood Press, 1980), and Lynn G. Stansbury and John R. Hess (2009) 'Blood transfusion in World War I: the roles of Lawrence Bruce Robertson and Oswald Hope Robertson' *Transfusion Medicine Reviews* 23: 232–6.

Back in America during WWI, Flexner described the Institute's role in 'War work of the Rockefeller Institute for Medical Research, New York' *The Military Surgeon* 47 (1920): 491–512, and Carrel's surgical work also figured prominently in 'Clinical Congress of Surgeons of North America — War Session' *JAMA* 69 (1917): 1538–41. The problem of post-influenza empyema is described in Carol R. Byerly, *Fever of War: The Influenza Epidemic in the U.S. Army during World War I* (New York: New York University Press, 2005), and in 'Empyema in base hospitals' *Review of War Surgery and Medicine* 1 (1918): 1–40. See also Peter D. Olch (1989) 'Evarts A. Graham in World War I: the Empyema Commission and service in the American Expeditionary Forces' *Journal of the History of Medicine and Allied Sciences* 44: 430–6.

The 1920s

This period in Carrel's career, and the life of the Institute in general, is poorly described, but there is an account of Flexner's work in Karen D. Ross's *Making Medicine Scientific: Simon Flexner and Experimental Medicine*, PhD thesis, University of Minnesota 2006. There is some background in Sinclair Lewis' novel *Arrowsmith* (1925) and in Saul Benison, *Tom Rivers — Reflections on a Life in Medicine and Science* (Cambridge: Massachusetts Institute of Technology, 1967). Carrel at work is described in R.W.G. Wyckoff (1984) 'Souvenirs d'Alexis Carrel à New-York' *Lyon Chirurgical* 80: 194–6, and Carrel's colleague du Noüy's career is found in Mary

Lecomte du Noüy, *The Road to "Human Destiny": A Life of Pierre Lecomte du Noüy* (New York: Longmans, Green and Co., 1955).

For the pre-1920s reductionist mood, see Jacques Loeb's *Mechanistic Theory of Life*, republished with an Introduction by Donald Fleming (Cambridge: Harvard University Press, 1964). The move away is found in Alexis Carrel (1925) 'The future progress of medicine' *The Scientific Monthly* 21: 54–8 and Simon Flexner (1922) 'Experimental epidemiology' *JEM* 36: 9–14. For accounts of the wider arrival of holistic thinking and therapy, see David Cantor (ed.), *Reinventing Hippocrates* (London: Ashgate, 2002) and Christopher Lawrence and George Weisz, *Greater than the Parts: Holism in Biomedicine 1920–1950* (Oxford: Oxford University Press, 1998).

The 1920s developments in tissue culture are found in Duncan Wilson (2005) 'The early history of tissue culture in Britain: the interwar years' *Social History of Medicine* 18: 225–43. Carrel's approach is closely analysed in J.A. Witkowski (1979) 'Alexis Carrel and the mysticism of tissue culture' *Medical History* 23: 279–96, and J.A. Witkowski (1980) 'Dr. Carrel's immortal cells' *Medical History* 24: 129–42. For a retrospective, see Albert H. Ebeling (1942) 'Dr. Carrel's immortal chicken heart' *Scientific American* 166: 22–4.

The anarchic state of tissue transplantation in the 1920s is noted in Waro Nakahara (1925) 'Tissue transplantation: real and bogus' *American Mercury* 17: 456–7 and in David Hamilton, *The Monkey Gland Affair* (London: Chatto & Windus, 1986).

Carrel and his 'Philosophers' appear in the novel *The Talkers* by Robert W. Chambers (New York: George H. Doran, 1923), and for two of Carrel's friends, see Virginia K. Veenswijk, *Coudert Brothers* (New York: Dutton, 1994), Paula Murray Coudert, Paul B. Jones and Lawrence Klepp, *Frederic R. Coudert Jr: A Biography* (P.M. Coudert, 1985) and Dorothy D. Bromley 'Nicholas Murray Butler: portrait of a reactionary' *The American Mercury*, March 1935, 286–98.

Man, the Unknown

In declinist thinking, an early New York work was Raymond B. Fosdick, *The Old Savage in the New Civilisation* (New York: Doubleday, Doran & Co,

1928). French introspection is examined in Robert Nye *Crime, Madness and Politics in Modern France: the Medical Concept of National Decline* (Princeton: Princeton University Press, 1984), Richard Overy, *The Twilight Years* (London: Viking, 2009) and William H. Schneider, *Quality and Quantity: The Quest for Biological Regeneration in Twentieth-Century France* (Cambridge: Cambridge University Press, 1990).

The background to Carrel's support for parapsychology is explored in Seymour H. Mauskopf and Michael R. McVaugh, *The Elusive Science: Origins of Experimental Psychical Research* (Baltimore: Johns Hopkins University Press, 1980) and M. Brady Brower, *Unruly Spirits: The Science of Psychic Phenomena in Modern France* (Urbana: University of Illinois Press, 2010). For popular culture at the time, see James Playsted Wood, *Of Lasting Interest: The Story of the Reader's Digest* (New York: Doubleday, 1967). For Carrel's high public profile, see Andrés H. Reggiani 'Drilling Eugenics into Peoples' Minds' in Susan Currell and Christina Cogdell (eds.), *Popular Eugenics* (Athens: Ohio University Press, 2006). 'Celebrity' scientists are identified in Rae Goodell, *The Visible Scientists* (Boston: Little, Brown and Company, 1975).

The Pump

For a historical review of organ perfusion, see W. Boettcher, F. Merkle and H.H. Weitkemper (2003) 'History of extracorporeal circulation' *Journal of Extracorporeal Technology* 35: 172–91. For some details of the pump in action, see Richard J. Bing (1987) 'Lindbergh and the biological sciences' *Historical Perspectives in Cardiovascular Medicine & Surgery* 14: 231–7 and R.J. Bing (1983) 'Carrel: a personal reminiscence' *JAMA* 250: 3297–8. Details of Carrel's links with Lindbergh are found in A. Scott Berg, *Lindberg* (New York: G.P. Putnam & Sons, 1998), Charles A. Lindbergh, *Autobiography of Values* (New York: Harcourt Brace Jovanovich, 1976), David M. Friedman, *The Immortalists: Charles Lindbergh, Dr. Alexis Carrel and their Daring Quest to Live Forever* (New York: HarperCollins, 2007), and Anne Morrow Lindbergh, *The Flower and the Nettle* (New York: Harcourt Brace Jovanovich, 1976). Other information on Carrel's small inner circle is found in James D. Newton, *Uncommon Friends: Life with Thomas*

Edison, Henry Ford, Harvey Firestone, Alexis Carrel and Charles Lindbergh (New York: Harvest Books, 1989).

Paris Events

For Vichy France, see Philip Nord, *France's New Deal: From the Thirties to the Postwar Era* (Princeton: Princeton University Press, 2010) and Coudert's wartime links with Vichy are described in Barbara Giles 'Coudert — Vichy lawyer' *The New Masses*, September 1, 1942: 13–15. Italian fascist bio-politics are examined in Francesco Cassata, *Building a New Man: Racial Studies in Twentieth Century Italy* (Budapest: Central European University Press, 2011) and Carl Ipsen, *Dictating Democracy: The Problem of Population in Fascist Italy* (Cambridge: Cambridge University Press, 1996). Vichy's gender politics at the time are highlighted in Francine Muel-Dreyfus, *Vichy and the Eternal Feminine* (Durham: Duke University Press, 2001).

For life in Paris, see David Pryce-Jones, *Paris in the Third Reich* (London: Collins, 1981) and Ian Ousby, *Occupation: The Ordeal of France 1940–1944* (London: John Murray, 1997). The work of Carrel's Fondation is covered in detail in Alain Drouard, *Une inconnue des sciences sociales: la Fondation Alexis Carrel 1941–1945* (Paris: Editions de la Maison des sciences de l'homme, 1992), and there is further important analysis in Andrés H. Reggiani, *God's Eugenicist: Alexis Carrel and the Sociobiology of Decline* (New York: Berghahn Books, 2007).

Aftermath

For the vitality of post-WWII French surgery, see Jean Natali (1992) 'Jacques Oudot and his contribution to surgery of the aortic bifurcation' *Annals of Vascular Surgery* 6: 185–92 and J.O. Menzoian, A.L. Kosher and N. Rodrigues (2011) 'Alexis Carrel, Rene Leriche, Jean Kunlin, and the history of bypass surgery' *Journal of Vascular Surgery* 54: 571–4.

For the rehabilitation of Carrel, see J.-J. Gillon 'Les aspects essentiels de l'oeuvre scientifique d'Alexis Carrel' *Le Concours Médical* vol. 73, October 11 and 17, 1951. The neo-Carrelians are described in Albert

Bessierres, *La destinée humaine devant la science — Alexis Carrel, Lecomte du Noüy, Charles Nicolle* (Paris: Editions Spes, 1950). Books by these authors include Lecomte du Noüy's *L'Homme et sa destinée* (Paris: La Colombe, 1947) and André Missenard's *In Search of Man* (New York: Hawthorn Books, 1957).

Published proceedings at celebratory Carrel conferences include J. Descotes (ed.), *Alexis Carrel 1873–1944: Pionnier de la chirurgie vasculaire et des transplantations d'organes* (Lyon: Simep editions, 1966) and Joseph T. Durkin (ed.), *Papers of the Alexis Carrel Centennial Conference* (Georgetown University, 1973).

For praise of Carrel from the Right, see Mark Wegierski (1993–4) 'The New-Right in Europe' *Telos* 98–99, 55–74. For Islamic interest in Carrel's *Man, the Unknown*, see Tariq Ali, *The Clash of Fundamentalisms: Crusades, Jihads and Modernity* (New York: Verso Books, 2002) and Ibrahim M. Abu-Rabi *Intellectual Origins of Islamic Resurgence* (New York: State University of New York Press, 1996).

Carrel's Publications

The first bibliography of Carrel's voluminous works was a thorough search carried out by Jean Sutter for Robert Soupault's *Alexis Carrel, 1873–1944* of 1952. More recently, Andrés H. Reggiani (see above) in *God's Eugenicist: Alexis Carrel and the Sociobiology of Decline* used Soupault's listing, adding some of Carrel's general works. Many of Carrel's publications, numbering nearly 300, are brief, and duplication of data was common. Listed below are his historically important publications, and many others are given in the main text.

1901

Le goitre cancéreux Paris: Baillière — a work based on his Lyon M.D. thesis.

1902

'La technique opératoire des anastomoses vasculaires et la transplantation des viscères' *Lyon Mèdical* 99: 859–62; there is a translation of this paper in Toni Hau, *Renal Transplantation* (Austin: Silvergirl, 1987): 4–5.

1905

with C.C. Guthrie, 'Functions of a transplanted kidney' *Science* 22: 473.
with C.C. Guthrie, 'Extirpation and replantation of the thyroid gland' *Science* 22: 535.

1906

with C.C. Guthrie, 'The reversal of the circulation in a limb' *Annals of Surgery* 43: 203–15.
with C.C. Guthrie, 'Results of replantation of the thigh' *Science* 23: 393–4.
with C.C. Guthrie, 'Anastomosis of blood-vessels by the Patching Method and transplantation of the kidney' *JAMA* 4: 1648–50.

1907

'The surgery of blood vessels' *Johns Hopkins Hospital Bulletin*, 1907, No. 190, 18–28.

1908

'Further studies on transplantation of vessels and organs' *Proceedings of the American Philosophical Society* 47: 677–98.
'Transplantation in mass of the kidneys' *JEM* 10: 98–140.
'Results of the transplantation of blood vessels, organs and limbs' *JAMA* 51: 1662–7.
'La transfusion directe du sange (Méthode de Crile)' *Lyon Chirurgie* 1: 13–19.

1909

'Note on the production of renal insufficiency by reduction of the arterial circulation of the kidney' *PSEBM* 6: 107.

1910

'Graft of the vena cava on the abdominal aorta' *Annals of Surgery* 52: 462–70.
'On the experimental surgery of the thoracic aorta and heart' *Annals of Surgery* 52: 83–95.
'Latent life of arteries' *JEM* 12: 460–65.

with M.T. Burrows, 'Cultivation of adult tissues outside of the body'
JAMA 55: 1379–81.
'The treatment of wounds' *JAMA* 55, 2148–50.

1912

with R. Ingebrigtsen, 'The production of antibodies by tissues living
outside of the organism' *JEM* 15: 287–91.
'The preservation of tissues and its applications in surgery' *JAMA* 59: 523–7.
'On the permanent life of tissue outside of the organism' *JEM* 15:
516–28.
'Suture of blood vessels and transplantation of organs' *Nobel Lectures,
Physiology or Medicine 1901–1921.* (Amsterdam: Elsevier Publishing
Company, 1967): 437–66.

1913

'Artificial activation of the growth in vitro of connective tissue' *JEM* 17:
14–19.

1914

with Theodor Tuffier, 'Anatomico-pathological study of the surgery of the
orifices of the heart' *Medical Press and Circular*, 539–42 and 566–9.
'The transplantation of organs' *New York Medical Journal* 99: 839–40.
'Experimental operations on the orifices of the heart' *American Journal of
Surgery* 60: 1–6.

1915

'Traitement abortif de l'infection des plais' (with others) *Bulletin de
l'Académie de Médecine* 74: 361–8.

1922

'Leucocyte secretions' *JEM* 36: 645–59.

1925

'Mechanism and formation of malignant tumours' *Annals of Surgery* 82:
1–13.
'The future progress of medicine' *Scientific Monthly* 21: 55–7.

1928

'Tissue cultures in the study of viruses' in Thomas M. Rivers (ed.), *Filterable Viruses* (London: Baillière Tindall & Cox, 1928): 97–112.

1931

'The new cytology' *Science* 73: 297–303.

1936

'The mystery of death' in Eugene H. Pool, *Medicine and Mankind* (New York: D. Appleton, 1936): 195–217.

1937

'The making of civilised men' *Dartmouth Alumni Magazine* 30: 6–10.
'Culture of whole organs' *JEM* 65: 515–26.

Books

Carrel and G. Dehelly, *The Treatment of Infected Wounds* (New York: P.B. Hoeber, 1919).
Carrel and Charles A. Lindbergh, *The Culture of Organs* (New York: Paul B. Hoeber, 1938).
Man, the Unknown (New York: Harper and Brothers, 1935), translated as *L'Homme cet inconnu* (Paris: Plon, 1935).
Le voyage de Lourdes (Paris: Plon, 1949), translated as *The Voyage to Lourdes* (New York: Harper & Brothers, 1950).
La Prière (Paris: Plon, 1944), translated as *Prayer* (London: Hodder & Stoughton, 1947).
Réflexions sur la conduite de la vie (Paris: Plon, 1950), translated as *Reflections on Life* (London: Hamish Hamilton, 1952).
Jour après jour: journal 1893–1944 (Paris: Plon, 1956).

Abbreviations Used

BMJ — British Medical Journal
CRSB — Comptes Rendus Hebdomadaires des séances et mémoires de la Société de Biologie

GULBFC — Georgetown University Library, Booth Family Center for Special Collections
JAMA — Journal of the American Medical Association
JEM — Journal of Experimental Medicine
MTU — *Man, the Unknown*
NAR — U.S. National Archives and Records
NYT — New York Times
PSEBM — Proceedings of the Society for Experimental Biology and Medicine
RUA RAC — Rockefeller University Archives, Rockefeller Archives Centre
YULMA — Yale University Library Manuscripts and Archives

Index